Y0-BXX-666

INTERNATIONAL PSYCHIATRY CLINICS

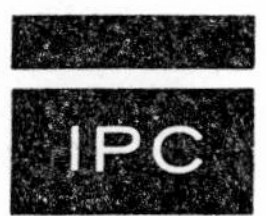

SUBSCRIPTION RATE $21.50 PER YEAR. FOREIGN RATE $24.00 PER YEAR.

SLEEP AND DREAMING

EDITED BY

Ernest Hartmann, M.D.
Boston State Hospital
Tufts University School of Medicine

BOSTON
LITTLE, BROWN AND COMPANY

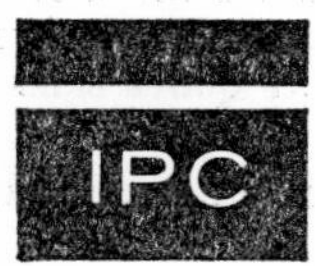

INTERNATIONAL PSYCHIATRY CLINICS
VOL. 7, NO. 2

COPYRIGHT © 1970 LITTLE, BROWN AND COMPANY (INC.)

ALL RIGHTS RESERVED. NO PART OF THIS BOOK MAY BE REPRODUCED IN ANY FORM, BY ANY ELECTRONIC OR MECHANICAL MEANS, INCLUDING INFORMATION STORAGE AND RETRIEVAL SYSTEMS, WITHOUT PERMISSION IN WRITING FROM THE PUBLISHER, EXCEPT BY A REVIEWER WHO MAY QUOTE BRIEF PASSAGES IN A REVIEW.

LIBRARY OF CONGRESS CATALOG CARD NO. 70-118265

PUBLISHED IN GREAT BRITAIN
BY J. & A. CHURCHILL LTD., LONDON

BRITISH STANDARD BOOK NO. 7000 0194 8

PRINTED IN THE UNITED STATES OF AMERICA

Contributing Authors

ERNEST HARTMANN, M.D., Editor

Associate Professor of Psychiatry,
Tufts University School of Medicine;
Director, Sleep and Dream Laboratory,
Boston State Hospital, Boston, Massachusetts

FREDERICK BAEKELAND, M.D., D.M.Sc.

Assistant Professor, Department of Psychiatry,
State University of New York, Downstate Medical Center, Brooklyn

RALPH J. BERGER, Ph.D.

Associate Professor of Psychology, University of California, Santa Cruz

ROGER J. BROUGHTON, M.D., Ph.D.

Associate Professor of Medicine and Pharmacology,
Faculty of Medicine, University of Ottawa;
Director, Department of Electroencephalography and Clinical
Neurophysiology, Ottawa General Hospital, Ottawa, Ontario, Canada

JOSEPH V. BYRNE

Laboratory Technician, Sleep Laboratory,
The Mount Sinai Hospital, New York

PATRICIA CARRINGTON, Ph.D.

Member of Faculty,
Postgraduate Center for Mental Health, New York;
Director of Child Therapy,
East Brunswick Guidance Clinic, East Brunswick, New Jersey

ROSALIND DYMOND CARTWRIGHT, Ph.D.

Professor of Psychology, University of Illinois;
Director, Sleep Laboratory,
Department of Psychiatry, Neuropsychiatric Institute,
Chicago, Illinois

EDMOND M. DEWAN, Ph.D.
Physicist and Biophysicist, Data Sciences Laboratory,
Air Force Cambridge Research Laboratories,
L. G. Hanscom Field, Bedford, Massachusetts

ADELE EDWARDS
Laboratory Supervisor, Sleep Laboratory,
The Mount Sinai Hospital, New York

HARMON S. EPHRON, M.D.
Associate Clinical Professor in Psychiatry,
New York Medical College;
Attending Clinical Associate in Psychiatry,
Flower–Fifth Avenue Hospital, New York

CHARLES FISHER, M.D., Ph.D.
Clinical Professor in Psychiatry,
Mount Sinai School of Medicine of The City University of New York;
Attending Psychiatrist, The Mount Sinai Hospital, New York

DAVID FOULKES, Ph.D.
Professor, Department of Psychology,
University of Wyoming, Laramie

GORDON G. GLOBUS, M.D.
Assistant Professor,
Department of Psychiatry and Human Behavior,
University of California, Irvine

RAMON GREENBERG, M.D
Assistant Clinical Professor in Psychiatry,
Tufts University School of Medicine;
Staff Psychiatrist and Director,
Sleep Physiology Laboratory, Psychiatry Service,
Boston Veterans Administration Hospital, Boston, Massachusetts

PETER HAURI, Ph.D.
Assistant Professor, Department of Psychiatry,
University of Virginia School of Medicine, Charlottesville

DAVID R. HAWKINS, M.D.
Professor and Chairman, Department of Psychiatry,
University of Virginia School of Medicine;
Psychiatrist-in-Chief, University of Virginia Hospital, Charlottesville

J. ALLAN HOBSON, M.D.
Assistant Professor, Department of Psychiatry,
Harvard Medical School;
Senior Psychiatrist and Director, Laboratory of Neurophysiology,
Massachusetts Mental Health Center, Boston

CAROLYN J. HURSCH, Ph.D.
Assistant Professor of Psychology,
J. Hillis Miller Health Center;
Department of Clinical Psychology and Department of Psychiatry,
University of Florida, Gainesville

RICHARD M. JONES, Ph.D.
Professor of Psychology,
State University of New York, Old Westbury

EDWIN KAHN, Ph.D
Research Associate, Department of Psychiatry,
Mount Sinai School of Medicine of the City University of New York;
Adjunct Assistant Professor, Department of Psychology,
Hunter College of the City University of New York, New York

ISMET KARACAN, M.D., (Med.) D.Sc.
Associate Professor of Psychiatry and Director of Sleep Laboratories,
Department of Psychiatry, University of Florida College of Medicine;
Psychiatrist, Shands Teaching Hospital and Clinics,
Gainesville, Florida

NATHANIEL KLEITMAN, Ph.D.
Professor Emeritus of Physiology,
University of Chicago, Chicago, Illinois

HELEN B. LEWIS, Ph.D.
Clinical Psychologist, Department of Psychiatry,
State University of New York, Downstate Medical Center, Brooklyn

EDWARD M. ORNITZ, M.D.
Assistant Professor of Psychiatry,
UCLA School of Medicine, Los Angeles, California

CHESTER A. PEARLMAN, JR., M.D.
Clinical Assistant in Psychiatry,
Harvard Medical School;
Clinical Investigator, Boston Veterans' Administration Hospital,
Boston, Massachusetts

EDWARD R. RITVO, M.D.
Assistant Professor of Psychiatry (in residence),
UCLA School of Medicine, Department of Psychiatry,
Division of Child Psychiatry;
Staff Psychiatrist, Neuropsychiatric Institute,
UCLA Center for Health Sciences,
Los Angeles, California

ARTHUR SHAPIRO, M.D.
Professor of Psychiatry,
University of Pennsylvania;
Senior Research Associate,
Institute of the Pennsylvania Hospital, Philadelphia

JAMES C. SKINNER, M.D.
Associate Professor in Psychiatry,
Boston University School of Medicine;
Visiting Physician in Psychiatry,
University Hospital, Boston, Massachusetts

WARREN C. STERN, Ph.D.
Research Fellow, Department of Psychiatry,
Tufts University School of Medicine;
Research Fellow, Sleep and Dream Laboratory,
Boston State Hospital, Boston, Massachusetts

JOHANN STOYVA, Ph.D.
Assistant Professor, Department of Psychiatry,
University of Colorado School of Medicine, Denver

ROBERT L. VAN DE CASTLE, Ph.D.
Professor of Clinical Psychology,
University of Virginia School of Medicine, Charlottesville

W. B. WEBB, Ph.D.
Professor and Chairman,
Department of Psychology, University of Florida, Gainesville

ROBERT L. WILLIAMS, M.D.
Professor and Chairman, Department of Psychiatry,
University of Florida College of Medicine;
Chief of Psychiatric Services, Shands Teaching Hospital and Clinics,
Gainesville, Florida

ROBERT T. WILKINSON, Ph.D.
Applied Psychology Unit,
Medical Research Council, Cambridge, England

HERMAN A. WITKIN, Ph.D.
Professor, Department of Psychiatry,
State University of New York, Downstate Medical Center, Brooklyn

ELIZABETH R. ZETZEL, M.D.
Associate Clinical Professor of Psychiatry,
Harvard Medical School;
Director, Psychotherapy Study Center,
Massachusetts Mental Health Center, Boston

WILLIAM W. K. ZUNG, M.D.
Assistant Professor of Psychiatry,
Duke University Medical Center, Durham, North Carolina

Preface

No matter what scientific area is under discussion, there is little doubt that its recent growth has been phenomenal. The last few years have seen a burgeoning in the development of plant morphogenesis and a mushrooming of interest in nuclear explosions, equaled only by the ballooning of meteorological surveys and the eruption and overflowing of studies in volcanology. Sleep and dream research is no exception. I do not mean that there has been great dozing and yawning among the students of sleep, or dreaming of oneirological findings, but simply that we too are growing; and that this is not a unique event and a cause for self-congratulation, but a natural part of the phenomenology of the age. Whether this scientific gigantism will make us supermen or will direct us in the footsteps of the dinosaur remains unclear.

We have passed the stage of the neonate (when anyone asking where it is all leading or what the use of it is can be silenced by the classic researcher's retort: "What use is a newborn child?"). We are arriving at a stage where questions of purpose, of specific direction, of theoretical implication and practical application must be asked. The present issue of *International Psychiatry Clinics* is at least the beginning of such a task.

I have not asked each sleep expert to review his particular area of study for the tenth or twentieth time. Instead, I have chosen some old, obvious, but obviously important questions, such as *What is good sleep? How much sleep is needed? What is the function of sleep? Of dreaming? What clinical relevance does this research have?* . . . and asked sleep researchers whose experience and experiments have been relevant to try to provide answers.

It is assumed that the reader has some acquaintance with the fundamentals of the field and has read at least one book or review article covering the area. For anyone who has not, a paper by the editor reviewing sleep and dream research up to 1965 has been included as Appendix A. In addition, a glossary containing terms peculiar to sleep research is found in Appendix B.

This issue of IPC is not an overall review of the entire field; some of the most exciting areas of basic sleep research—the detailed biochemistry underlying the stages of sleep, single cell recordings—are referred to but certainly not surveyed in depth. Also, several of the more theoretical questions originally formulated received no answers whatever from researchers and therefore are not included. Among these were: *Do sleep patterns begin to fit into an evolving science of man? Are there important interrelationships between sleep-dream research and other fields of research related to the mind and mental illness, or is sleep-dream research just one more fascinating wild goose chase?* Actually several of the essays included are at least relevant to these topics.

In the areas covered, accumulated knowledge is reviewed, but generally the papers do not stop where the data stop; hypotheses are offered and amended and even pure speculation is included at times. I consider this proper and healthy, as long as the distinction between facts and speculation remains visible. I believe and sincerely hope that such is the case for this volume.

Ours is neither a circumscribed nor a unified field; contributors to sleep-dream research include biochemists, neurophysiologists, psychophysiologists, research and clinical psychiatrists, psychologists of many backgrounds and viewpoints, and psychoanalysts. In this volume contributions from all these areas and more are called on to provide a view of where we are and where we are going in terms of significant theoretical and practical questions. On looking over the articles included I am struck by the fact that many of the questions which now already have answers or solid attempts at answers could hardly even have been asked ten years ago.

The questions considered are relatively independent and can be read entirely separately, but there is a sort of progression from beginning to end in two senses: from more physiological questions to more psychological ones, and from relatively specific and empirical questions to more general and theoretical ones. Some readers will find it worthwhile to read all the papers in consecutive order, but this is by no means necessary: answers to a given question are seldom predicated on answers to earlier ones, and where material of interest to one question is contained elsewhere in the book, a cross-reference is included, referring the reader to the appropriate section.

ERNEST HARTMANN

Contents

SLEEP AND DREAMING

Contributions of Sleep Research to Neurophysiology

---

*What has sleep and dream research of the past fifteen years contributed to the development of basic neurophysiology?**

Sleep Research and Basic Neurophysiology

J. ALLAN HOBSON

Sleep is a behavioral state characterized by immobility and diminished but reversible sensitivity to external stimuli. To these postural and threshold criteria of sleep have recently been added electrographic criteria which permit the objective differentiation of waking and two distinctive stages of sleep.

The relative reliability of the definition of sleep and the global nature of the behavioral change from waking to sleep have made it a popular subject of basic biological research, especially for neurophysiologists and biochemists. Many have felt that if the biological bases of sleep were understood, the way to understanding other behaviors, normal and abnormal, might become more clear.

* The reader interested in this question may wish to refer also to the papers by Zung (p. 123) and by Berger (p. 277).

It is the purpose of this paper to review in broad outline the divergence, parallel development, and recent convergence of electrographic and cellular neurophysiological techniques in their relation to the study of sleep and dreaming. Emphasis is placed on the role of technical developments in opening new areas of investigation. The cellular physiology of sleep is reviewed in detail and some possible future developments are indicated.

PARALLEL DEVELOPMENTS IN THE GENERAL ELECTROPHYSIOLOGY OF SLEEP AND CELLULAR NEUROPHYSIOLOGY

As is well known, the discovery of the electroencephalogram (EEG) by the psychiatrist Berger [3], in 1930, first revealed the presence of the electrical activity of the human brain and showed that that electrical activity underwent a change from low voltage, fast (desynchronized) activity to high voltage, slow (synchronized) activity when subjects passed from waking into sleep. This finding, of course, depended upon a relatively simple application of the string galvanometer, developed by Einthoven and already successfully used to reveal physiological potentials in muscle. It is not so widely appreciated that general acceptance of Berger's discovery, thought by many to be an artefact, came only when it was confirmed by two neurophysiologists, Adrian and Matthews [1], using the oscilloscope that they developed to record action potentials in isolated nerve fibers. At this point, in 1934, two lines of work diverged.

The reason that most neurophysiologists, following Adrian and Matthews, turned away from the EEG was that the physiological basis of the potentials recorded was not known. Two simple theories were initially advanced: (1) the EEG potential is a sum or envelope of cellular (somatic) action potentials, and (2) the EEG potentials represent dendritic depolarization. Neither of these theories has proved adequate and the matter is still in doubt, but current theory emphasizes the contribution of postsynaptic potentials which have been discovered as a result of the development of techniques in cellular neurophysiology.

These techniques include essentially: (1) the cathode ray oscilloscope which substituted an electron beam for a pen and enabled events as rapid as the action potentials of nerve cells to be recorded; (2) the microelectrode (developed by Ling and Gerard [22], 1949) which allowed the activity of individual units to be resolved in situ; and (3) the use of these two instruments in preparations chosen because the cells were large, easily isolated, or easily stabilized. It is beyond the scope of this paper to outline the knowledge that has accrued from the application of these techniques, but they constitute one of the most exciting chapters in modern science and have recently been summarized in an excellent short book by Katz [21]. In later discussion I will describe experiments on naturally sleeping animals in which some of the cellular mechanisms proposed by biophysicists have been demonstrated.

The application of the EEG to the study of sleep did not advance significantly until 1938 when Loomis and his colleagues [23] showed that there was considerable variability in the degree of synchronization of human brain waves in sleep. This variability was quantified as stages, but their ordered sequence and psychophysiological significance were not fully appreciated until 1953 when Aserinsky and Kleitman [2], who were attempting to study eye movements in children, showed (1) a periodic alternation of EEG synchronization and desynchronization in sleep; (2) association of rapid eye movements (REMs) with the EEG desynchronization of sleep; and (3) the concomitance of dreaming with the desynchronized phase of sleep. The modern history of sleep psychophysiology began at that point in time and is the subject of detailed treatment elsewhere in this issue.

APPLICATION OF CELLULAR TECHNIQUES TO THE PHYSIOLOGY OF SLEEP

Spontaneous Cortical Unit Activity

The first step in recombining cellular and EEG technologies was made by Jasper, Ricci, and Doane [18] who in 1953 developed a mechanical micromanipulator to study cortical unit activity during conditioning in restrained but unanesthetized monkeys. This effort was inspired in part by the discovery of the phenomenon of reticular activation of the cortex by Moruzzi and Magoun [26] which suggested that sleep and waking or waking and arousal might be differentiated by distinctive rates or patterns of cortical unit activity. In addition to their central focus, the authors also observed the relation of unit activity to the EEG waves.

The direct results of this study were disappointing. The EEG was apparently independent of unitary firing (probably because averaging techniques were not used). Some units speeded up while others slowed in the transition from waking to sleep; the effects of arousal on unit firing were equally various and no simple physiological interpretation was possible. An indirect result, however, was the demonstration that unit activity could be recorded in mammals under entirely physiological conditions. This has led to several important developments.

It was through an attempt in the cat to extend Jasper's results that Hubel developed the hydraulic micromanipulator and tungsten microelectrodes that he and Wiesel [17] have since used so profitably in studies of the visual system in acute (short-term use) preparations. Hubel [16] was the first to report the tendency of cells to fire in bursts in sleep. It was through the combination of a modification of Hubel's hydraulic micromanipulator and the glass insulated platinum-iridium electrodes developed by Wolbarsht [27] that Evarts [9] was able to conduct his extensive studies of cortical unit activity in sleep and waking on freely moving animals. The truly chronic (long-term use) microelectrode had to be made by electropolishing hard metals to permit transdural penetrations of the brain. Thus the first systematic study of the activity of clearly defined units under entirely physiological conditions was made.

Evarts's systematic results, for sleeping and waking, qualitatively confirmed the anecdotal findings of Jasper et al. and of Hubel but went further toward an interpretation of them. Establishing the relative size of cells by the method of antidromic activation, Evarts [8] was able to show that relatively large cells tended to discharge slowly in waking and to speed up in synchronized sleep, whereas small cells discharged rapidly in waking and slowed down in sleep. All cells, whether large or small, tended to increase their rates in desynchronized sleep, which had not been studied by earlier work.

In addition to changes in rate, Evarts noted that irregularity of firing pattern progressed with the succession of states: waking, synchronized, and desynchronized sleep. He postulated that progressive disinhibition was responsible for the increase in rate of some cells and for the pattern changes; this was the first theory of sleep to be stated in the terms of cellular neurophysiology. Unfortunately it is not now directly testable because the inhibitory interneurons which Evarts supposes to become progressively less active in sleep are too small to be resolved with the chronic microelectrode technique. Whether it is correct or not, however, the theory is limited in that it does not attempt to account for the periodicity of sleep stages and its probably central control.

The recognition that size differentiates a cell's spontaneous activity and thus determines the change in that activity with change in state under natural conditions is, however, an important extension of the "size principle" enunciated by Henneman et al. [15] on the basis of experiments in acute spinal preparations. This fundamental principle relates morphological and functional properties in the following way: Large cells have lower membrane resistance and hence higher thresholds (i.e., require more current to effect a given change in membrane potential) than do small cells. Consequently the smaller the cell, the more easily excitable it will be [14]. Small cells should therefore have higher resting discharge rates than large cells, given the same transmembrane current. Evarts's work shows this to be true. Evarts points out that smaller cells are not only more active but also more liable to fatigue as a function of size; they expend relatively more energy in generating action potentials because the ratio of surface area (membrane) to volume (energy source) is higher than that of large cells. Hence a function of sleep may be to rest those cells below a critical size. The problem with this theory is that the capacity of the sodium pump in even the smallest cells is far greater than the demands of the highest recorded firing rates.

The bursts of cortical cell discharge that characterize desynchronized sleep are temporally correlated with each other and have a definite relation to other events in that state. For this reason, and others deriving from lesion work, it is necessary to postulate a central, active control mechanism, whether or not diffuse, passive disinhibition is playing a role. McCarley and I have recently confirmed Evarts's results on rate and pattern of unit discharge in all respects and have detailed the temporal sequence of phasic events in desynchronized sleep. In brief summary, we found that eye movement is always the initial event, followed at relatively long intervals by a peak of surface positivity (75 msec.) in the EEG and a burst of unit firing (72 msec.). The unit firing has no obvious relationship to direction or velocity of eye movement. The results seem to imply that the cortex is receiving greatly delayed and nonspecific information about eye movement or its central correlates.

Further investigation of this phenomenon in sleeping animals may contribute to our understanding of the occulomotor system and its integration with the perceptual side of the visual apparatus. Direct extension of the Evarts technique to other cortical and subcortical areas will allow (1) testing of the generality of his findings with respect to sleep, and (2) the first direct tests of "center theory" of sleep and waking—a theory which has depended until now rather heavily on the indirect results of lesion experiments. An example of the latter approach would be to examine the spontaneous activity of brainstem units for evidence of pacemaker function.

Spinal Reflex Activity

After Dement [7] described EEG desynchronization and REMs in sleeping cats, Jouvet and Michel [20] noted the concomitant disappearance of tonic nuchal electromyographic potentials. Extensive investigation of this phenomenon has been made by Pompeiano and his co-workers [11], who have established the inhibitory nature of the phenomenon. They first demonstrated that the spinal monosynaptic reflex activity, measured by stimulating cutaneous afferent nerve and recording from homonymous muscles, was tonically diminished during desynchronized sleep and underwent further phasic diminution during the bursts of REM.

Two additional experiments indirectly implicated descending inhibition (as against disfacilitation) as the mechanism for these reflex modulations: (1) The activity of cells in brainstem centers responsible for facilitation of the reflex in question was enhanced, not diminished, in desynchronized sleep [5]; and (2) selective section of the dorsolateral funiculus of the cord, by which fibers from the inhibitory reticular formation descend, resulted in abolition of reflex modulation below the level of the lesion [13].

It remained to demonstrate directly that the synapse in question was inhibited and to elucidate the mechanism(s) of the inhibition. Postsynaptic inhibition (of the anterior horn cell) was implicated by the finding that the recurrent discharge elicited by antidromic stimulation of the efferent ventral root fibers [12] and the direct response of alpha motoneurons to stimulation [24] were tonically diminished in desynchronized sleep. Presynaptic inhibition was also implicated by the finding [25] that the amplitude of the antidromic response in the afferent dorsal root nerves was phasically enhanced during REMs. (The increase in excitability of the primary afferent terminals is thought to be caused by activation by descending fibers and to result in effective inhibition by depolarizing the terminals so that impulses arising within the reflex pathway release less than usual amounts of transmitter.)

Pompeiano's results suggest therefore that tonic postsynaptic inhibition and phasic presynaptic inhibition are responsible for the modulation of spinal reflex activity in sleep. These experiments are the first to demonstrate presynaptic inhibition under entirely natural conditions. Since their completion, presynaptic inhibition has been shown to occur in the geniculate [4] and cuneate nuclei [6] during sleep. Chronic extracellular techniques could now be used to examine the activity of units in the bulbar inhibitory reticular formation during desynchronized sleep. Their activity should increase. Direct proof of postsynaptic inhibition must, however, await the development of chronic intracellular recording of spinal cord units.

POSSIBLE FUTURE DEVELOPMENTS

One combination of existing methods that has yet to be tried is that of unit recording in certain anatomical preparations. After midbrain transection (as in the cerveau isolé), the EEG of the forebrain is predominantly synchronized, presumably as a result of elimination of reticular activation, but the cortical cellular activity of this preparation has never been studied for comparison with that of natural sleep. The muscle tone of such a preparation, or one from which all structures anterior to the section are removed (such as the pontine cat), continues to show periodic suppression together with eye movement, supporting the notion that timekeeping and triggering mechanisms of desynchronized sleep are in the brainstem. Because of its relative immobility it should be easier, if less physiological, than it is in the intact animal to explore the brainstem units of such a preparation for evidence of pacemaker activity.

The implications of recent results using pharmacological and biochemical techniques should also be tested with chronic recording techniques. If it is true that the raphe system of serotonergic neurons is active in sleep, as Jouvet [19] suggests, it should be possible to show consistent increases in firing rates of neurons in that region before and during sleep. Such an approach is based on the assumption (which should also be tested experimentally) that the release of transmitters and so-called neuromodulators is related to cell discharge. This assumption is based on an analogy with the neuromuscular junction where the quantal release of acetylcholine in conjunction with miniature end-plate potentials has been demonstrated [21]. Actually it should be remembered that chemical transmission has yet to be demonstrated in the central nervous system, and that even if it were, chemical clocks within cells might control the level of available transmitter and thereby effectively uncouple the supposed rapport between action potential generation in the somata of cells and release of transmitter from its endings.

Most of the experiments described in this paper were motivated by functional questions about sleep, but it is clear that questions about basic neurophysiology might equally well motivate experiments in sleeping animals. This is so because the sleeping animal shares an advantage of other commonly used mammalian preparations, namely, immobility, but avoids a disadvantage, anesthesia. This is perhaps the greatest contribution of sleep research to basic neurophysiology.

It is clearly only a matter of time before the chronic microelectrode is sufficiently refined to allow intracellular recording. This will allow the neurophysiologist to extend his fundamental studies of membrane potential and its variability to unanesthetized mammals, to test physiological theories of sleep (such as the disinhibition hypothesis), and to study plastic changes in nerve cells that may be related to the phenomenon of learning.

The perfection of chronic recording techniques in sleeping animals can soon be expected to permit the waking state, with its elaborate behavioral details, to be examined from the vantage point of cellular physiology. A step in this direction has been taken by Evarts [10] in his studies of unit activity in relation to movement in monkeys. Another example of this approach is found in the work of Wurtz [28]: an animal is reinforced for maintaining a fixed posture and for fixating on a tangent screen while visual field mapping is carried out, or trained to move its eyes in a certain direction to study the responsivity of units to a stationary stimulus.

These experiments combine chronic microelectrode technique with operant control of the behavior in question. The possibilities opened by this advance are numerous. In essence they all depend upon the capability of producing gross immobility so that input–output relationships can be precisely defined. Even more naturalistic experiments will be possible when "floating" microelectrodes, which will move with the brain instead of being fixed to the skull, are perfected.

It seems to me intuitively and empirically unlikely that *the* mechanism or *the* function of a complex behavior such as sleep is forthcoming. Rather, mechanisms and functions will emerge according to the level of analysis and techniques used. The integration of the results of behavioral, EEG, and neurophysiological research depends upon communication between the several disciplines.

REFERENCES

1. Adrian, E. D., and Matthews, B. H. C. The interpretation of potential waves in the cortex. *J. Physiol.* (London) 81:440, 1934.
2. Aserinsky, E., and Kleitman, N. Regularly occurring periods of eye motility and concurrent phenomena during sleep. *Science* 118:273, 1953.
3. Berger, H. Ueber das Elektroenkephalogramm des Menschen. *J. Psychol. Neurol.* 40:160, 1930.
4. Bizzi, E. Changes in the orthodromic and antidromic response of optic tract during the eye movements of sleep. *J. Neurophysiol.* 29:861, 1966.
5. Bizzi, E., Pompeiano, O., and Somogyi, I. Vestibular nuclei: Activity of single neurons during natural sleep and wakefulness. *Science* 145:414, 1964.
6. Carli, G., Diete-Spiff, K., and Pompeiano, O. Transmission of sensory information through the lemniscal pathway during sleep. *Arch. Ital. Biol.* 105:31, 1967.
7. Dement, W. C. The occurrence of low voltage, fast, electroencephalogram patterns during behavioral sleep in the cat. *Electroenceph. Clin. Neurophysiol.* 10:291, 1958.
8. Evarts, E. V. Neuronal Activity in Visual and Motor Cortex During Sleep and Waking. In M. Jouvet (Ed.), *Aspects Anatomo-Fonctionnels de la Physiologie du Sommeil.* Centre National de la Recherche Scientifique, Paris: 1965.
9. Evarts, E. V. Methods for Recording Activity of Individual Neurons in Moving Animals. In R. F. Rushmer (Ed.), *Methods in Medical Research.* Chicago: Year Book, 1966.
10. Evarts, E. V. Pyramidal tract activity associated with a conditioned hand movement in the monkey. *J. Neurophysiol.* 29:1011, 1966.
11. Gassel, M., Marchiafava, P. L., and Pompeiano, O. Tonic and phasic inhibition of spinal reflexes during deep, desynchronized sleep in unrestrained cats. *Arch. Ital. Biol.* 102:471, 1964.
12. Gassel, M., Marchiafava, P. L., and Pompeiano, O. An analysis of the supraspinal influences acting on motoneurons during

sleep in the unrestrained cat: Modification of the recurrent discharge of the alpha motoneurons during sleep. *Arch. Ital. Biol.* 103:25, 1965.

13. Giaquinto, S., Pompeiano, O., and Somogyi, I. Descending inhibitory influences on spinal reflexes during natural sleep. *Arch. Ital. Biol.* 102:282, 1964.
14. Henneman, E., Somjen, G., and Carpenter, D. O. Excitability and inhibitibility of motoneurons of different sizes. *J. Neurophysiol.* 28:599, 1965.
15. Henneman, E., Somjen, G., and Carpenter, D. O. Functional significance of cell size in spinal motoneurons. *J. Neurophysiol.* 28:560, 1965.
16. Hubel, D. H. Single unit activity in striate cortex of unrestrained cats. *J. Physiol.* (London) 147:226, 1959.
17. Hubel, D. H., and Wiesel, T. N. Receptive fields, binocular interaction and functional architecture in the cat's visual cortex. *J. Physiol.* (London) 160:106, 1962.
18. Jasper, H., Ricci, G. F., and Doane, B. Patterns of Cortical Neuron Discharge During Conditioned Responses in Monkeys. In G. E. W. Wolstenholme and C. M. O'Connor (Eds.), *Neurological Basis of Behavior.* Boston: Little, Brown, 1957.
19. Jouvet, M. Biogenic amines and the states of sleep. *Science* 163:32, 1969.
20. Jouvet, M., and Michel, F. Correlation electromyographiques du sommeil chez le chat decortiqué et mésencephalique chronique. *C. R. Soc. Biol.* (Paris) 153:422, 1959.
21. Katz, B. *Nerve, Muscle and Synapse.* New York: McGraw-Hill, 1966.
22. Ling, G., and Gerard, R. W. The normal membrane potential of frog sartorius fibers. *J. Cell. Comp. Physiol.* 34:383, 1949.
23. Loomis, A. L., Harvey, E. N., and Hobart, G. A. Cerebral states during sleep as studied by human brain potentials. *J. Exp. Psychol.* 21:127, 1937.
24. Morrison, A. R., and Pompeiano, O. An analysis of the supraspinal influences acting on motoneurons during sleep in the unrestrained cat: Responses of the alpha motoneurons to direct electrical stimulation during sleep. *Arch. Ital. Biol.* 103:497, 1965.
25. Morrison, A. R., and Pompeiano, O. Central depolarization of group 1-a afferent fibers during desynchronized sleep. *Arch. Ital. Biol.* 103:517, 1965.

26. Moruzzi, G., and Magoun, H. W. Brain stem reticular formation and activation of the EEG. *Electroenceph. Clin. Neurophysiol.* 1:455, 1949.
27. Wolbarsht, M. L., MacNichol, E. F., Jr., and Wagner, H. G. Glass insulated platinum iridium microelectrode. *Science* 132:1309, 1960.
28. Wurtz, R. H. Visual cortex neurons: Response to stimuli during rapid eye movements. *Science* 162:1148, 1968.

Implications of the Rest-Activity Cycle

What are the implications of the 90-minute "sleep-dream" cycle, or "basic rest-activity" cycle (the periodicity itself, as distinct from the work on sleep and dreaming)?

Implications for Organization of Activities

NATHANIEL KLEITMAN

The 90-minute "sleep-dream" cycle represents a basic rest-activity cycle (BRAC) which is easily discerned during sleep, but which probably represents a fundamental periodicity in the activity of the central nervous system of homoiothermic animals, without any particular relation to the alternation of sleep and wakefulness. The length of the cycle seems to vary directly with the size of the animal species, running from 10 to 13 minutes in the rat to 2 hours in the elephant. Ontogenetically, too, the BRAC lengthens from infancy to maturity—in the human subject from 50–60 minutes up to 85–95 minutes, parallel with the lengthening of the cardiac and respiratory cycles, as pointed out by Hartmann [3].

Unlike plants and certain animal parasites, the majority of animal species have to stir into activity from time to time to procure food and fill the stomach. The activity phase of the BRAC serves to initiate feeding, as shown by the data of Marquis [4] on interfeeding periods of newborn infants on a "self-demand" feeding schedule. Mean interfeeding intervals during the daytime hours were equal to four BRACs, but lengthened to five BRACs at night, when it was quiet in the nursery. Mild hunger contractions, as reported by Wada [5], occur at the end of each BRAC, and an infant, when not demanding to be fed at the end of the third or fourth BRAC, would do so at the end of the fifth. For adults, oral activity cycles (eating, drinking, smoking) have been observed during midday waking hours, with a mean cycle length of 96 minutes for normal subjects [2] and 88 minutes for mild chronic schizophrenic patients [1].

There is probably very little one can—or should—do with respect to the operation of the BRAC in sleep. In wakefulness, however, we can perhaps utilize the existence of this "biological hour" to schedule classes in schools, stints of work in factories and offices, coffee breaks and, in general, arrange our activities on a rational physiological basis. Therein lie the implications of the BRAC, as distinct from the work on sleep and dreaming.

REFERENCES

1. Friedman, S. Oral activity cycles in mild chronic schizophrenia. *Amer. J. Psychiat.* 125:743, 1968.
2. Friedman, S., and Fisher, C. On the presence of a rhythmic, diurnal, oral instinctual drive cycle in man. *J. Amer. Psychoanal. Ass.* 15:317, 1967.
3. Hartmann, E. The 90-minute sleep-dream cycle. *Arch. Gen. Psychiat.* (Chicago) 18:280, 1968.
4. Marquis, D. F. Learning in the neonate: The modification of behavior under three feeding schedules. *J. Exp. Psychol.* 29:263, 1941.
5. Wada, T. Experimental study of hunger in its relation to activity. *Arch. Psychol.* 8:1, 1922.

Rhythmic Functions during Sleep

GORDON G. GLOBUS

When following the fantastic calligraphy of the electroencephalogram tracing during sleep, one of the most impressive phenomena is the waxing and waning of amplitude and frequency. Just as adult human sleep as a whole tends to follow a circadian or near circadian rhythm, recurring approximately every 24 hours [11], faster frequency rhythms (ultradian) occur within sleep itself. It seems that an understanding of the biological significance of sleep has to encompass not only the functions taking place in the cross section of a given phase of sleep, but the temporal organization of sleep as well. Since little data on sleep has been reported from the vantage point of rhythmicity, this paper examines some vicissitudes of the REM-NREM (non-rapid eye movement) sleep cycle under a number of conditions, as culled from the literature.

BINARY AUTOCORRELATION METHOD

In order to examine sleep rhythmicity, a binary autocorrelation method has been applied to sleep data. This method will be reported in detail elsewhere [4]. Essentially, a night of sleep data scored for sleep stage (see Glossary: Stages of Sleep) is converted to a binary system by labeling each minute of REM sleep "1" and every other minute "0" or, pari passu, each minute of stage 4 sleep "1" and every other minute "0." An autocorrelation is then performed on the binary time series so constructed. A high correspondence of the time series with itself following a time displacement (lag), as indicated by the presence of a high percentage agreement between the base and lagged time series, reveals the presence of a periodic function.

Ninety-two all night sleep recordings from 10 normal subjects collected by Dr. William Dement were subjected to the binary autocorrelation. The mean percentage agreement at successive time displacements at 1 minute was computed for all nights of each subject and then pooled across subjects. Although a periodic function would be expected to be apparent for the REM-NREM sleep cycle, it does not necessarily follow that the other sleep stages also would be periodic—i.e., stage 2 sleep vs. non-stage 2 sleep and stages 3 and 4 sleep vs. non-stages 3 and 4 sleep. For example, it might be predicted that if stage 2 sleep is simply a transitional stage between the more important REM sleep and slow wave (stages 3 and 4) sleep, i.e., a kind of "filler," then it would not be rhythmic.

Table 1 contains the results, grouped in 10-minute intervals for economy of presentation. Scanning down the vertical columns of Table 1, which indicate the percentage agreement at a given time displacement, it is apparent that periodicity is present for all three comparisons and that the periods which best fit the data are quite similar. For stage REM vs. NREM, the period is 99 minutes; for

TABLE 1. *Normative sleep data*

Lag (minutes)	Percentage Agreement		
	REM vs. NREM	Stage 2 vs. Non-stage 2	Stages 3–4 vs. Non-stages 3–4
1– 10	76.11	77.35	77.89
11– 20	44.68	54.92	52.40
21– 30	22.30	46.27	36.83
31– 40	9.38	43.76	26.82
41– 50	4.64	43.09	22.19
51– 60	5.21	43.05	23.56
61– 70	11.41	44.29	28.12
71– 80	22.39	45.99	31.52
81– 90	34.06	47.78	32.72
91–100	39.51	50.36	33.29
101–110	38.13	52.29	31.27
111–120	31.48	52.19	27.83
121–130	24.12	50.39	25.29
131–140	18.43	46.95	23.60

stage 2 vs. non-stage 2, 110.5 minutes; and for stages 3 and 4 vs. non-stages 3 and 4, 95 minutes. Although the percentage correspondence indicates that the stage REM vs. NREM periodicity is more clearly expressed, the various sleep stages all seem to follow periodic functions on the order of 100 minutes.

STABILITY OF SLEEP RHYTHMICITY

Given this ultradian rhythmicity during sleep, the question then arises as to the stability of this rhythm under different conditions. Following prolonged total sleep deprivation, it might be anticipated that the pressure for slow wave sleep would be so great that the rhythmicity of stages 3 and 4 vs. non-stages 3 and 4 sleep would be disrupted. Gulevich et al. [5] reported a study of a 17-year-old boy who remained awake continuously for 264 hours. Analysis of the data presented in Table 2 reveals a periodicity for stages 3 and 4

TABLE 2. *Sleep loss*

Lag (minutes)	Percentage Agreement: Stages 3–4 vs. Non-stages 3–4
1.0– 8.6	82.53
8.6– 17.2	59.72
17.2– 25.8	42.28
25.8– 34.4	32.28
34.4– 43.0	28.31
43.0– 51.6	27.91
51.6– 60.2	30.34
60.2– 68.8	40.59
68.8– 77.4	49.28
77.4– 86.0	54.28
86.0– 94.6	51.02
94.6–103.2	42.86
103.2–111.8	37.76
111.8–120.4	35.71

sleep of 86 minutes, which is well within one standard deviation of the means of the 10 normal subjects noted above. Thus severe total sleep deprivation does not appear to alter the fundamental rhythmicity of slow wave sleep.

Turning to the opposite of sleep deprivation, Rechtschaffen [10] studied a subject who slept excessively on two occasions for over 21 and 22 hours. It might be anticipated that such unusually prolonged sleep would lead to a breakdown of the REM sleep cycle from simple surfeit of REM sleep, but this proved not to be the case, as shown in Table 3. Periods of 104 and 113 minutes for the two extended sleep sessions again approximate the normative data. Sleep excess apparently does not effect the REM-NREM sleep cycle.

The syndrome of narcolepsy provides an unusually interesting

TABLE 3. *Sleep excess*

Lag (minutes)	Percentage Agreement (REM vs. NREM)			
	Prolonged Sleep		Narcolepsy	
	Night 1	Night 2	Sleeping	Waking
1– 10	80.83	80.97	76.92	71.81
11– 20	47.75	43.87	39.89	32.72
21– 30	19.15	14.17	7.21	4.73
31– 40	4.57	1.82	6.02	0.00
41– 50	0.77	0.00	0.10	0.00
51– 60	2.85	0.01	0.91	0.00
61– 70	11.44	3.96	15.08	0.00
71– 80	24.84	15.42	15.08	0.00
81– 90	34.69	25.10	26.63	3.42
91–100	41.96	32.04	31.33	6.22
101–110	47.27	43.30	26.77	4.76
111–120	41.19	48.78	25.52	9.95
121–130	31.99	40.83	21.11	37.62
131–140	20.98	27.63	25.14	51.09
141–150	16.19	15.44	27.69	40.42
151–160	15.89	10.19	35.68	19.69

opportunity to study the REM sleep cycle, as narcolepsy apparently consists of attacks of REM sleep [1]. Narcolepsy is also characterized by REM periods at sleep onset [10]. The question here is whether or not attacks of narcolepsy follow a rhythm. Passouant [9] reported a case studied for 24 hours which is of interest in this regard. The binary autocorrelation for REM vs. NREM sleep is contained in Table 3 for both sleep and waking. During a 9¼-hour sleep period at night, the subject had five REM sleep occurrences (108 minutes total). The period is between 91 and 100 minutes. During the 14¾-hour waking period, there were six intrusions of REM sleep (85 minutes total), three of which were followed by NREM sleep. The period is between 131 and 140 minutes. The percentage agreement indicates that the REM sleep periodicity during waking is even more clearly expressed than during sleep.

These data, which tentatively suggest a periodicity of the REM sleep process during waking as well as sleep, are of special interest in the light of hypotheses that the REM sleep cycle continues throughout the 24 hours [2, 3, 6–8]. It has previously been suggested by this writer [3] that REM "sleep" may be a misnomer, REM periods having nothing intrinsically to do with sleep itself; rather it simply may be easier to measure manifestations of the process against the quiet background of sleep. Further comparable studies on narcoleptics and also on possible manifestations of REM sleep reflected in the behavior of normal waking subjects are needed to test this hypothesis.

The rather long period of over two hours during waking should be noted in passing. One difficulty in analyzing the REM-NREM sleep cycle as an ultradian rhythm over long time spans is that the length of the period may vary as a function of the circadian rhythm, so that data derived from nighttime sleep hours may not be entirely representative. A systematic analysis cannot be obtained from the present data, but in looking at the intervals between REM sleep periods at different times of day in the narcoleptic and hypersomniac subjects who were followed over long time spans, there appears to be a marked 24-hour component, and also possibly a 12-hour component.

FUNCTION OF PHYSIOLOGICAL PERIODICITY

It is apparent from the above analyses that the temporal organization during sleep is highly characteristic and resistant to change. Rhythms for REM sleep, stage 2 sleep, and stages 3 and 4 sleep are similar. Total sleep deprivation, sleep excess, and intrusion of REM sleep into waking in the form of narcoleptic attacks do not appear to alter greatly the fundamental periodicity. Such a highly buffered system seems designed to insure some biological advantage, but it is not apparent immediately just what that advantage is. Kleitman's notion [7] of a basic rest-activity cycle as a building block for the temporal structure of waking and sleeping seems particularly cogent. If rest and activity were only a function of transient environmental demands and internal needs, then this behavior might be highly variable, in response to the immediate situation. Temporal organization of rest and activity might serve to modulate the behavior considerably, increasing autonomy from stimulus demands and providing more efficient functioning. It is clear, however, that at present much too little information is available about ultradian rhythms for their biological function to be confidently set forth.

ACKNOWLEDGMENT

The writer thanks Dr. William Dement for providing sleep data on normal subjects and Dr. Alan Rechtschaffen for providing sleep data on the hypersomniac subject.

REFERENCES

1. Dement, W. C., Rechtschaffen, A., and Gulevich, G. The nature of the narcoleptic sleep attack. *Neurology* (Minneap.) 16:18, 1966.
2. Friedman, S., and Fisher, C. On the presence of a rhythmic, diurnal, oral instinctual drive cycle in man: A preliminary report. *J. Amer. Psychoanal. Ass.* 15:317, 1967.
3. Globus, G. Rapid eye movement cycle in real time: Implica-

tions for a theory of the D-state. *Arch. Gen. Psychiat.* (Chicago) 15:654, 1966.
4. Globus, G. Quantification of the sleep cycle as a rhythm. In press.
5. Gulevich, G., Dement, W. C., and Johnson, L. Psychiatric and EEG observations on a case of prolonged (264 hours) wakefulness. *Arch. Gen. Psychiat.* (Chicago) 15:29, 1966.
6. Hartmann, E. The 90-minute sleep-dream cycle. *Arch. Gen. Psychiat.* (Chicago) 18:280, 1968.
7. Kleitman, N. *Sleep and Wakefulness* (2d ed.). Chicago: University of Chicago Press, 1963.
8. Kripke, D. F., and O'Donoghue, J. P. Perceptual deprivation, REM sleep, and an ultradian biological rhythm (abstract). *Psychophysiology* 5 (No. 2):231, 1968.
9. Passouant, P., Cadilhac, J., and Baldy-Moulinier, M. Physiopathologie des hypersomnies. *Rev. Neurol.* (Paris) 116 (No. 6): 585, 1967.
10. Rechtschaffen, A., Wolpert, E., Dement, W., Mitchell, S., and Fisher, C. Nocturnal sleep of narcoleptics. *Electroenceph. Clin. Neurophysiol.* 15:599, 1963.
11. Sollberger, A. *Biological Rhythm Research.* Amsterdam: Elsevier, 1965.

Comments on the 90-Minute Sleep-Dream Cycle

ARTHUR SHAPIRO*

The 90-minute sleep-dream cycle is a concept derived initially from observations by Dement and Kleitman [1]. They found that the time between the onset of one REM period and the next, observed over many nights and many subjects, was 85.5 minutes. Later it was recognized that this was precisely the same as the average time between one nocturnal penis erection and the next, as reported by Ohlmeyer et al. [2] in 1944. Many other physiological variables have since been found to be generally associated with this periodicity.

* Deceased.

There have been several attempts to provide a theoretical mechanism to account for this recurring periodicity. Most of them have assumed that the approximately 90-minute interval represented the time taken to accumulate some toxic substance requiring REM sleep to discharge it or to use up some necessary substance that required REM sleep to accumulate it. It has also been proposed that the cycle was a manifestation of some underlying time-keeping mechanism which divided the 24-hour period into sixteen 1 ½-hour segments coupled to clock time. Still another type of proposal assumed the interaction of brain states associated with nearly complete deafferentation and those in which stimulation from within the brain produced a kind of protective arousal.

FACTS THE THEORIES CANNOT IGNORE

It must be admitted that at the present time there is insufficient evidence for any of these theoretical proposals. But there are some specific and important facts that must be accounted for by any theory.

1. While statistically the 85.5-minute periodicity has been repeatedly confirmed as the average value, individual intervals occur as short as 20 minutes and as long as 120 minutes. Even when average values alone are considered they are not constant over time of night, nor are they necessarily related to the duration of the REM period which begins each cycle, or to the duration of preceding sleep stages.

2. While the onset of eye movements in stage 1 sleep provides a fairly precise marker for time measurements, there are no reliable data establishing a periodicity for onset or termination of other stages of sleep. Even for REM sleep, the average accompanying physiological phenomena (e.g., penis erection, irregular breathing, faster irregular heart rate) often begin as much as 10 minutes before or 10 minutes after the beginning of the REM period and may last well past the end of the REM period or terminate long before it. Disappearance of submental electromyogram potentials in unse-

lected human REM periods correlates even less well with the actual onset and termination of each REM period.

3. There is very strong evidence that dreaming may occur in non-REM sleep and that some REM periods are not associated with dreaming.

In the light of the real complexity of the data for which it must account, it is not surprising that we do not yet have an established theoretical mechanism for the 90-minute sleep-dream cycle. It is perhaps worth noting that 85.5 minutes is also the value of Schuler's constant for the gyrocompass and is equal to $\frac{1}{2\pi}\sqrt{\frac{R}{g}}$ where R is the radius of the earth and g is the acceleration due to gravity at the earth's surface. Ninety minutes is also the approximate period of revolution of artificial satellites fairly close to the surface of the earth.

A GEOPHYSICAL THEORY

Could it be that somewhere in our brains a mechanism is still operating to preserve the perceptual image of a flat stationary earth, when we are actually living on the surface of a rotating sphere which moves at a tangential velocity of about 1000 miles per hour and reverses its direction every 12 hours? Such a fundamental rhythm, perhaps dating phylogenetically to the time of first emergence of vertebrates from the sea, could conceivably be used as a coordinating timing mechanism for different processes in different species. Some evidence suggests its presence in the heart rate records of arctic foxes telemetered in their natural environments. At the present stage of our knowledge, the geophysical origins of the 90-minute cycle are no less plausible than any of the others that have been proposed.

REFERENCES

1. Dement, W., and Kleitman, N. Cyclic variations in EEG during sleep and their relation to eye movements, body motility, and dreaming. *Electroenceph. Clin. Neurophysiol.* 9:673, 1957.
2. Ohlmeyer, P., and Brilmayer, H. Periodische Vorgaenge im Schlaf. *Pflueger Arch. Ges. Physiol.* 249:50, 1947.

The Effects of Age on Sleep

---

*In what ways does age affect sleep patterns and sleep requirements? What mechanisms or intervening variables may be involved?**

Age-related Changes in Sleep Characteristics

EDWIN KAHN

An increasing number of empirical investigations [1–11] on different age groups are providing some answers to questions regarding the relationship of sleep and age. In collaboration with Charles Fisher, I have completed investigations on the sleep of the aged male [4] and the aged female [6] and have recently collected data on the sleep of children, aged 2 to 5 years, which have not as yet been analyzed.

SLEEP PATTERNS OF THE AGED

From preliminary observation the most striking difference between the sleep records of the aged and those of children is the

* The reader interested in these questions may wish to refer also to another paper in this issue by Webb (p. 44) and to the paper by Hawkins (p. 85).

amplitude and duration of slow wave activity, a difference first noted by Roffwarg, Dement, and Fisher [9]. For the child, stage 4 delta waves may easily reach 400 to 500 μv. or more, but for the aged the amplitude rarely exceeds 200 to 250 μv. Stretches of high voltage, slow activity also continue for considerably longer periods [3, 8–10]. Young adult findings reflect the gradual reduction in amounts of stage 4 sleep from childhood to old age [3]. In the elderly we have found that the time from sleep onset to the first REM period is often shorter than that reported for younger age groups. This shortened latency is probably a direct result of the decrease in stage 4 sleep. Some increase in slow wave activity for the aged may be associated with the beginnings of pathological brain change [3]. One of our oldest subjects, aged 91, had the highest proportion of stages 3 and 4 sleep of all subjects studied. Since an increase in slow wave activity has been reported in the awake EEG of the aged, both findings may reflect the influence of a similar mechanism.

Another change in the sleep patterns of the aged is increased wakefulness. For men and women between the ages of 66 and 95 years, we found significant correlations between age and sleep disturbance (as measured by number of awakenings and percentage of time awake). This confirms a finding of Feinberg, Koresko, and Heller [3], who also found significant correlations between age and number of awakenings for adults between the ages of 19 and 36 years. Thus there appears to be a progressive increase in number of awakenings from sleep, starting at young adulthood and lasting through the life span. Sleep time, however, is not necessarily reduced as a result of the increased wakefulness; that is, the older person may spend more time in bed to get the same amount of sleep as the young adult [3].

In early observations, Roffwarg, Dement, and Fisher [9] reported that REM sleep time of the aged was reduced to 13 to 18 percent of total sleep time, from the 22 percent of the young adult. More recent investigations indicate that this reduction is not that marked, at least until extreme old age. For instance, we found REM percentages of 20.1 for the male (aged 71 to 95 years) and 18.0 for the female (aged 66 to 87 years). However, amounts of REM sleep were quite low in four of the oldest individuals studied, aged 95, 95, 91, and 87 years. The mean REM percentage for these four was 13.0; REM periods were frequently interrupted by short stretches of stage 2 sleep and, for two, were foreshortened by abrupt awakenings.

POSSIBLE CAUSES OF AGE-RELATED CHANGES

Several hypotheses have been advanced regarding the function of sleep states, and especially REM sleep. Perhaps the most thoroughly developed explanation of age-related changes in sleep characteristics has been presented by Feinberg and his associates [2, 3]. Feinberg studied in detail the sleep characteristics and intellectual abilities of normal, aged subjects, patients with chronic brain syndrome, and mentally retarded patients. He found that within each group studied, sleep variables, and in particular amounts of REM sleep, correlated with measures of level of intellectual functioning. He took these findings as support for the view that during sleep the brain carries out processes required for cognition. However, he did offer an alternate hypothesis that brain pathology may impair sleep mechanisms and intelligence in the absence of any direct relationship between the latter two variables.

The findings obtained by us on the sleep characteristics of the normal aged seem to favor the latter alternative. For the aged male we found [5] that amounts of REM sleep did tend to correlate with aspects of cognitive functioning. However, we also observed that amounts of REM sleep tended to correlate with noncognitive measures, such as amount of REM-period erection and strength of grip. Feinberg found that cognitive performance in the normal aged was estimated at least as well by REM sleep measures as by the age of the subject. We were unable to replicate this finding; that is, we found that cognitive measures correlated consistently higher with age than with amounts of REM sleep. Thus we have not been able fully to confirm Feinberg's results in the normal aged.

An experiment may be suggested which would be of further theoretical interest. In the patient groups studied by Feinberg the relationships between amounts of REM sleep and noncognitive measures, such as amount of nocturnal erection and strength of grip, would be compared to the correlations between amounts of REM sleep and the cognitive measures obtained for these patients. Such an investigation might help further clarify whether the relationship between REM sleep and intelligence is or is not a causal one.

REFERENCES

1. Agnew, H. W., Jr., Webb, W. W., and Williams, R. L. Sleep patterns in late middle age males: An EEG study. *Electroenceph. Clin. Neurophysiol.* 23:168, 1967.
2. Feinberg, I., Braun, M., and Shulman, E. EEG sleep patterns in mental retardation. *Electroenceph. Clin. Neurophysiol.* 27: 128, 1969.
3. Feinberg, I., Koresko, R. L., and Heller, N. EEG sleep patterns as a function of normal and pathological aging in man. *J. Psychiat.* Res. 5:107, 1967.
4. Kahn, E., and Fisher, C. The sleep characteristics of the normal aged male. *J. Nerv. Ment. Dis.* 148:477, 1969.
5. Kahn, E., and Fisher, C. Some correlates of REM sleep in the normal aged male. *J. Nerv. Ment. Dis.* In press.
6. Kahn, E., Fisher, C., and Lieberman, L. The sleep characteristics of the aged female. *J. Nerv. Ment. Dis.* 148:495, 1969.
7. Kales, A., Wilson, T., Kales, J. D., Jacobson, A., Paulson, M. J., Kollar, E., and Walter, R. D. Measurements of all-night sleep in normal elderly persons: Effects of aging. *J. Amer. Geriat. Soc.* 15:405, 1967.
8. Kohler, W. C., Coddington, R. D., and Agnew, H. W., Jr. Sleep patterns in 2-year-old children. *J. Pediat.* 72:228, 1968.
9. Roffwarg, H. P., Dement, W. C., and Fisher, C. Preliminary Observations of the Sleep-Dream Pattern in Neonates, Infants, Children and Adults. In E. Harms (Ed.), *Monographs on Child Psychiatry,* No. II. New York: Pergamon, 1964.
10. Ross, J. J., Agnew, H. W., Jr., Williams, R. L., and Webb, W. B. Sleep patterns in pre-adolescent children: An EEG-EOG study. *Pediatrics* 42:324, 1968.

11. Williams, R. L., Agnew, H. W., Jr., and Webb, W. B. Sleep patterns in young adults: An EEG study. *Electroenceph. Clin. Neurophysiol.* 17:376, 1964.

Length and Distribution of Sleep and the Intrasleep Process

W. B. WEBB

Sleep is age-linked in at least three ways: length, distribution, and the intrasleep process. The relationship between sleep length and age has been reviewed elsewhere [6]. In brief, it is reported that average sleep length decreased from 16½ hours at birth [3] to 15 hours at 4 weeks of age and 14 hours by the twenty-sixth week [1]. Between the ages of 2 and 3, sleep averaged 12½ hours plus a 1-hour nap; between 4 and 5 years of age, sleep length was 11 hours with a 1-hour nap [4]. Two reports on sleep length in two older groups presented an interesting point. Terman and Hocking [5] in 1913 reported average times of sleep approximately 10 hours for 8- to 12-year-olds and approximately 9 hours for 12- to 17-year-old subjects. Data collected nearly fifty years later reported [2] sleep length averages about one hour less in comparable age groups. It is our opinion that the data are equally valid and that sleep length averages have decreased by an hour over the fifty years.

The above articles also review the matter of sleep distribution. Again in brief, sleep of the neonate was quite polyphasic and in the third week only 57 percent of the sleep occurred between 9:00 P.M. and 8:00 A.M. However, by the twenty-sixth week some 73 percent of the sleep occurred during this period with a perceptible tendency for the day sleep to become biphasic around the periods of 10:00 A.M. to noon and 2:00 P.M. to 4:00 P.M. [1]. By the first year naps tended to consolidate into a single afternoon nap and to drop out of the subjects' sleep behavior by the age of 5 [4]. There seems to be some evidence of a deterioration of the single consolidated night sleep period in the aged.

There are systematic changes in the intrasleep patterns of subjects as reflected by the electroencephalogram. Table 1, which was reported in the review article by Webb and Agnew [6], displays these changes. There are three prominent aspects of this table: (1) REM sleep is quite stable from the preteen group through the elderly group (the slight decrease in the older group is not statistically significant). The higher REM in the youngest group appears to reflect the transition from the typically reported amounts of approximately 50 percent in the infant. (2) There is a clear general reduction of stage 4 sleep with age, with no stage 4 in some older subjects. (3) There is an increase in light and interrupted (stage 1 and stage 0) sleep.

TABLE 1. *Sleep stage percentages for age groupings*

Age of Group (years)	Stages of Sleep						Mean Sleep Length (minutes)	No. of Subjects
	0	1	REM	2	3	4		
21–31 mos.	2	8	29	43	—	18	596	16
8–11	2	6	24	44	6	18	565	18
16–19	1	5	23	47	6	18	454	32
20–29 (m)	1	5	24	50	7	13	418	28
20–29 (f)	1	6	22	48	7	16	451	16
30–39	2	8	22	53	5	10	443	12
50–59	4	11	23	51	8	3	436	16
60–69	9	12	20	51	5	3	440	16

Source: From Webb and Agnew [6].

As for the interpretation of these age-linked characteristics, I suspect that the length and distribution aspects are primarily determined by hereditary–ecological interactions (in short, evolution), although I remain convinced that in the human, at least, these characteristics are malleable within limits (see my discussion of individual differences in sleep length, p. 44 of this issue). More certain answers are likely to emerge from the comparative studies of sleep across species and in varied environments.

REFERENCES

1. Kleitman, N., and Englemann, T. G. Sleep characteristics of infants. *J. Appl. Physiol.* 6:269, 1953.
2. O'Connor, A. L. Questionnaire Responses About Sleep. University of Florida (Gainesville) M.A. Thesis, 1964.
3. Parmalee, A. H., Schultz, H. R., and Disbrow, M. A. Sleep patterns of the newborn. *J. Pediat.* 58:241, 1961.
4. Reynolds, M. M., and Mallay, H. The sleep of children in a 24-hour nursery school. *J. Genet. Psychol.* 43:322, 1933.
5. Terman, L. M., and Hocking, A. The sleep of school children: Its distribution according to age and its relation to physical and mental efficiency. *J. Educ. Psychol.* 4:138, 1913.
6. Webb, W. B., and Agnew, H. W., Jr. Measurement and Characteristics of Nocturnal Sleep. In L. A. Abt and B. F. Riess (Eds.), *Progress in Clinical Psychology,* Vol. 8. New York: Grune & Stratton, 1969.

The Need for Sleep

---

*What determines how much sleep a person needs? How much dreaming? Are there persons who need far more sleep or less sleep than most of us? If so, what characterizes their sleep? And what are they like psychologically?**

Sleep Requirements and the Characteristics of Some Sleepers

FREDERICK BAEKELAND AND
ERNEST HARTMANN

One of the most important problems connected with sleep is that of sleep requirements. It is often assumed that an individual's sleep time *is* his sleep requirement. Defined in this sense, sleep can be thought of as a response and studied in relation to changes in environmental variables. Another paper in this issue (p. 49) describes

* The reader interested in these questions may wish to refer also to papers in this issue by Webb (p. 29) and Hauri (p. 70) and to other papers by Baekeland (p. 49) and Hartmann (p. 59).

recent experiments of this kind where the emphasis has been primarily on sleep composition rather than on sleep length or postsleep functioning. Clinical studies [14, 20] indicate that sleep may be shortened in a variety of psychopathological conditions associated with elevated levels of anxiety or arousal, such as anxiety reactions, impending or acute psychosis, neurasthenia, and depression. Conversely, increased sleep times occur in conditions where anxiety is low and sleep can provide an escape from intrapsychic and interpersonal conflicts, as in mild depressions and chronic schizophrenia [20].

Although an individual's sleep time could be equated with his sleep requirement, it seems just as plausible to suppose that some people may sleep more and others less than they "need" to. For the concept of *sleep need* in this second sense to become operationally definable, sleep requirements must be thought of in relation to specific functions during wakefulness, such as learning and memory, problem solving, stability, and kind of affect, somatic functioning, and the like. Investigations of sleep requirements in this second sense have taken the direction of studying the effects either of total or of partial sleep deprivation.

SLEEP DEPRIVATION

The extensive literature on total sleep deprivation agrees on a number of points [36]: The effects on behavioral tasks are a function both of amount of deprivation and of time of day, and they are reversible. They include reduced levels of arousal associated with periodic lapses in performance efficiency, especially in tasks which are boring or unduly complex. Beyond 40 hours of sleep deprivation, subjects show increased irritability, lack of perseverance, and often (especially during periods of relative inactivity) perceptual (visual, temporal, and cognitive) distortions. After 100 hours of sleep deprivation some subjects may show disordered behavior resembling paranoid psychosis. On recovery nights, lost slow wave (stages 3 and

4) sleep is preferentially made up before REM sleep (D-state). Interesting as such experiments have been, their main use has been to define upper limits for toleration of sleep deprivation.

On the other hand, the results of studies of the effects of partial sleep deprivation, which involve sleep times in the normal range for some people, have been contradictory. Some have claimed impaired performance or mood, while others have reported no impairment [20]. Conflicting results have also come from studies of restricted sleep regimens where the subject's sleep was broken into two short periods of sleep with an intervening waking interval [20] or where the subject slept only once every 40 to 48 hours [20, 23, 24]. Most of these studies are hard to evaluate since they have tended to be short term, to use few subjects, and to involve rather insensitive tasks. However, they show striking individual differences among subjects with respect to their ability to tolerate partial sleep deprivation. The best study of this kind to date is that of Wilkinson [37, 38], who used a number of different restricted sleep routines in 24 subjects and studied their performance on a demanding, lengthy, and very monotonous vigilance task. He found that after one night of restricted sleep, performance was not impaired until sleep had been reduced to 2 hours, while after two nights of restricted sleep, performance was impaired at the 5-hour level. He interpreted his data as indicating that until the first 3 hours of his subjects' sleep were intruded upon, there was no change in their capacity, as opposed to willingness, to perform.

Several recent EEG sleep studies [9, 27, 33] have focused on the effects of extended restricted sleep regimens on sleep patterns rather than on postsleep performance. They indicate that nightly amounts of stage 4 sleep increase in the course of such experiments and that if they are continued long enough [9] there are no compensatory increases in stage 4 sleep on recovery nights. On the other hand, on recovery nights there are compensatory increases in REM sleep-time (D-time) a classic sign of REM deprivation [3, 7, 18]. These studies indicate that subjects can learn to preserve slow wave sleep at the expense of other stages of sleep. Like Wilkinson's experiment [36,

37], they also suggest that the lower limits of tolerance to restricted sleep regimens are set by the individual's basic requirements for slow wave sleep.

OBLIGATORY SLEEP

Amounts of slow wave sleep are negatively related to age [4, 5, 16, 19, 22, 25–27], vary positively with exercise levels [2, 6], growth hormone secretion during sleep [28, 29], and perhaps thyroid function [17]. Such findings suggest that amounts of slow wave sleep are related to levels of biological energy expenditure. It therefore seems possible that a night's sleep might be in principle divided into two portions. The first, earlier portion, necessary for unimpaired biological health and performance, is composed largely of slow wave sleep and might be called *obligatory sleep*. The second and later portion, consisting mostly of REM and stage 2 sleep, is less clearly obligatory and could be termed *facultative sleep,* at least in this biological sense. The partial sleep deprivation experiments described suggest that this second portion of sleep may be in part a function of habit and that under appropriate circumstances, which remain to be spelled out, much of it might safely be dispensed with. That such a notion is not entirely chimerical is suggested by a recent report of Jones and Oswald [15], who studied the sleep patterns of two healthy and apparently normal subjects who had for years slept less than three hours per night. Their sleep recordings showed amounts of REM and slow wave sleep about the same as those reported for the first three hours of sleep in subjects with normal sleep times. The importance of the composition of the earlier obligatory portion of sleep in determining the need for additional hours of sleep is underscored by a report of Williams and Williams [39]. They studied "restless" and "quiet" sleepers and found that the restless group, who had less slow wave sleep, showed the greatest performance decrements in response to acute sleep deprivation.

However, this scheme is certainly oversimplified. It is probable that a certain amount of REM sleep is also required, perhaps for proper psychological functioning; early reports on the effects of REM deprivation suggested considerable psychological disruption [8] and some recent studies have reported defects in short-term memory [1, 10] and in defense effectiveness [11]; however, results are still controversial and no very solid effects of REM deprivation have been demonstrated [32].

"LONG" AND "SHORT" SLEEPERS

Clearly the question of defining the kinds of sleep required by man in general, and the amount of each kind, has not been resolved. But if we are willing to assume tentatively that an individual's habitual sleep time approximates his sleep requirement, it becomes pertinent to ask whether there are persons who obtain far more or less sleep than most of us; and if there are, what characterizes their sleep, and what characterizes them psychologically. The average person sleeps about 7.5 hours, but there are some individuals (around 5 percent of the population at each extreme) who sleep less than 6 hours (short sleepers) or more than 9 hours (long sleepers) per night [20, 30, 35]. Studying a population at the extremes could help answer some of the questions discussed above. For instance, a young average sleeper gets about 70 minutes per night (16 percent of sleep) of stage 4 sleep, and about 100 minutes (23 percent) of REM time. Will a person who sleeps 300 minutes per night instead of the usual 440 still obtain 70 minutes of stage 4, though this would now be 24 percent of sleep? Or 100 minutes of REM time, though this would now represent 33 percent of sleep? Either of these results would suggest an approximate universal requirement for a certain length of time spent in a given stage of sleep. On the other hand, if "short sleepers" are found to spend considerably less time than average in stage 4, say, or in REM, suggesting a lower "requirement," can this be explained in terms of greater "intensity"—i.e., higher arousal threshold during stage 4, or more eye movements in REM?

We are currently studying the sleep and personality patterns of long and short sleepers [13] in the hope of getting some clues about the sources of individual differences in sleep requirements. Before being accepted for laboratory study, prospective subjects are screened by a battery of psychological tests and a psychiatric interview. After two nights of adaptation to the laboratory, the subjects sleep for 3 consecutive nights whose length is equal to their mean sleep times at home. As a check on whether they are actually partially sleep deprived on their usual sleep schedules, short sleepers spend a fourth consecutive night in the laboratory on which they can sleep as long as they wish.

Analysis of the sleep records of the first 20 subjects (10 long and 10 short sleepers, mean ages 24.5 and 24.6 years) showed that the long sleepers accumulated significantly more wakefulness, REM, stage 1, and stage 2 sleep during their laboratory nights, but did not have significantly different amounts of stages 3 and 4 sleep (Table 1).

TABLE 1. *Sleep of "long sleepers" and "short sleepers" compared*[a]

Stage	Long Sleepers		Short Sleepers		Significance of Difference between LS & SS, based on minutes
	Minutes	Percent of Total Sleep[b]	Minutes	Percent of Total Sleep[c]	
Waking	41.4	—	11.2	—	$p < .02$
REM sleep (D-state)	122.5	23.2	64.5	19.5	$p < .001$
Stage 1 sleep	31.5	6.0	15.8	4.8	$p < .05$
Stage 2 sleep	261.3	49.6	161.1	48.8	$p < .002$
Stage 3 sleep	23.6	4.5	25.7	7.8	n.s.
Stage 4 sleep	47.0	8.9	51.7	15.7	n.s.

[a]Based on three nights of sleep (nights 3, 4, and 5 in the laboratory) for each subject.
[b]527 minutes.
[c]330 minutes.

Our findings agree with those of Webb and Agnew [34], who studied a smaller, younger, and less extreme group of long and short sleepers, except that their long sleepers accumulated somewhat more stage 3 than did their short sleepers.

Although our short sleepers slept slightly longer on their ad lib sleep nights (6.28 vs. 5.50 hours, $.05 < p < .10$) than on those preceding them, these final nights did not show significantly shorter sleep latencies or REM latencies, less intercurrent wakefulness, or increases either in REM or slow wave sleep. Any one of these changes, had it occurred, would have been considered evidence of prior sleep deprivation. Hence it appears that our short sleepers were not partially sleep deprived but rather were well adapted to their self-imposed sleep routines.

The fact that the two groups had equivalent amounts of slow wave sleep but differed in respect to the other stages of sleep is consistent with previous evidence [40] that virtually all slow wave sleep is accumulated in the first half of the night, while REM [31, 40] and stage 2 sleep [40] are positive functions of sleep length. Our results support the idea that a certain fairly constant amount of slow wave sleep is needed by all persons, while requirements of REM sleep may vary considerably among individuals.

It might be supposed that the short sleepers had a lesser need for sleep on a constitutional basis. However, their interviews indicated that their sleep times had been in the average range or even above average until their late teens when, under increasing time pressure (school, work, extracurricular activities), they began to curtail their sleep without apparent distress. The long sleepers, on the other hand, tended often to have slept more than their age mates since childhood. Hence it seems that aspects of personality development and psychological style may be involved in the differences, in addition to any simple physiological constitutional basis.

Indeed we found a number of personality differences between the two groups: The short sleepers tended to view sleep as an unfortunate necessary intrusion on the scope of their desired waking activities, and they did not worry about possible effects of occasional sleep deprivation. As a rule they appeared ambitious, active, energetic (often holding multiple jobs or going to school full time while holding half- to full-time jobs), cheerful, conformist in their opinions, and sure about their career choices. They were poorer home dream recallers than the long sleepers. Their typical way of dealing with problems was to deny the problem and keep busy in the hope that it would go away. On the other hand, the long sleepers enjoyed their sleep, protected it, and were concerned about the possible deleterious effects of sleep deprivation. A number of them complained or were embarrassed about the fact that they had to sleep so much. They tended to be shy, introverted, slightly anxious or inhibited, mildly depressed, passive, and unsure of themselves. A number of them, for instance, had had no sexual experience at age 25 to 30. They had a wide variety of minor social and psychological problems. Several of them openly stated that sleep was an escape from problems, and most seemed to us to be using sleep in this way.

Formal psychological testing (Minnesota Multiphasic Personality Inventory and California Psychological Inventory) suggested that the short sleepers had a greater need to appear normal or acceptable than the long sleepers and were higher on factors such as sociability, tolerance, and flexibility.

The short sleepers could be described psychologically as tending to be hypomanic, with a great deal of energy and self-confidence and a tendency to the use of denial as a defense. Their physiological sleep patterns are quite similar to, though less extreme than, those described for manic patients [12]. Is it possible that the less troubled days characteristic of the short sleepers, with rapid, painless, relatively unemotional decisions, require less of the integration or reprograming which may occur during the REM state at night?

These findings raise a number of other interesting questions. Do the action-oriented short sleepers need to avoid introspection and fantasy, and hence the subjective experience of dreaming? On the other hand, do the more inhibited and introspective long sleepers have a preferential need for conflict resolution via fantasy and dreaming? Would they therefore more poorly tolerate the effects of REM sleep deprivation? The answers to such questions must await the results of future experiments.

SUMMARY

Our study has delineated some physiological characteristics of long and short sleep, and some psychological characteristics of the respective sleepers. These studies suggest to us that sleep need consists of two portions: a remarkably constant need for slow wave sleep, and a far more variable need for REM (and perhaps stage 2). However, neither this nor other recent sleep research has yet provided any definitive answers to the question of exactly what factors determine individual sleep requirements. This state of affairs is hardly surprising if one realizes that asking what determines sleep requirements is really equivalent to asking what is the function of sleep.

REFERENCES

1. Adelman, S., and Hartmann, E. Psychological Effects of Amitryptyline-induced Dream-Deprivation. Paper read at Association for the Psychophysiological Study of Sleep (APSS), Denver, 1968.
2. Adey, W. R., Bors, E., and Porter, R. W. EEG sleep patterns after high cervical lesions in man. *Arch. Neurol.* (Chicago) 19: 377, 1968.
3. Agnew, H. W., Jr., Webb, W. B., and Williams, R. L. Comparison of stage 4 and 1-REM sleep deprivation. *Percept. Motor Skills* 24:851, 1967.
4. Agnew, H. W., Jr., Webb, W. B., and Williams, R. L. Sleep Patterns of 30–39-Year-Old Subjects. Paper read at APSS, Denver, 1968.
5. Agnew, H. W., Jr., Webb, W. B., and Williams, R. L. Sleep Patterns of the Normal Elderly. Paper read at APSS, Denver, 1968.
6. Baekeland, F., and Lasky, R. Exercise and sleep patterns in college athletes. *Percept. Motor Skills* 23:1203, 1966.
7. Dement, W. The effect of dream deprivation. *Science* 131: 1705, 1960.
8. Dement, W. Recent studies on the biological role of rapid eye movement sleep. *Amer. J. Psychiat.* 122:404, 1965.
9. Dement, W. C., and Greenberg, S. Changes in total amount of stage-4 sleep as a function of partial sleep deprivation. *Electroenceph. Clin. Neurophysiol.* 20:523, 1966.
10. Feldman, R., and Dement, W. Possible Relationships Between REM Sleep and Memory Consolidation. Paper read at APSS, Denver, 1968.

11. Greenberg, R., Pearlman, C., Kawlische, S., Kantrowitz, J., and Fingar, R. The Effects of Dream Deprivation. Paper read at APSS, Denver, 1968.
12. Hartmann, E. Longitudinal studies of sleep and dream patterns in manic-depressive patients. *Arch. Gen. Psychiat.* 19:312, 1968.
13. Hartmann, E., Baekeland, F., Zwilling, G., and Hoy, P. Long Sleepers and Short Sleepers: Preliminary Results. *Psychophysiology* 6:255, 1969.
14. Hawkins, D. R., and Mendels, J. Sleep disturbances in depressive syndromes. *Amer. J. Psychiat.* 123:682, 1966.
15. Jones, H. S., and Oswald, I. Two cases of healthy insomnia. *Electroenceph. Clin. Neurophysiol.* 24:378, 1968.
16. Kahn, E., and Fisher, C. The Sleep Characteristics of the Aged. Paper read at APSS, Denver, 1968.
17. Kales, A., Heuser, G., Jacobson, A., Kales, J. D., Hanley, J., Zweizig, J. R., and Paulson, M. J. All night sleep studies in hypothyroid patients. *J. Clin. Endocr.* 27:1593, 1967.
18. Kales, A., Hoedemaker, F. S., Jacobson, A., and Lichtenstein, E. L. Dream deprivation: An experimental reappraisal. *Nature* 204:1337, 1964.
19. Kales, A., Wilson, T., Kales, J. D., Jacobson, A., Paulson, M. J., Kellar, E., and Walter, R. D. Measurements of all-night sleep in normal elderly persons: Effects of aging. *J. Amer. Geriat. Soc.* 15:405, 1967.
20. Kleitman, N. *Sleep and Wakefulness.* Chicago: University of Chicago Press, 1963.
21. Kohler, W. C., Coddington, R. D., and Agnew, H. W., Jr. Sleep patterns in 2-year-old children. *J. Pediat.* 72:228, 1968.
22. Lairy, B. F., Cormordret, M., Faure, R., and Ridjanovic, S. Electroencephalographic study of sleep in the aged, normal and pathologic. *Rev. Neurol.* (Paris) 107:188, 1962.
23. Meddis, R. Human circadian rhythms and the 48-hour day. *Nature* 218:964, 1968.
24. Oswald, I. *Sleeping and Waking.* New York: Elsevier, 1962. Pp. 172–173.
25. Roffwarg, H. P., Muzio, J. N., and Dement, W. C. Ontogenetic development of the human sleep-dream cycle. *Science* 152:604, 1966.
26. Ross, J. J., Agnew, H. W., Jr., Williams, R. L., and Webb, W. B. Sleep patterns in pre-adolescent children: An EEG-EOG study. *Pediatrics* 42:324, 1968.

27. Rush, J., Muzio, J. N., and Roffwarg, H. P. The Sleep Stage Pattern Under the Influence of Controlled Sleep Limitation. Paper read at APSS, Gainesville, Fla., 1966.
28. Sassin, J. F., Parker, D. C., Mace, J. W., Gotlin, R. W., Johnson, L. C., and Rossman, L. G. Human Growth Hormone Release During Sleep. Paper read at APSS, Boston, 1969.
29. Takahashi, Y., Kipnis, D. M., and Daughaday, W. H. Growth hormone secretion during sleep. *J. Clin. Invest.* 47:2079, 1968.
30. Tune, G. S. Sleep and wakefulness in normal human adults. *Brit. Med. J.* 2:269, 1968.
31. Verdone, P. Sleep satiation: Extended sleep in normal subjects. *Electroenceph. Clin. Neurophysiol.* 24:417, 1968.
32. Vogel, G. W. REM deprivation. III. Dreaming and psychosis. *Arch. Gen. Psychiat.* (Chicago) 18:312, 1968.
33. Webb, W. B., and Agnew, H. W., Jr. Sleep effects of a restricted regime. *Science* 150:1745, 1965.
34. Webb, W. B., and Agnew, H. W., Jr. Sleep Patterns of Long and Short Sleepers. Paper read at APSS, Denver, 1968.
35. Webb, W. B., and Stone, W. A note on the sleep responses of young college adults. *Percept. Motor Skills* 16:162, 1963.
36. Wilkinson, R. T. Sleep Deprivation. In O. G. Edholm and A. L. Bacharach (Eds.), *Physiology of Human Survival.* New York: Academic, 1965. Pp. 399–430.
37. Wilkinson, R. T. Sleep Deprivation: Performance Tests for Partial and Selective Sleep Deprivation. In L. A. Abt and B. R. Riess (Eds.), *Progress in Clinical Psychology,* Vol. VII. New York: Grune & Stratton, 1969.
38. Wilkinson, R. T., Edwards, R. S., and Hanes, E. Performance following a night of reduced sleep. *Psychonomic Science* 5:471, 1966.
39. Williams, H. L., and Williams, C. L. Nocturnal EEG profiles and performance. *Psychophysiology* 3:164, 1966.
40. Williams, R. L., Agnew, H. W., Jr., and Webb, W. B. Sleep patterns in young adults: An EEG study. *Electroenceph. Clin. Neurophysiol.* 17:376, 1964.

Individual Differences in Sleep Length

W. B. WEBB

This paper is confined to the subject of relatively stable and persistent individual differences in sleep length. I believe that the studies of partial and total sleep deprivation involve a presently uninterpretable issue: To what extent are measured effects of sleep restriction due to the interruption of a stabilized biological program and to what extent are the effects due to the loss of sleep itself? Nor shall I be concerned here with the antecedents of individual nights of sleep. On the one hand, in the human subject the determinants of sleep length are most likely to be complex extrapersonal social determinants such that prediction is chancy beyond research capability at the present time. On the other hand, intermittent variations of an hour or so are not likely, in my opinion, to yield measurable effects.

From neonates to the aged there is a wide range of individual differences in persistent "natural" sleep lengths. Parmalee and associates [4] reporting on observations from 75 full-term neonates during the first 3 days of sleep noted a range of 10.5 to 23 hours of sleep per 24 hours. The Kleitman and Engelman study [2] of 19 infants, observed from the third to the twenty-sixth week, reports that 1 subject had a mean sleep length of 16 hours while another had a mean sleep length of 22 hours per 24 hours. A study by Reynolds and Mallay [5] of 2- to 3-year-old children showed a range of difference of 3 hours, and of about 2 hours in 3- to 5-year-old children. Table 1 shows the distribution of reported sleep time for a group of 18-year-olds entering the University of Florida in 1968. These ranges of difference in sleep length extend into old age. Indeed there is some evidence that they increase in the older population [3].

These differences are quite stable. As noted by Reynolds [5], ". . . the variations in amount of sleep taken by a child from day to day were large: . . . the variations in weekly, biweekly, or triweekly

TABLE 1. *Sleep length responses from students aged 18 and under entering University of Florida, Fall 1968*

	Sleep Length (hours)				
Sex	< 5½	5½–6½	6½–7½	7½–8½	> 8½
Males	17	78	359	653	171
Females	5	92	353	492	149
Total	22	170	712	1145	320

averages for the same child were suprisingly small . . . ." Self-reports show a reliable difference in length [7].

What causes these differences in length? Here data is almost nonexistent. Probably the determinants of stable sleep length differences represent a constellation of causes. I conceive of at least six potential, undoubtedly interacting, sources which may serve as sleep length determinants:

1. Stable biophysiological substrata such as metabolism, central nervous system states, biochemical conditions, and temperature determinants—genetically or environmentally derived, or both
2. Transient biophysiological state variables such as malnutrition, alcohol and drug consumption, chronic low-grade infections, and the like
3. Early environmental conditioning determined by parental attitudes and control, economic and cultural determinants, and the like
4. Personal and environmental-induced stress (or lack of stress) levels over periods of time
5. Task (or lack of) demands
6. Voluntarily imposed regimens

What are the consequences of these various sleep diets? Again data are almost totally absent. We are at the present time studying a population of short and long sleepers, drawn from the population cited in Table 1, in terms of achievement, aptitudes, personality measures, and physical variables.

There are some grounds to suspect that these variations in sleep length will not show substantial effects. If there were substantial and consistent effects correlated with long and short sleep, it is reasonable to suppose that these would have been observed during man's long history of sleep and subsequent performance of varied duties. More critical perhaps is the increasing evidence from electroencephalographic studies that sleep tends to "adjust" to different sleep regimens. In an earlier study by Webb and Agnew [6], we reported that short sleepers (6 hours or less) obtained the same absolute amounts of stage 4 and REM sleep as average sleepers (7½ hours). More striking is the report of Jones and Oswald [1]. They studied 2 subjects who chronically slept less than 3 hours per 24 hours. There was no apparent pathology associated with these regimens. The EEG indicated that the sleep had adjusted to these regimens by showing a high proportion of stages 3 and 4 sleep (49 percent) and a higher amount of REM than would normally be expected in the first 3 hours of a normal sleep regimen (24 percent vs. 7 percent).

One last comment: How much dreaming does a person need? Our own thinking in this matter is that the amount of REM (which we are identifying as dreaming sleep) appears to be a function primarily of the length of sleep rather than the characteristics of the individual or the waking activities of the individual.

REFERENCES

1. Jones, H. S., and Oswald, I. Two cases of healthy insomnia. *Electroenceph. Clin. Neurophysiol.* 24:378, 1968.
2. Kleitman, N., and Englemann, T. G. Sleep characteristics of infants. *J. Appl. Physiol.* 6:269, 1953.
3. O'Connor, A. L. Questionnaire Responses about Sleep. University of Florida (Gainesville) M.A. Thesis, 1964.
4. Parmalee, A. H., Schultz, H. R., and Disbrow, M. A. Sleep patterns of the newborn. *J. Pediat.* 58:241, 1961.

5. Reynolds, M. M., and Mallay, H. The sleep of children in a 24-hour nursery school. *J. Genet. Psychol.* 43:322, 1933.
6. Webb, W. B., and Agnew, H. W., Jr. Sleep patterns of long sleepers and short sleepers (abstract). *Psychophysiology* 5:215, 1968.
7. Webb, W. B., and Stone, W. A note on the sleep responses of young college adults. *Percept. Motor Skills* 16:162, 1963.

Effects of the Day's Events on Sleep

---

*Do the activities and events of the day—physical effort, mental effort, stress, mood—affect that night's sleep pattern in a predictable way?**

Laboratory Studies of Effects of Presleep Events on Sleep and Dreams

FREDERICK BAEKELAND

Clinical experience tells us that the activities of the day certainly do affect that night's sleep and dreams. Precisely how and to what extent they do so have only recently begun to be spelled out in the laboratory.

PRESLEEP EXPERIENCES AND SLEEP PATTERNS

EFFECTS OF PHYSICAL ACTIVITY. It is commonly thought that exercise promotes "sound" or "deep" sleep. Indeed, the author [6]

* The reader interested in this question may wish to refer also to papers by Webb (p. 44), Karacan and Williams (p. 93), Van de Castle (p. 171), Fisher (p. 183), Broughton (p. 188), Cartwright (p. 227), and Berger (p. 277).

showed in a group of college athletes that exercise increased the nightly contribution of delta (slow wave, stages 3 and 4) sleep. Delta sleep, by a number of criteria [10, 19, 38, 39, 50, 56], may be thought of as deep sleep. The delta sleep–promoting effect of exercise has been confirmed in the cat [29] and the rat [33]. The time at which the exercise is taken seems important and also whether the individual is used to it. Even in athletes, if taken near bedtime, exercise tends to disturb sleep [6]. In sedentary nonathletes, prolonged exercise taken before bed did not affect speed of sleep onset, probably because of the extreme fatigue induced, but did produce signs of physiological activation which persisted for several hours [25].

ANXIETY AND VIGILANCE EFFECTS. It is well known clinically that anxiety, expectation (such as of a trip the next day), or even a novel sleep situation may disturb sleep. The effects of these factors are routinely seen on first nights in the laboratory [1, 22, 32, 37, 40, 41]. First-night effects include longer sleep latencies, increased first REM period latencies (D-latencies), diminished REM sleep, more awakenings and time spent awake, and increased spontaneous electrodermal response rates—all disturbances of normal sleep patterns which quickly subside in most subjects as they become used to the laboratory. Such changes in sleep patterns are most parsimoniously interpreted as evidence of a state of increased vigilance and arousal. They are similar to, but less pronounced than, those reported in depressed patients [13, 20, 23, 26, 34, 35, 42]. While changes in slow wave sleep are not usually included among first-night effects, reduced stage 4 sleep has been observed as the result of daytime life stresses in normal persons [31].

EFFECTS OF EXPERIMENTAL PRESLEEP PROCEDURES. A potentially fruitful approach to studying the effects of daytime experiences on sleep patterns has been to examine the effects of specific presleep experimental procedures. Hauri [25], for example, found that intensive studying before bed delayed sleep onset, presumably because it is a mentally stimulating and alerting activity. In this laboratory, a stressful film shown to subjects just before bed increased both rapid eye movement activity during REM periods and the number of spontaneous awakenings associated with REM periods [5]. However, NREM sleep was not significantly affected. The author has suggested that the stress film had a specific REM sleep-disturbing effect via film-generated anxiety which carried over into the subjects' sleep and dreams, and that it increased rapid eye movement activity secondary to nonspecific (i.e., both sexual and aggressive) drive enhancement.

A number of experiments suggest that drive deprivation may increase amounts of both REM sleep and REM activity during REM periods. Bokert [9], for example, deprived his subjects of water and found that thirst increased REM activity in REM periods, an effect which may be attributed to increased drive pressure during sleep due to reduced opportunities for drive discharge during wakefulness. Similarly, the author [4] has found that exercise deprivation increased REM activity in athletes. Van der Kolk and Hartmann [48], who subjected subjects to several hours of sensory deprivation before sleep, found that this procedure decreased first REM period latencies and increased both the length of the first REM period and amounts of REM sleep throughout the night. They suggested that the organism needs a certain amount of external stimulation and that if this is lacking, internal sources of stimulation (such as REM sleep, a state of physiological and neurophysiological activation) may increase. Wood [55] found that subjects confined to a room and subjected to prolonged social isolation had increased amounts of REM sleep. Deprivation experiments such as the above, like that with the presleep films, are consistent with the notion that REM sleep has an important drive-discharge function.

PRESLEEP EXPERIENCE AND DREAM CONTENT

It has long been known that daytime experiences, especially "indifferent" ones, are frequently represented in the manifest content of that night's dreams [17]. However, it is only recently that this phenomenon has been studied experimentally. A number of investigators [3, 8, 13, 14, 21, 50, 52–54] have noted that the experimental situation itself is an important determinant of the content of laboratory dreams, in which it is perceived as threatening by female and annoying and exhibitionistic by male subjects [3, 14, 50]. Fewer sexual and aggression-misfortune elements were found in laboratory than in home dreams [14]. In subjects who underwent a presleep association period there was significantly more representation of the laboratory in the dreams of those who were extreme in cognitive style (field-dependent or -independent), and this effect was more pronounced in later than earlier REM period reports [3]. Finally, field-dependent subjects are most likely to have dreams containing the experimenter [3, 53, 54].

A number of studies have shown that the day's residue is more prominent in earlier than in later REM period reports, which have more distant temporal referents than do earlier ones [7, 28, 49].

An early study in this laboratory [8] indicated that both a hypnagogic presleep association period, in which subjects were asked to free associate, and presleep films could influence subsequent dream content, usually via transformation rather than direct incorporations. A more extensive study, still in progress, of the effects of stressful and neutral presleep films [18, 52–54] is examining the subject's cognitive style as a determinant of how and to what extent he transforms his presleep experiences in his dreams. In this study it was found that the stress film reduced dream recall, presumably via repression, since on stress film nights there was an increase in "no dream" (ND) reports in which the subject said he was dreaming but couldn't remember any content, while on the other hand there were no more than usual dreamless sleep reports, in which the subject denies any prior mental activity. The author [7] studied the relationship between the content of a presleep association period and the dreams of the night. The degree of contiguity of the association period to sleep, the subject's cognitive style, and time of night all affected the extent to which the presleep association period material was represented in their REM period reports. In field-dependent subjects, but not in field-independents, the amount of material related to the association period steadily declined in the course of the night. Field-independent subjects' dreams contained the most transformations of material derived from the association period.

The effects of presleep films have also been studied in other laboratories. In adults Foulkes and Rechtschaffen [16] found a greater nonspecific arousal in dream content after a violent film than after a romantic comedy. Foulkes et al. [15] studied the effects in male latency-age children of the presleep viewing of an aggressive film stimulus (a western film) as compared to a more neutral baseball film. The western produced less vivid dreams with less hostile-unpleasant content. The authors interpreted their results in terms of the theory of a cathartic function for the vicarious viewing of hostility. However, the western film produced dreams with more female age-mates and wild animals, a result suggesting a film-induced stimulation of aggressive and sexual drives which carried over into sleep. Obviously wish-fulfilling dreams were rare. Collins et al. [11] studied the effects of a threat film used by other workers [5, 8, 52–54], a depiction of pubertal circumcision rites in Australian aborigines. They found that the degree of incorporation of film elements was related both to first viewing mood reactions to the film and to adaptation to the psychological threat posed by the film.

The effects of other kinds of presleep experiences have been studied as well. In a study by Hunter and Breger [30], the subject was "focused" upon in a presleep group therapy session. One-third of the subjects' dreams on therapy nights directly included other members of the group, while all their dreams were directly related to major thematic material dealt with in the preceding therapy session. Their therapy night dreams also showed more unpleasant interactions between characters, inadequate-unsuccessful roles for the dreamer, and undesirable outcomes. Bokert [9] examined the extent to which a somatic drive (thirst) and a thirst-related auditory stimulus could influence dream content. He found more thirst-related content on days when subjects were water-deprived. The dreams of one group of subjects suggested drive satisfaction, while those of a second group suggested frustration or avoidance of drive gratification. Subsequently, the latter subjects felt thirstier and drank more water. This experiment supports the notion of a drive-discharge function for dreaming, as does that of Hauri [25], who found less content concerned with thinking or problem-solving activities after intensive presleep studying, and less content concerned with physical activity after an extensive presleep exercise period.

Recent preliminary work [47] indicates that long-standing perceptual alterations (e.g., colored lenses), may systematically alter the hallucinatory content of dreams.

Both Stoyva [43, 44] and Tart [45, 46] have studied the effects of presleep posthypnotic suggestions that subjects have dreams with specific content. Both investigators found that certain subjects will dream about a suggested topic in every REM period of the night, but that the suggestion does not enter the dream as a separate entity but is rather embellished and modified by the addition of nonsuggested dream content. Similarly, Arkin et al. [2] have reported that sleep talking may be posthypnotically induced and often is related to REM period dream content.

CLINICAL IMPLICATIONS

The clinical implications of these recent laboratory studies are much more obscure than their theoretical ramifications and remain to be worked out. However, they do suggest important drive-discharge and adaptive functions for dreaming. Hence, one might question the psychological wisdom of the wholesale use of hypnotics, most of which depress REM sleep, in hospitalized patients who are socially isolated and confined to bed and thus have limited opportunities for discharging their sexual and aggressive drives during wakefulness. In view of the experimentally documented sleep-disturbing effect of emotional presleep experiences it would seem prudent to advise patients not to undertake emotion-laden discussions before bed and, of course, to avoid late evening psychotherapy sessions. Similarly, exercise taken before bed seems inadvisable. The hypnotic studies underscore the well-known fact that patients tend to have dreams whose content is in accord with their therapists' theoretical expectations, something which raises important technical questions with respect to dream interpretation for clinical purposes.

REFERENCES

1. Agnew, H. W., Jr., Webb, W. B., and Williams, R. L. The first night effect: An EEG study of sleep. *Psychophysiology* 2:263, 1966.
2. Arkin, A. M., Hastey, J. M., and Reiser, M. F. Posthypnotically stimulated sleep-talking. *J. Nerv. Ment. Dis.* 142:293, 1966.
3. Baekeland, F. Dreams with laboratory references: Effects of cognitive style and time of night. Unpublished manuscript.
4. Baekeland, F. The effect of exercise deprivation on sleep patterns in college athletes. Unpublished manuscript.
5. Baekeland, F., Koulack, D., and Lasky, R. Effects of a stressful presleep experience on electroencephalograph-recorded sleep. *Psychophysiology* 4:436, 1968.
6. Baekeland, F., and Lasky, R. Exercise and sleep patterns in college athletes. *Percept. Motor Skills* 23:1203, 1966.
7. Baekeland, F., Resch, R., and Katz, D. Presleep mentation and dream reports. I. Cognitive style, contiguity to sleep, and time of night. *Arch. Gen. Psychiat.* (Chicago) 19:300, 1968.
8. Bertini, M., Lewis, H. B., and Witkin, H. A. Some preliminary observations with an experimental procedure for the study of hypnagogic and related phenomena. *Arch. Psicol. Neurol.* 25: 493, 1964.
9. Bokert, E. The Effects of Thirst and a Related Auditory Stimulus on Dream Reports. New York University Doctoral Dissertation, 1965.
10. Coleman, P. D., Gray, F. E., and Watanabe, K. EEG amplitude and reaction time during sleep. *J. Appl. Physiol.* 14:397, 1959.
11. Collins, G., Davison, L. A., and Breger, L. The Function of Dreams in Adaptation to Threat: A Preliminary Study. Paper read at Association for the Psychophysiological Study of Sleep (APSS), Santa Monica, Cal., 1967.
12. Dement, W. C., Kahn, E., and Roffwarg, H. P. The influence of the laboratory situation on the dreams of the experimental subject. *J. Nerv. Ment. Dis.* 140:119, 1965.

13. Diaz-Guerrero, R., Gottlieb, J., and Knott, J. The sleep of patients with manic-depressive psychoses, depressed type: An electroencephalographic study. *Psychosom. Med.* 8:399, 1946.
14. Domhoff, B., and Kamiya, J. Problems in dream content study with objective indicators. II. Appearance of experimental situation in laboratory dream narratives. *Arch. Gen. Psychiat.* (Chicago) 11:525, 1964.
15. Foulkes, D., Pivik, T., Steadman, H. S., Spear, P. S., and Symonds, J. D. Dreams in the male child: An EEG study. *J. Abnorm. Psychol.* 72:457, 1967.
16. Foulkes, D., and Rechtschaffen, A. Presleep determinants of dream content: Effects of two films. *Percept. Motor Skills* 19: 983, 1964.
17. Freud, S. The interpretation of dreams (1900). In *The Standard Edition of the Complete Psychological Works of Sigmund Freud,* tr. and ed. by J. Strachey with others. London: Hogarth and the Institute of Psycho-Analysis, 1953. Vols. IV, V.
18. Goodenough, D. R. Some Recent Studies of Dream Recall. In H. A. Witkin and H. B. Lewis (Eds.), *Experimental Studies of Dreaming*. New York: Random House, 1967. Pp. 128–147.
19. Goodenough, D. R., Lewis, H. B., Shapiro, A., Jaret, L., and Sleser, I. Dream reporting following abrupt and gradual awakenings from different types of sleep. *J. Personality Soc. Psychol.* 2:170, 1965.
20. Gresham, S. C., Agnew, H. W., Jr., and Williams, R. L. The sleep of depressed patients: An EEG and eye movement study. *Arch. Gen. Psychiat.* (Chicago) 13:503, 1965.
21. Hall, C. S. Representation of the laboratory setting in dreams. *J. Nerv. Ment. Dis.* 144:198, 1967.
22. Hartmann, E. Adaptation to the Sleep Laboratory and Placebo Effect. Paper read at APSS, Santa Monica, Cal., 1967.
23. Hartmann, E. Longitudinal Sleep Studies in Manic-Depressive Patients. Paper read at APSS, Denver 1968.
24. Hauri, P. Effect of Evening Activities on Subsequent Sleep and Dreams. University of Chicago Doctoral Thesis, 1965.
25. Hauri, P. Effects of evening activity on early night sleep. *Psychophysiology* 4:267, 1968.
26. Hawkins, D. R., and Mendels, J. Sleep disturbance in depressive syndromes. *Amer. J. Psychiat.* 123:682, 1966.
27. Hawkins, D. R., Mendels, J., Scott, J., Bensch, G., and Teachey, W. The psychophysiology of sleep in psychotic depression: A longitudinal study. *Psychosom. Med.* 24:329, 1967.

28. Herman, J., Roffwarg, H., and Tauber, E. Color and Other Perceptual Qualities of REM and NREM Sleep. Paper read at APSS, Denver, 1968.
29. Hobson, J. A. Sleep after exercise. *Science* 162:1503, 1968.
30. Hunter, I., and Breger, L. The Effect of Pre-sleep Group Therapy Upon Subsequent Dream Content. Paper read at APSS, Santa Monica, Cal., 1967.
31. Lester, B. K., Burch, N. R., and Dossett, R. C. Nocturnal EEG-GSR profiles: The influence of presleep states. *Psychophysiology* 3:238, 1967.
32. McDonald, D. G., Shallenberger, H. D., Stoller, R. H., Tamsky, L. I., and Oshry, S. B. Correlates of Autonomic Activity in Sleep. Paper read at APSS, Denver, 1968.
33. Matsumoto, J., Nishisho, T., Suto, T., Sadahiro, T., and Miyoshi, M. Influence of fatigue on sleep. *Nature* 218:177, 1968.
34. Mendels, J., and Hawkins, D. R. The psychophysiology of sleep in depression. *Ment. Hyg.* 51:501, 1967.
35. Mendels, J., and Hawkins, D. R. Sleep and depression: A controlled EEG study. *Arch. Gen. Psychiat.* (Chicago) 16:344, 1967.
36. Mendels, J., and Hawkins, D. R. Sleep and depression: A follow-up study. *Arch. Gen. Psychiat.* (Chicago) 16:536, 1967.
37. Mendels, J., and Hawkins, D. R. Sleep laboratory adaptation in normal subjects and depressed patients ("first night effect"). *Electroenceph. Clin. Neurophysiol.* 22:556, 1967.
38. Okuma, T., Nakamura, K., Hayashi, A., and Fujimori, M. Psychophysiological study on the depth of sleep in normal human subjects. *Electroenceph. Clin. Neurophysiol.* 21:140, 1966.
39. Rechtschaffen, A., Hauri, P., and Zeitlin, M. Auditory awakening thresholds in REM and NREM sleep stages. *Percept. Motor Skills* 22:927, 1966.
40. Rechtschaffen, A., and Verdone, P. Amount of dreaming: Effect of incentive, adaptation to laboratory, and individual differences. *Percept. Motor Skills* 19:947, 1964.
41. Schmidt, H. S., and Kaelbling, R. Laboratory Adaptation Effect on Sleep Patterns: A Comparison of Six Consecutive Nights. Paper read at APSS, Denver, 1968.
42. Snyder, F., Anderson, D., Bunney, W., Kupfer, D., Scott, J., and Wyatt, R. Longitudinal Variation in the Sleep of Severely

Depressed and Acutely Schizophrenic Patients with Changing Clinical Status. Paper read at APSS, Denver, 1968.

43. Stoyva, J. M. Posthypnotically suggested dreams and the sleep cycle. *Arch. Gen. Psychiat.* (Chicago) 12:287, 1965.
44. Stoyva, J., and Budzynski, T. The Nocturnal Hypnotic Dream: Fact or Fabrication? Paper read at APSS, Denver, 1968.
45. Tart, C. T. A comparison of suggested dreams occurring in hypnosis and sleep. *Int. J. Clin. Exp. Hypn.* 12:263, 1964.
46. Tart, C. T. Some effects of posthypnotic suggestion on the process of dreaming. *Int. J. Clin. Exp. Hypn.* 14:30, 1966.
47. Tauber, E. S., Roffwarg, H. P., and Herman, J. The Effects of Longstanding Perceptual Alterations on the Hallucinatory Content of Dreams. Paper read at APSS, Denver, 1968.
48. Van der Kolk, B., and Hartmann, E. Sensory Deprivation and Subsequent Sleep. Paper read at APSS, Denver, 1968.
49. Verdone, P. Temporal reference of manifest dream content. *Percept. Motor Skills* 20:1253, 1965.
50. Whitman, R. M., Pierce, C. M., Maas, J. W., and Baldridge, B. J. The dreams of the experimental subject. *J. Nerv. Ment. Dis.* 134:431, 1962.
51. Williams, H. L., Hammack, J. T., Daly, R. L., Dement, W. C., and Lubin, A. Responses to auditory stimulation, sleep loss and the EEG stages of sleep. *Electroenceph. Clin. Neurophysiol.* 16:269, 1964.
52. Witkin, H. A. Experimental Manipulation of the Cognitive and Emotional Content of Dreams. In M. Kramer and R. M. Whitman (Eds.), *Dream Psychology and the New Biology of Dreaming.* Springfield, Ill.: Thomas, 1969.
53. Witkin, H. A., and Lewis, H. B. The relation of experimentally induced presleep experiences to dreams: A report on method and preliminary findings. *J. Amer. Psychoanal. Ass.* 13:819, 1965.
54. Witkin, H. A., and Lewis, H .B. Presleep Experiences and Dreams. In H. A. Witkin and H. B. Lewis (Eds.), *Experimental Studies of Dreaming.* New York: Random House, 1967. Pp. 148–202.
55. Wood, P. B. Dreaming and social isolation. University of North Carolina Doctoral Dissertation, 1962.
56. Zung, W. W. K., and Wilson, W. P. Response to auditory stimulation during sleep. *Arch. Gen. Psychiat.* (Chicago) 4:548, 1961.

Good Sleep

*What is good sleep? We can now define approximately what an average night of sleep looks like physiologically. But what determines when a person really feels he has slept well? What determines how he feels in the morning?**

What Sleep Is Good Sleep?

ERNEST HARTMANN

I shall consider here the straightforward question of what physiological characteristics of a night's sleep are related to how well a person feels in the morning and how well he thinks he has slept. I shall not be concerned with tests of waking performance, which can be made very objective but are not necessarily related to the subject's impression of sleep. I shall simply define a night of *good sleep* as a night after which a person claims he has slept well and after which he reports feeling well in the morning; the problem then is to describe such a night in terms of its physiology. This

* The reader interested in these questions may wish to refer also to papers by Kahn (p. 25), Baekeland and Hartmann (p. 33), Zung (p. 123), Hartmann (p. 308), and Wilkinson (p. 369).

paper summarizes one study from my laboratory relating directly to this question and discusses a number of other studies which appear relevant, although they were not directed to this point specifically.

A STUDY OF SUBJECTIVE EVALUATIONS OF LABORATORY SLEEP

We have been studying the sleep of normal volunteer subjects for a number of years. The most frequent design involves the subject's appearing for a night of laboratory study—all night polygraphic recording—once per week over a number of weeks. We have been interested chiefly in changes in physiological sleep and dream parameters over time, and their changes after certain drugs, but among other things each subject fills out a brief form in the morning after each night of uninterrupted laboratory sleep (starting only with his sixth night in the laboratory, so that he will have a basis for comparison). The form asks two simple questions:

1. How well did you sleep last night compared to the way you usually sleep in the laboratory?
2. How well do you feel this morning compared to other times you have slept in the laboratory?

For each question the subject has five choices: (1) Much worse than usual. (2) A little worse. (3) About the same. (4) A little better. (5) Much better than usual. We have tried including subtler questions, adjective checklists, and so on, but it seems most individuals are not very good at describing their state in this way and the subcategories have not been useful. The simpler questions have seemed more meaningful; this is consistent with the results of a study by Hauri [9].

This is an intrasubject study—we are interested in times when a given subject feels better or worse than he usually does, and our object is then to relate this to various parameters of his recorded night's sleep, again *relative to* his own mean values for these variables.

To convey an overall impression, I am reporting here on all laboratory nights for which we have questionnaires available, a total of 120 nights on a total of 16 subjects. About 50 percent of these nights were on placebo and 50 percent on a variety of drugs. The individual drugs used* showed no clear relationship to answers on questions 1 and 2.

Table 1 presents results for question 1 for three physiological variables: total sleep, total D-time, and number of awakenings—i.e., each subject gives his subjective sense of how well he slept relative to his usual laboratory sleep, and the three variables are categorized as to whether they are above or below that subject's mean for placebo nights in the laboratory. The results indicate that how well the subject feels he has slept is definitely related to total sleep obtained, shows little relationship to total D-time for the night, and shows a slight inverse relationship with number of awakenings during the night.

Table 2 presents the same data for question 2. It appears that how well the subjects feels in the morning again bears some relationship to total sleep but shows a direct relationship to total D-time as well.† Again, feeling well in the morning was inversely related to the number of awakenings.

Thus total sleep recorded for the night correlates strongly with how well the subject feels he has slept, and to some extent with how well he feels in the morning, while total D-time for the night appears more closely related to how well the subject feels in the morning, and bears almost no relationship to how well he feels he has slept. Unfortunately stages 2, 3, and 4 were not scored separately for all of these records, so that correlations for these variables cannot be made.

Thus this study suggests that good sleep in the sense of questions

* Amitriptyline, diphenylhydantoin, chlordiazepoxide, pentobarbital, chloral hydrate, L-tryptophane.

† This finding appeared even more clearly when only placebo nights were considered, though the number was much smaller.

TABLE 1. *Physiological patterns (sleep time, D-time, number of awakenings) related to question 1: How well did you sleep last night, compared to the way you usually sleep in the lab?*

Answers to Question 1	Total Sleep: No. of Answers in Each Category When Total Sleep Was			
	Below S's Mean	Above S's Mean	Below Mean[a]	Above Mean[a]
1. Much Worse	3	2	18	19
2. Slightly Worse	15	17		
3. Same	30	44		
4. Slightly Better	10	40	10	61
5. Much Better	0	21		

Answers to Question 1	Total D-Time: No. of Answers in Each Category When Total D-Time Was			
	Below S's Mean	Above S's Mean	Below Mean[a]	Above Mean[a]
1. Much Worse	3	2	18	17
2. Slightly Worse	15	15		
3. Same	47	27		
4. Slightly Better	24	25	38	32
5. Much Better	14	7		

Answers to Question 1	Number of Awakenings: No. of Answers in Each Category When No. of Awakenings Was			
	Below S's Mean	Above S's Mean	Below Mean[a]	Above Mean[a]
1. Much Worse	1	1	7	19
2. Slightly Worse	6	18		
3. Same	17	23		
4. Slightly Better	18	14	23	18
5. Much Better	5	4		

[a]The figures on the right combine answers 1 and 2, omit answer 3, and combine answers 4 and 5. The numbers should be taken as indicating trends. X^2 and similar tests of significance are not applicable since the data are not all independent.

TABLE 2. *Physiological patterns (sleep time, D-time, number of awakenings) related to question 2: How do you feel this morning compared to other times you have slept in the lab?*

Answers to Question 2	Total Sleep: No. of Answers in Each Category When Total Sleep Was			
	Below S's Mean	Above S's Mean	Below Mean[a]	Above Mean[a]
1. Much Worse	3	4	21	29
2. Slightly Worse	18	25		
3. Same	31	58		
4. Slightly Better	6	23	7	36
5. Much Better	1	13		

Answers to Question 2	Total D-Time: No. of Answers in Each Category When Total D-Time Was			
	Below S's Mean	Above S's Mean	Below Mean[a]	Above Mean[a]
1. Much Worse	6	1	33	18
2. Slightly Worse	27	17		
3. Same	40	38		
4. Slightly Better	12	16	21	21
5. Much Better	9	5		

Answers to Question 2	Number of Awakenings: No. of Answers in Each Category When No. of Awakenings Was			
	Below S's Mean	Above S's Mean	Below Mean[a]	Above Mean[a]
1. Much Worse	0	2	8	14
2. Slightly Worse	8	12		
3. Same	22	36		
4. Slightly Better	13	11	17	11
5. Much Better	4	0		

[a] The figures on the right combine answers 1 and 2, omit answer 3, and combine answers 4 and 5. The numbers should be taken as indicating trends. X^2 and similar tests of significance are not applicable since the data are not all independent.

1 and 2 depends on adequate total sleep length and on not having too many awakenings during the night, while good sleep in the second sense (feeling well in the morning) also depends on D-time.

OTHER STUDIES OF GOOD SLEEP

There are a number of other studies which may be relevant. The relationship of sleep length to "euphoria" was studied in 1935 by Barry and Bousfield [2]. A large number of college students were asked to rate how well they felt on arriving in class, and after they had made the rating (a global rating on a 10-point scale) they were asked a number of questions about the past 24 hours, including how much sleep they had obtained. There was a definite and significant increase in "euphoria" as sleep time rose from 5 hours to 8 to 9 hours, but a slight decrease with sleep of over 9 hours.

A study in our laboratory involves awakenings for dream recall 5 or 10 minutes after the start of each D-period. Besides reporting their dreams, the subjects are also asked to grade on an adjective checklist how they felt at the time of awakening. It turns out that, overall, subjects tend to feel successively better (less depressed) as the night progresses. There are a number of possible explanations for this, but if there is any relationship to the amount of various kinds of sleep that the subject has had before the awakening, delta sleep would not be involved—the records indicate that most delta sleep was obtained before any of the awakenings—but more D-time (and stage 2) will clearly have accumulated between awakenings. Though a very tentative finding, it may be worth investigating further since the results are in the direction opposite to what one would expect—that a subject would become increasingly unhappy and annoyed with each successive awakening during a night when his sleep is being interrupted four, five, or six times by the experimeter. A study by Foulkes [3] in which subjects rated their dreams by a number of adjectives similarly showed that later dreams of the night were rated as more "pleasant" than earlier ones.

The studies in my laboratory investigated variability in subjective estimates of good and poor sleep *within* subjects. One can also do a comparison of good and poor sleep *between* groups of subjects, by finding persons who habitually complain that they sleep poorly and comparing them with subjects who claim that they sleep well. A careful investigation of this kind has been done by Monroe [12]. He defined two groups, chosen from a large sample of college students, as extreme "good sleepers" or "poor sleepers" in terms of their answers to a number of sleep questions, such as: How well do you sleep? How long does it take you to get to sleep? Do you awaken often during the night? Several nights of laboratory sleep were then recorded for each subject. The findings were first of all that, as expected, the good sleepers spent significantly more time asleep than the poor sleepers; poor sleepers spent more time lying in bed awake. There were no significant differences between the groups in amount of delta sleep, but the good sleepers had considerably more D-time. Again, a relationship was suggested between subjective "good sleep" and both total sleep and total D-time. (This also agrees with our findings in long and short sleepers that amount of delta sleep is relatively constant among subjects, whereas D-time varies greatly.)

Some other studies are relevant to the same points: Interviews with normal subjects who sleep for many nights in our laboratory, and others, indicate that the first night is typically described as a night of poor sleep relative to later nights. Physiologically the first night is usually characterized by slightly decreased total sleep and stage 4 time, and considerably decreased D-time.

From a number of different laboratory studies I have come to the perhaps obvious conclusion that a subjective feeling of poor sleep may be produced by almost any disturbing environmental condition, such as a noisy room, uncomfortable bed, poor air-conditioning system, random awakenings by the experimenter, and so on. In terms of physiological recording, we have shown that such nights are similar to the "first night"—they contain decreased D-time and usually decreased stage 4 and total sleep.

Tune [15] reports on an unpublished French study of night-shift workers who slept in the daytime for a number of days and then switched back to night sleep, usually on weekends. They almost always complained that their daytime sleep was poor sleep, even though of adequate length. EEG studies showed a great deal of descending stage 1, approximately normal delta sleep time, but clearly decreased D-time.

Kales et al. [11] report preliminary results concerning daytime mood changes (on adjective checklists) during periods of sleeping medication administration. One drug, which produced no change in D-time during the night, was associated with increased "vigor, surgency, alertness" and low "aggression, fatigue, depression," while a drug which decreased D-time often produced lowered feelings of "energy." Again, amount of D-time appears to be implicated in subjective assessments of sleep.

Psychotically depressed patients characteristically complain of very poor sleep. Most laboratory studies report that these patients' sleep contains greatly decreased stage 4 time and D-time [4, 10, 14].* However, a group of manic-depressive patients studied in my laboratory was found not to complain particularly of poor sleep during depressed periods; in the laboratory these patients showed only a slight reduction in stage 4 time, normal or increased D-time, and a normal or almost normal total sleep time [6, 7]. This again suggests that a feeling of poor sleep is associated with reduced D-time and perhaps with a reduced stage 4.

A very striking situation is found in mania. A typical manic patient may sleep 4 or 5 hours a night for weeks or even months on end, but usually feels he has slept well and does not feel tired; at least he claims to feel fine in the morning. We have shown that the sleep of the manic is characterized by low D-time though not very low stage 4. However, evidence from our study of manic patients has led us to conclude that specifically in this condition "D-pressure" (need for D-time) is reduced—there is no evidence of

* A decreased arousal threshold during sleep has also been reported in such patients; this suggests that it might also be fruitful to attempt to relate "good sleep" to arousal threshold during sleep. So far little work has been done in this area.

recovery afterward—so that here the patient may be fulfilling his "need for D" although his absolute D-time is low [6, 7].

Thus it is probably not the absolute amount of time spent in stage 4 or in the D-state that affects feelings of good sleep, but the time relative to the requirement of that particular subject in a particular state. Our studies of long and short sleepers, described elsewhere [8] (see also Baekeland and Hartmann, pp. 33–43) suggest that actually the delta sleep requirement is quite constant among subjects, while the requirement for D-time may differ considerably. In our study the short sleepers, a group who generally slept for only about 5½ hours per night, had only 60 minutes of D-time per night. But these were subjects who felt they slept well and never complained of poor sleep. Apparently these subjects have a low requirement for D-time, somewhat like the manic patients. (And in fact, characterologically these persons are somewhat hypomanic.)

Other changes within subjects may also be associated with an altered requirement for D-time or other portions of sleep: I have reported that women had more D-time and earlier D-periods during the progestational and especially the premenstrual phase of the menstrual cycle [14]. I suggested that more D-time might be required at these times and that in part the psychological symptoms of premenstrual tension might be related to this requirement, which could best be fulfilled by sleeping longer. There was no controlled study of the subjective symptoms, but a number of women told me that indeed allowing more sleep during the week before menses improved their mood considerably.

One would think that the question of whether the D-state or stage 4, or both, are required for a feeling of good sleep might be settled by investigating the effects of depriving subjects of one or the other of these stages. Only one study [1] exists which used similar tests on two groups of subjects, one group stage 4–deprived for 7 days, and the other group D–deprived for 7 days. Stage 4 deprivation produced some bodily discomfort, decreased aggressiveness, and a depression or hypochondriac picture. D-deprivation led to the subject's being "psychologically less well integrated, and having less interpersonal effectiveness." Apparently both groups felt uncomfortable; specific feelings about sleep were not reported, but the suggestion is that both groups felt worse than usual in the morning during the experiment.

Wilkinson [16] has performed a number of studies of daytime functioning after deprivation of varying amounts of sleep, though without using EEG recordings (see also pp. 369–381). He found that when enough deprivation was involved to disturb delta sleep early in the night, *ability to perform* on behavioral tasks was impaired. When he used a deprivation schedule such that most D-time would probably be eliminated but delta sleep left alone, the subjects showed a pattern that could be attributed to a decreased *motivation to perform* though ability was unaffected. Perhaps this motivation is also an aspect of good sleep in the sense of depending on the subject's feeling well and ready to work in the morning.

These studies, and our studies of long and short sleepers, suggest that delta sleep time as well as D-time is involved in the impression of good sleep, though delta sleep, which preempts the early hours of sleep, is reduced only in very unusual circumstances.

My conclusion from all these studies, a conclusion that must be considered tentative at this stage of our knowledge, is as follows: Good sleep, subjectively experienced, does bear a relationship to the sleep patterns that can be recorded in the laboratory. Good sleep results from having fulfilled a sleep requirement which can be divided into two portions: a requirement for delta sleep, which is remarkably constant among subjects, and a requirement for D-time, which varies greatly among subjects and sometimes within the same subject at different times. Personality factors and mood appear to be involved in this second requirement, and it is the second requirement which probably is most related to how we feel in the daytime.

REFERENCES

1. Agnew, H. W., Jr., Webb, W. B., and Williams, R. L. Comparison of stage 4 and 1-REM sleep deprivation. *Percept. Motor Skills* 24:851, 1967.

2. Barry, H., Jr., and Bousfield, W. A. A quantitative determination of euphoria and its relation to sleep. *J. Abnorm. Soc. Psychol.* 29:385, 1935.
3. Foulkes, D. *The Psychology of Sleep.* New York: Scribner's, 1966.
4. Gresham, S., Agnew, H., Jr., and Williams, R. The sleep of depressed patients. *Arch. Gen. Psychiat.* (Chicago) 13:503, 1965.
5. Hartmann, E. Dreaming sleep (the D-state) and the menstrual cycle. *J. Nerv. Ment. Dis.* 143(5): 406, 1966.
6. Hartmann, E. Sleep and Dream Patterns in Manic-Depressive Patients. Paper read at the Association for the Psychophysiological Study of Sleep (APSS), Gainesville, Fla., 1966.
7. Hartmann, E. Longitudinal studies of sleep and dream patterns in manic-depressive patients. *Arch. Gen. Psychiat.* (Chicago) 19:312, 1968.
8. Hartmann, E., Baekeland, F., Zwilling, G., and How, P. Long and Short Sleepers: Preliminary Results. Paper read at APSS, Boston, 1969. Abstract in *Psychophysiology* 6:255, 1969.
9. Hauri, P. Effects of Evening Activity on Subsequent Sleep and Dreams. University of Chicago Doctoral Dissertation, 1966.
10. Hawkins, D., and Mendels, J. Sleep disturbance in depressive syndromes. *Amer. J. Psychiat.* 123:682, 1966.
11. Kales, A., Malmstrom, E. J., and Tan, T. Drugs and Dreaming. In *Progress in Clinical Psychology,* Vol. 9. New York: Grune & Stratton, 1969. Chap. 9, pp. 154–167.
12. Monroe, L. Psychological and Physiological Differences Between Good and Poor Sleepers. University of Chicago Doctoral Dissertation, 1965.
13. Monroe, L., Rechtschaffen, A., Foulkes, D., and Jensen, J. Discriminability of REM and non-REM reports. *J. Personality Soc. Psychol.* 2:456, 1965.
14. Oswald, I., Berger, R., Jamarillo, R., Keddie, K., Olley, P., and Plunkett, G. Melancholia and barbiturates: Controlled EEG, body and eye movement study of sleep. *Brit. J. Psychiat.* 109:66, 1963.
15. Tune, G. S. The human sleep debt. *Sci. J.* (London) 4:67, 1968.
16. Wilkinson, R. T. Sleep Deprivation and Behavior. In B. F. Riess and L. A. Abt (Eds.), *Progress in Clinical Psychology,* Vol. 8. New York: Grune & Stratton, 1968.
17. Zung, W. W. K., Wilson, W. P., and Dodson, W. E. Effect of depressive disorders on sleep EEG responses. *Arch. Gen. Psychiat.* (Chicago) 10:439, 1964.

What Is Good Sleep?

PETER HAURI

It seems that we sleep to recover from previous wakefulness, to restore our physical and mental energy. In this paper a good night's sleep is therefore defined as one after which we function well, both in terms of performance and mood, while a poor night's sleep is defined as one which is followed by a lesser level of functioning.

A search of the literature indicates that so far nobody has successfully correlated measures taken during sleep with the subtle fluctuations in performance and mood that occur throughout the subsequent day. This means that we do not yet know directly what types of sleep are good or poor. However, there are a number of studies which yield indirect information on this point. Studies will be reviewed in this paper which suggest that good or poor sleep is related to personality variables, mood changes, amount of wakefulness during the night, and to delta (slow wave) sleep. Finally, two studies will be mentioned which suggest that sleep quality might even be related to the type of dreams one experiences during a certain night.

PERSONALITY VARIABLES

A connection between poor sleep and certain types of psychopathology has long been observed by clinicians. Othmer [16] recently investigated answers from 120 students and reported a correlation coefficient of .46 ($p < .001$) between the feeling of sleeping poorly and scores on a neuroticism scale derived from Eysenck's work. Monroe [13] found that people who described themselves as poor sleepers scored significantly higher on many Minnesota Multiphasic Personality Inventory scales than people who felt that they were good sleepers. Thus personality variables clearly relate to sleep quality ratings.

Both Othmer and Monroe selected extreme groups for further study in the laboratory. Othmer found that his "psychically labile subjects" (essentially neurotics) had less stage 2 sleep and more REM time than his "psychically stabile subjects." Monroe's results go in the opposite direction: his poor sleepers show more stage 2 and less REM time than his good sleepers. Obviously Othmer's "psychically labile subjects" were not equivalent to Monroe's "poor sleepers" even though both complained of poor sleep.

MOOD VARIABLES

Trying to evaluate whether the mood before going to sleep or after awakening was related to the feeling of having slept well or poorly, this author used the Nowlis Mood Adjective Check List [14]. For one week, 10 volunteers completed the Nowlis each evening before retiring and each morning upon arising. Upon awakening these volunteers also evaluated the quality of their sleep on a separate sleep questionnaire. Based on these latter ratings, the best and the worst night for each subject were selected from among the seven nights tested. Surprisingly, the best night was not significantly different from the worst night in any of the twelve mood factors assessed on the Nowlis scale. This suggests that there is probably no set mood during either the previous evening or during the morning which is directly associated with the feeling of having slept well or poorly. However, when mood *changes* were investigated by subtracting morning mood scores from evening scores, three significant relationships emerged. The best night's sleep was significantly related to a greater mood change in the direction of more elation (Wilcoxon test, $p < .02$), more ability to concentrate ($p < .01$), and less fatigue ($p < .05$). Thus this pilot study suggests that the feeling of having slept well might be related not to absolute mood levels but to fluctuations within that level. Where these fluctuations stem from, however, cannot be answered from the study described.

WAKEFULNESS AND BODY MOVEMENTS

Poor sleep is often assumed if one cannot fall asleep easily or shows restless sleep and many body movements. However, when I asked normal volunteers after each night in the lab how well they had slept, the volunteers' answers correlated more (— .39) with how long they *thought* it had taken them to fall asleep and less (— .18) with how long it had taken them according to EEG criteria [5]. This suggests that ratings of sleep quality may be more dependent on our subjective recall of a night's sleep and less dependent on "objective" measures.

The number and duration of gross body movements was also assessed in this study. Much to our surprise there was *no* relationship whatsoever between body movements during sleep and the ratings of sleep quality made by the sleepers in the morning. Rather than finding body movements to be indicators of poor sleep, Othmer [15] even came to the conclusion that there is an optimal number of body movements and that a lack of such "sleep interruptors" might be as detrimental to sleep as an overabundance of them.

DELTA SLEEP AND PHYSIOLOGICAL RECOVERY

Somatic recovery goes on continuously throughout waking and sleeping. However, evidence reviewed in this section suggests that such recovery might be particularly efficient during delta sleep. Indeed, there seems to be ground for speculation that one hour of concentrated delta activity might be equivalent in physiological "recovery potential" to a much longer period spent in other stages of sleep. This speculation is best illustrated by the case of Miss G., a 37-year-old nurse recently studied in our laboratory. Miss G. usually sleeps only 2 to 6 hours per night, and her sleep during this period is characterized by as much as 20 percent to 30 percent delta activity. However, during recurrent depressive episodes she "escapes" into sleeping about 12 to 18 hours per night, and during these nights she shows *no* regular delta sleep, but spends most of her sleep time either in stage 2 sleep or in REM periods.

Isolated case studies are rarely convincing. However, when volunteers were studied [1] who habitually slept either 6 hours or less, or 9 hours or more, it was found that the short sleepers obtained more minutes of stage 4 sleep per night than the long sleepers. Similarly, when the sleep of normal subjects was artificially curtailed from the usual 7 or 8 hours per night to a 3-hour period per night, the percentages of delta sleep (especially stage 4) increased in a highly significant manner [19]. It seems that the organism "learns" to spend a disproportionately high amount of time in delta sleep when time allotted for sleeping is short or when the need for recovery is great. This latter idea is supported by the concentration of delta sleep early in the night, when pressure for recovery from previous wakefulness seems high. The longer this wakefulness lasts, the longer the amount of time spent in delta sleep [20].

Even though my earlier study [6] did not directly confirm it for a variety of reasons, it appears probable that the amount of delta sleep obtained during a given night is directly related to the amount of physical activity engaged in during previous wakefulness [3, 8]. Physiologically, delta sleep seems to be a particularly appropriate stage of sleep for recovery from exercise. The rate of body movements per minute is significantly lower in delta sleep than in any other stage [17]. Although most physiological variables thus far measured in the laboratory show a very stable, low level of functioning during delta sleep, it has nevertheless been found [6, 18] that both respiratory rate and blood volume in skeletal muscles are significantly higher during delta sleep than during stage 2 sleep taken from similar times of the night. Brebbia and Altschuler [4] found that delta sleep shows the lowest metabolic level of all sleep stages, but that carbon dioxide retention in the body was *less* during delta sleep than during stage 2 sleep. Thus the overall pattern during delta sleep shows low metabolism, but a facilitation of "waste removal" by a large blood volume in the skeletal muscles, high respiratory rate, and low CO_2 retention—an ideal situation for recovery from physical exercise.

Delta sleep is often reduced or lacking in states known to be associated with poor sleep, such as depression [7], fever [10], or old age [9]. This fact prompted many researchers to speculate that delta sleep is associated with a feeling of having slept well. However, in a preliminary investigation [5] using 15 healthy young males who each slept three nights in the lab, a correlation coefficient close to zero was found between the amount of delta sleep during the first half of the night, and the early morning feeling of having slept well or poorly. Thus it seems that the amount of delta sleep obtained might be important when rating long-range quality of sleep, but that it is much less crucial for healthy subjects when judging night by night fluctuations of sleep quality.

Psychological test data [2] support the idea that delta sleep is connected with somatic recovery. When volunteers were deprived of stage 4 sleep they became "physically uncomfortable, . . . and manifested concern over vague physical complaints and changes in bodily feelings." When similar volunteers were deprived of REM sleep, they showed much less somatic concerns and more phychological difficulties (e.g., confusion, suspicion, withdrawal, anxiety, insecurity).

Delta sleep, then, seems to be "good, efficient" sleep in terms of physiological recovery. It remains to be seen if the total time needed for sleep could be shortened by artificially increasing the time spent in delta sleep—e.g., through the administration of drugs such as chloralose, which increases delta sleep [12]; through the electrical superimposition of an artificial delta rhythm on the sleeping brain; through conditioning, or some other means.

DREAM CONTENT

The fascinating studies on the homeostatic mechanisms involved in REM sleep and REM deprivation are well known. The relationship of REM deprivation to a daytime mood of anxiousness, insecurity, confusion, suspicion, and so on, has just been alluded to. Recent evidence now suggests that not only is the amount of REM sleep important for a person's well-being during subsequent wakefulness, but that the *type of dreams* a person experiences during REM sleep might be important as well. For example, as part of a larger study on the interrelationship between waking and sleeping [5], 15 volunteers slept in the laboratory for three nights each. Among other things, they were awakened twice during REM sleep to collect dream narratives. These narratives were later rated by an outside judge on the amount of personal involvement that the dreamer seemed to experience. Upon awakening in the morning, the volunteers rated the quality of their sleep on a number of dimensions, such as how comfortably they had slept and how well rested they now felt. Based on these ratings, the best night in the lab and the worst one were selected for each subject while the third night was discarded. It was found that during their worst night the sleepers had been much more involved in their dreams than during their best night (matched t-test, $p < .05$). No direct cause and effect relationships can be demonstrated from this study, but I find it intriguing to speculate that on some mornings people may awaken in a groggy state because they were so involved in their dreams during that night, while on other mornings they may awaken much more refreshed because they experienced a series of noninvolving dreams.

Further evidence suggesting the importance of dream *content* for psychological recovery during sleep comes from the work done by Kramer et al. [11]. These investigators found that imipramine (an antidepressant) increased hostility in the dreams of normal subjects and depressed patients, and that after a few nights of such drug-induced hostile dreaming, some depressed patients improved clinically. Could it be that the rest of us do not become depressed because we are usually able to discharge pent-up hostility in our dreams?

SUMMARY

Evidence reviewed in this paper suggests that delta sleep is "good, efficient" sleep in terms of physiological recovery from previous wakefulness. While some such recovery goes on throughout all waking and sleeping, it appears that more of it is achieved in delta sleep, per unit time, than in any other state. Not only is delta sleep increased when physiological recovery is particularly pressing (e.g., after prolonged wakefulness, after exercise, or when sleep is curtailed), but the combination of low metabolism coupled with relatively high blood volume in the skeletal muscle, relatively high respiratory rate, and low CO_2 retention, seems ideal for physiological recovery.

The feeling of having slept well or poorly during a certain night seems multidetermined. It is influenced by, among other things, personality variables, changes in mood from evening to morning, amount of wakefulness remembered, and possibly even dream content.

REFERENCES

1. Agnew, H. W., Jr., and Webb, W. B. The Sleep Patterns of Long and Short Sleepers. Paper presented at the meeting of the Association for the Psychophysiological Study of Sleep, Santa Monica, Cal., 1967.
2. Agnew, H. W., Jr., Webb, W. B., and Williams, R. T. Comparison of stage 4 and 1-REM sleep deprivation. *Percept. Motor Skills* 24:851, 1967.
3. Baekeland, F., and Lasky, R. Exercise and sleep patterns in college athletes. *Percept. Motor Skills* 23:1203, 1966.
4. Brebbia, D. R., and Altschuler, K. Z. Stage Related Patterns and Nightly Trends of Energy Exchange During Sleep. In Kline and Laska (Eds.), *Computers and Electronic Devices in Psychiatry*. New York: Grune & Stratton, 1968. Pp. 319–335.
5. Hauri, P. Effects of evening activity on subsequent sleep and dreams. University of Chicago Doctoral Dissertation, 1966.
6. Hauri, P. Effects of evening activity on early night sleep. *Psychophysiology* 4:267, 1968.
7. Hawkins, D. R., and Mendels, J. Sleep disturbance in depressive syndromes. *Amer. J. Psychiat.* 123:682, 1966.
8. Hobson, J. A. Sleep after exercise. *Science* 162:1503, 1968.
9. Kales, A., Wilson, T., Kales, J. D., Jacobson, A., Paulson, M. J., Kollar, E., and Walter, R. D. Measurements of all-night sleep

in normal elderly persons: Effects of aging. *J. Amer. Geriat. Soc.* 15:405, 1967.

10. Karacan, I., Wolff, S. M., Williams, R. L., Hursch, C. J., and Webb, W. B. The effects of fever on sleep and dream patterns. *Psychosomatics* 9:331, 1968.
11. Kramer, M., Whitman, R. M., Baldridge, B., and Ornstein, P. H. Drugs and dreams. III. The effects of imipramine on the dreams of depressed patients. *Amer. J. Psychiat.* 124:79, 1968.
12. Lester, B., and Guerrero-Figueroa, R. Effects of some drugs on electroencephalic fast activity and dream time. *Psychophysiology* 2:224, 1966.
13. Monroe, L. J. Psychological and physiological differences between good and poor sleepers. *J. Abnorm. Psychol.* 72:255, 1967.
14. Nowlis, V. Research with the Mood Adjective Checklist. In S. Tomkins and E. Izard (Eds.), *Affect, Cognition and Personality.* New York: Springer, 1965.
15. Othmer, E. *Persönlichkeit und Schlafverhalten.* Meisenheim am Glan, West Germany: Anton Hain, 1965.
16. Othmer, E. Pathophysiologie des gestörten Schlafes und dessen psychopharmakologische Beeinflussung. *Arzneimittel-Forschung* [Drug Research] 16:300, 1966.
17. Sassin, J. F., and Johnson, L. C. Body motility during sleep and its relation to the K-complex. *Exp. Neurol.* 22:133, 1968.
18. Synder, F., Hobson, J. A., Morrison, D. F., and Goldfrank, F. Changes in respiration, heart rate, and systolic blood pressure in human sleep. *J. Appl. Physiol.* 19:417, 1964.
19. Webb, W. B., and Agnew, H. W., Jr. Sleep: Effects of a restricted regime. *Science* 150:1745, 1965.
20. Williams, H. L., Hammack, J. T., Daly, R. L., Dement, W. C., and Lubin, A. Responses to auditory stimulation, sleep loss and the EEG stages of sleep. *Electroenceph. Clin. Neurophysiol.* 16:269, 1964.

Sleep Duration and Feeling State

GORDON G. GLOBUS

In attempting to answer the question "What is good sleep?" it may be useful to resolve the question into two parts: "What sleep is good?" and "What good is sleep?" Recent evidence has helped to answer the former question, but at the present time only speculations can be offered with respect to the latter. This paper presents data relating sleep duration to subsequent feeling state and uses these data as a springboard for speculations on the function of sleep.

It is a banal observation that one does not feel "good" after sleep deprivation. Decreases in psychomotor performance have been extensively documented following sleep loss [11]. A report [8] of two cases of "healthy insomnia" in which individuals habitually slept only about 3 hours per night for many years but felt well seems to be the exception rather than the rule.

A question generally not raised is the effect of "too much" rather than "too little" sleep on the way an individual feels. This question probably does not occur to the sleep researcher who is too active and busy to obtain extra sleep and in general tends to be somewhat sleep-deprived. However, the more sluggardly investigator may have noted, as has this writer, that if on occasion one takes advantage of the opportunity to sleep late on Sunday morning, rather than feeling refreshed and restored on awakening, paradoxically one often feels tired, washed out, and finds it difficult to get going with the activities of the day.

A study to be reported in detail elsewhere describes evidence for a syndrome of feeling "worn-out" associated with "extra sleep"—which each subject defined for himself in terms of his own habitual sleep duration. The syndrome was most striking when the extra sleep lasted for 10 or more hours in a situation where the student subjects were not making up lost sleep, 87 percent reporting having experienced the syndrome as against 22 percent having experienced a dummy syndrome (to control for suggestion). The worn-out syndrome was experienced on 47 percent of extra sleep occurrences as opposed to 5 percent for the dummy syndrome. These differences were highly significant. For subjects whose extra sleep tended to be 10 or more hours in a situation where they were not making up lost sleep, the worn-out syndrome was experienced a significantly greater percentage of the time than a syndrome of feeling "just great." The worn-out syndrome lingered for an average of 4.4 hours.

METHODS AND RESULTS

In this initial study, the syndrome was defined for the subjects by the experimenter. In the data to be reported here, the syndrome was undefined and the subjects were asked to define it. One hundred and one female nursing students with an age range of 17 to 51 years were screened by questionnaire to provide a sample of 49 subjects who reported that they sometimes had nights on which they obtained "extra sleep," either by going to bed earlier than usual or getting up later than usual, and sometimes felt "worse" after such an extra sleep night. This was, therefore, a highly selected sample for which there was reason to believe that the subjects might have experienced a syndrome associated with extra sleep. The usual sleep night of this group averaged 7.0 hours, they felt that they "needed" 7.6 hours, and their average extra sleep night was 9.2 hours with a mean number of 4.2 nights per month.

These subjects were asked to fill out an adjective checklist of 74 items. This included all the items from Raskin's adjective checklist [14], and 23 items taken from the McNair-Lorr adjective checklist [12]. Subjects were asked to describe their feelings after an extra sleep night when they were not making up lost sleep, as compared with a night in which they had the amount of sleep they felt they typically need (which had already been defined for each individual earlier in the questionnaire) in terms of a 7-point scale (extremely less, quite a bit less, a little less, the same, a little more, quite a bit more, extremely more).

Each adjective was scored across all subjects as 3 for "extremely,"

2 for "quite a bit," and 1 for "a little" in the direction of feeling worse; the remaining ratings were scored as 0 for not feeling worse. Table 1 lists the rank order, grouped in 34 ranks, for all 74 adjectives with those highest in the list scoring highest in terms of negative feelings. Most striking are the high ranks in adjectives

TABLE 1. *Rank order of adjectives used to describe feelings after an "extra sleep night" compared to a "needed sleep night," in decreasing order of usage*

1. Sleepy
2. Less full of pep
3. Worn-out
4. Tired
5. Headache, inactive
6. Bushed, weary
7. Less well-rested
8. Slowed down, exhausted, washed out
9. Sluggish, less lively
10. Listless, less efficient
11. Less alert
12. Less vigorous, annoyed, foggy
13. Less able to concentrate, less able to work, depressed
14. Muscle ache
15. Grouchy
16. Impatient, less satisfied, worthless
17. Irritable
18. Less able to think clearly, less carefree
19. Less relaxed, bad-tempered, discouraged
20. Less sociable, less friendly, useless
21. Less dependable, blue, angry, less good-natured, sarcastic, moody
22. Restless, nervous, less happy, on edge, less cheerful
23. Peeved, muddled
24. Anxious, troubled by conscience, tense
25. Worried, shaky
26. Loss of appetite, less pleasant
27. Downhearted, forgetful, nausea, upset stomach, lonely
28. Less kind, bewildered, jittery
29. Unhappy, less at ease, troubled, less certain about things
30. Sorry for things done
31. Ashamed
32. Sad
33. Less warmhearted, less considerate
34. Rude

which might be broadly classified as "anergic," e.g., less full of pep, bushed, sluggish. It is an interesting paradox that despite the extra sleep, "sleepy" has the highest rank. Adjectives relating to cognitive difficulties, e.g., less alert, less able to concentrate, and performance difficulties, e.g., less efficient, less able to work, also tend to rank high. On the other hand, adjectives relating to anxiety, guilt, and depression rank on the low side, with adjectives relating to hostility perhaps ranking a bit higher.

DISCUSSION

Several alternative explanations of these data can be proffered to explain the effects of excess sleep on subsequent mood state. For example, it may be related to breaking a habitual routine [2], going without food or being inactive for long periods, sleeping at the wrong phase of one's circadian rhythm, being depressed *prior* to sleep, therefore sleeping longer and waking up still depressed, and so on. Clinical experience suggests, however, that the crucial variable may be simply duration of sleep. Fortunately, the question can be explored in the laboratory under controlled conditions.

In the context of the above data, it is of interest to consider sleep duration in terms of homeostatic regulation. There are very powerful mechanisms at work following sleep deprivation which impel the organism to sleep. Even though individuals have remained awake for monumental durations, e.g., 264 hours [7], they must struggle mightily against sleep. No comparable mechanism seems to function in relation to waking where interfering stimuli, such as hunger, thirst, or excretory demands, tend to disrupt sleep but can be easily remedied; with a glass of juice and a quick trip to the bathroom in the morning, many individuals are capable of returning to sleep. Verdone's subjects [15], allowed to sleep as long as they wished, averaged 10 hours in bed (not including initial and terminal wakefulness). In Aserinsky's study [1], subjects managed to sleep 14½ hours out of 24. Patients, particularly depressed adolescents and young adults, not infrequently report going through periods of weeks when they sleep half the 24 hours. Apparently the imperative to stop sleeping is not as strong as the imperious need to sleep.

Assuming that sleep has something to do with generally anabolic function (cf. the work of Hess [5] and recent work on increased growth hormone production in slow wave sleep [13]), it is in the interest of survival that powerful brain mechanisms actively insure the behavior of sleeping [10]. That the organism terminates sleep in order to carry out behaviors such as obtaining food—behaviors which are generally catabolic functions—is also highly adaptive. But modern man generally goes to sleep well fed, well hydrated, and even well rested—*his main imperatives for terminating sleep are social rather than biological.* He tends to arise grudgingly to work and steadfastly remain in bed when there is nothing for which to get up. If he continues sleeping, the reciprocal relationship between sleeping inactivity and waking activity apparently becomes tipped more in favor of the former, leading to the anergic syndrome described above.

Implicit in this view of sleep as adaptive "behavior" rather than a "state" is a notion about the role of brain activity. The question might be posed, does the brain actively pursue sleep in its own behalf as well as for the rest of the organism? Hobson [6], for example, following Evarts [3], suggests that the function of sleep is related to the "rest" of inhibiting nerve cells, in addition to enforcing inactivity on the somatic musculature. Although in terms of everyday *experience* it certainly seems as if our brains "need" to sleep, there is no direct evidence to suggest that the brain is in some way at rest during sleep. It seems more parsimonious to assume that sleep is simply a change in the organization of the brain—a change which serves to disconnect the organism from both sensory input and motor output. As Jouvet [9] has dramatically demonstrated, when motor inhibition is released during REM sleep in cats, extensive behaviors can take place. There is apparently mental activity in humans during both REM and NREM sleep [4], but it does not get connected to behavior. This suggests that the brain is "working" quite as hard in sleep as in waking, although in the former case imposing an inhibition of overt energy-consuming behavior on the organism.

It may be, then, that the answer to the question, "What good is sleep?" is really "not so good as we might think," at least in an affluent society. Because of a number of factors such as less physical work to accomplish and better nutrition, our bodies may not need anywhere near as much sleep as we actually obtain, but our brains continue to impose this evolutionary anachronism upon us. The immense practical importance of basic research in sleep is clear, as it is a tenable hope that we may someday be able considerably to decrease our time asleep by pharmacological means, freeing us for more intrinsically human activities.

REFERENCES

1. Aserinsky, E. Assessment of the Normal Sleep Requirement. Presentation to Society of Biological Psychiatry, Washington, D.C., 1968.
2. Bousfield, W. A. Further evidence of the relation of the euphoric attitude to sleep and exercise. *Psychol. Rec.* 2:334, 1938.
3. Evarts, E. In M. Jouvet (Ed.), *Aspects Anatomo-Fonctionnels de la Physiologie du Sommeil.* Paris: Centre National de la Recherche Scientifique, 1965. P. 397.
4. Foulkes, D. Nonrapid eye movement mentation. *Exp. Neurol.* Suppl. No. 4, p. 28, 1967.
5. Hess, W. R. The Diencephalic Sleep Center. In *Brain Mechanisms and Consciousness.* Oxford: Blackwell, 1954. P. 117.
6. Hobson, A. Exercise and sleep. *Science* 162:1503, 1968.
7. Johnson, L. C., Slye, E. S., and Dement, W. Electroencephalographic and autonomic activity during and after prolonged sleep deprivation. *Psychosom. Med.* 27:415, 1965.
8. Jones, H. S., and Oswald, I. Two cases of healthy insomnia. *Electroenceph. Clin. Neurophysiol.* 24:378, 1968.
9. Jouvet, M. Mechanisms of the States of Sleep: A Neuropharmacological Approach. In S. Kety, E. Evarts, and H. Williams (Eds.), *Sleep and Altered States of Consciousness.* Baltimore: Williams & Wilkins, 1967.
10. Jouvet, M. Biogenic amines and the states of sleep. *Science* 163:32, 1969.

11. Lubin, A. Performance Under Sleep Loss and Fatigue. In S. Kety, E. Evarts, and H. Williams (Eds.), *Sleep and Altered States of Consciousness*. Baltimore: Williams & Wilkins, 1967.
12. McNair, D. M., and Lorr, M. An analysis of mood in neurotics. *J. Abnorm. Soc. Psychol.* 69:620, 1964.
13. Parker, D. C., Sassin, J. F., Mace, J. W., Gotlin, R. W., and Rossman, L. G. Human Growth Hormone Release During Sleep: Electroencephalographic Correlation. Unpublished manuscript.
14. Raskin, A., Schulterbrandt, J., and Reatig, N. Factors of psychopathology in interview, ward behavior, and self-report ratings of hospitalized depressives. *J. Consult. Psychol.* 31:270, 1967.
15. Verdone, P. Sleep satiation: Extended sleep in normal subjects. *Electroenceph. Clin. Neurophysiol.* 24:417, 1968.

Sleep, Dreaming, and Clinical Psychiatry

*Does the new knowledge of sleep and dreaming have any relevance to clinical psychiatry? Can the sleep-dream patterns of a night be of use in diagnosis, prognosis, or treatment planning?**

Implications of Knowledge of Sleep Patterns in Psychiatric Conditions

DAVID R. HAWKINS

Is there relevance for clinical psychiatry in recent sleep studies? In a general way the answer must be unreservedly yes. If the question means "Is the clinical management of a single patient enhanced by our new knowledge of sleep?" or if we ask the second question, "Can the sleep-dream pattern of the night be of use in the prognosis or diagnosis of mental illness?" then I think the answer at this time must be generally no.

* The reader interested in this question may wish to refer also to papers by Baekeland and Hartmann (p. 33), Baekeland (p. 49), Hauri (p. 70), Zung (p. 123), Foulkes (p. 147), Witkin (p. 154), Greenberg (p. 258), and Stoyva (p. 355).

The discovery of the D-state of sleep, indicating a different type of sleep than previously conceived of, and a connection of the D-state with the intriguing phenomenon, dreaming, have led to an undue focus on the D-state and not enough consideration of both states of sleep, their relationship to each other and to the total function of the organism.

Whenever a new technique or method for studying patients is developed, in order to be clinically useful it must be capable of obtaining information of diagnostic or prognostic import that is either more precise, more quickly available, or less expensive than by other means. Data which detail sleep problems that occur in connection with psychiatric illness are accumulating rapidly. However, evidence to date suggests that sleep disturbances are generally not precise enough to be of diagnostic value. For example, the type of sleep disturbance found in depressive illness is somewhat similar to that found in schizophrenia in an acute phase, suggesting that the sleep disturbance is more a function of general psychological disruption than related to specific disease. The finding in narcolepsy of the occurrence of D-state sleep at sleep onset is highly specific unless there has been previous sleep deprivation or amphetamine addiction; but the diagnosis can easily be made on clinical grounds, and in usual practice the expense of study in the sleep laboratory would not be justified.

CONDITIONS MANIFESTING SLEEP ABNORMALITIES

In order to clarify these statements, I will briefly discuss some conditions in which studies of sleep have shown abnormalities.

Insomnia

First let us consider insomnia, whether it be chronic and unrelated to specific disease processes or occurring as part of a specific clinical condition. At this point in time I see little to be gained from sleep laboratory studies of the individual patient unless done by an investigator with great experience in this area. In most instances all that would be demonstrated would be the extent of wakefulness. The question that sleep research may soon answer is which drugs, under which circumstances, can be effective as hypnotics, and which ones distort the usual sleep pattern the least.

Because of the enormous time and expenses necessary to execute proper pharmacological evaluation of hypnotic drugs utilizing the sleep laboratory, we only have preliminary and tentative data. We do have indications that some drugs predominantly suppress D-sleep, and others stages 3 and 4 sleep. Unfortunately we don't understand sufficiently the function or necessity of different sleep stages to know which we must be most careful not to suppress in most instances.

In light of our present knowledge of the marked diminution of stages 3 and 4 sleep in depressive patients, I would be very reluctant to use a hypnotic which itself decreases stage 3 or 4 sleep.

Kales and Jacobson [11] and their colleagues are particularly concerned with these matters. Their studies to date strongly suggest that in the chronic insomniac, hypnotic drugs do not have any substantive value and indeed may compound the problem. It should be possible soon to have more definitive knowledge of which hypnotic drugs are least disruptive of the usual sleep pattern or come closest to helping induce normal sleep.

Within the last few months much of the literature circulated by drug companies with regard to hypnotics indicates some preoccupation with and awareness of the importance of drug effects on sleep stages. Some of the brochures may indicate little interference with REM sleep but say nothing of stage 4 sleep or vice versa. At this point it behooves the clinician to be very skeptical of these results until he can get independent comparative studies of many drugs which include all dimensions of sleep.

Psychosomatic Disorders

Let us next consider psychosomatic disorders in which the disease process may have some relation to phases of sleep. There is some indication that patients with peptic ulcer have a greatly increased gastric acid secretion during D-periods, though in normal individuals gastric function does not seem to vary with sleep [1]. Not enough subjects have yet been studied and for the moment one is perplexed as to what use to make of this knowledge. However, it is an area to be closely watched.

A number of investigations have suggested that patients with coronary artery disease may have episodes of myocardial-ischemia in relation to D-state sleep, though the data at this point are somewhat contradictory. Study of an individual patient with nocturnal angina in the sleep laboratory might be a worthwhile undertaking even in our present state of limited knowledge [14]. Nocturnal asthmatic attacks do not apparently correlate with stages of sleep [10]. To date, what we have learned about sleep in relationship to epilepsy does not suggest that study of sleep beyond the sort of sleep test that was for a long time standard in EEG laboratories is of value. Recent studies suggest that abnormal spike-and-wave discharges are considerably less frequent in D-state than in S-state (NREM) sleep [15].

Mental Retardation and Aging

There are two areas where there is some promise for a diagnostic capability for sleep studies. These are mental retardation and aging. Feinberg et al. [4] have shown that as compared with normal subjects, mental retardates of the mongolian type show low D-time (amounts of D-state sleep) with an extreme reduction in the amount of eye movements. Subjects with phenylketonuria show a trend toward low D-time. There are other sleep EEG abnormalities as well. Brain-damaged subjects have normal amounts of D-time but little stage 4 sleep as compared to normal subjects or other retardates.

Feinberg et al. [5] have found increased sleep onset latency and more wakefulness in the aged. They also find less stage 4 sleep as compared with normal young adults. Whether the diminution in stage 4 is a regular aspect of the aging process or whether it reflects pathological changes in the central nervous system which occur frequently but not inevitably in an aged population is still problematical. In our studies [13] we find considerable interaction of aging and depression in that stage 4 sleep in elderly depressives is extremely low as compared with younger depressives; our elderly controls did not show any evidence of diminution of stage 4 as compared with young adults in our laboratory. However, we did not study any extremely aged individuals nor a large population of the aged.

The above findings suggest that sleep may reflect the integrity of the central nervous system and that the psychophysiological study of sleep may aid diagnostically in evaluating degree of damage or loss of function in the brain. Feinberg [2], in studying patients with chronic brain syndrome, postulates the "possibility that total sleep time is related to the overall rate of cerebral metabolism."

Schizophrenia

There have been many studies of sleep in schizophrenia, most of which have tended to focus on the D-state of sleep. A recent example is a study by Stein et al. [16] which can serve as a bibliographical source for other work in this area. Essentially, they found no major differences in the sleep of their schizophrenics except for some shortening of the latency to REM onset. They did not pay close attention to other sleep stages. Some investigators in some patients have found diminution in D-time percentage. Feinberg and his colleagues, who have a series of studies of the sleep of schizophrenics, are finding that absence or diminution of stage 4 is usual and marked in schizophrenics [3]. As in depression, as will be detailed in the next section, many more careful longitudinal studies with attention to the type of patient, duration and stage of illness are indicated before we can use sleep studies as a diagnostic or prognostic tool in schizophrenia.

Depression

The connection of sleep disturbance and depression or melancholia has been noted as long as the recorded history of medicine. In general, precise knowledge of the sleep pattern is not needed to make the basic diagnosis of depression, though the possibility exists that as we know more about sleep, study of an individual's sleep might suggest the basic mechanism of depression in somebody with mixed symptomatology. The possibility that precise knowledge of an individual sleep pattern might distinguish types of depression has been and still is to a limited extent a hope. To date psychophysiological studies of sleep and depression have confirmed what was long assumed clinically: that there are profound sleep disturbances accompanying depression. However, it would appear to date that the sleep disturbance has more to do with the degree of emotional distress than the specific variety of depressive illness. Of course, if we knew more about depression and could, with confidence, separate different depressive syndromes, we might be in a position to find subtle differences in sleep.

Studies in our laboratory [6, 8, 9, 12] and other laboratories find disturbances in many dimensions of sleep. The depressed patient takes longer to fall asleep, has more wakefulness during the sleep period, wakes earlier, and has abnormal wave forms in his sleep EEG pattern. In general, D-state time is decreased, though on occasional nights it may be increased, probably as a rebound phenomenon from previous deprivation. Hartmann [7] alone among investigators has indicated in his findings an increase in D-time in some depressives. The most consistent and persistent abnormality in the sleep of depressed patients is diminution or absence of stage 4 and sometimes even stage 3 sleep. Perhaps the more accurate way to put this may be that there is a lack of delta wave sleep. There is some suggestion that the degree of delta wave sleep disturbance might be a measure of the presence of a factor which has been reflected by the term *endogenous* as applied to depression. However, this is far from established.

What may be more hopeful is that careful study of the sleep of depressed patients might be of prognostic value or could be a guide to the management of therapy. It may be possible as we come to understand more completely the relationship of sleep and depression that a careful analysis of a patient's sleep may give us insight into the extent of somatic disturbance, which might suggest the type of treatment or the likely prognosis.

We have found that with successful treatment, sleep tends to improve earlier than most aspects of behavior, and not infrequently the improvement in sleep may be dramatic. With successful treatment in the depressive all parameters of sleep tend toward normal, but the improvement in stage 3 or 4 delta sleep is only slight. To date we do not have long-term followup sleep studies of longitudinally studied depressed patients. Our assumption had been that there would be a gradual return to normal values of delta wave sleep. A preliminary unpublished study in our laboratory of a small group of subjects in the fifth decade of life with previous histories of recurring depressions showed an almost total absence of delta wave sleep. At the time of the study these subjects were asymptomatic and reported no subjective sleep difficulties. Findings such as this suggest the possibility that sleep studies could identify subjects with a predisposition to depression.

Use of Sleep Studies

Crystal ball gazing is hazardous. My prediction is that continued psychophysiological study of sleep will contribute greatly to an understanding of central nervous system functioning and its role in many diseases but will be unlikely to contribute much directly to our diagnostic capacity. The use of sleep studies as a prognostic tool or guide for management of a patient seems to me more likely to be useful. There is much promise in the use of sleep studies as a guide to the usefulness and side effects of drugs given either as hypnotics, tranquilizers, or for other central nervous system effects.

REFERENCES

1. Armstrong, R. H., Burnap, D., Jacobson, A., Kales, A., Ward, S., and Golden, J. Dreams and gastric secretions in duodenal ulcer patients. *New Phycn.* (Chicago) 14:241, 1965.
2. Feinberg, I. Sleep electroencephalographic and eye movement patterns in patients with schizophrenia and with chronic brain syndrome. *Sleep and Altered States of Consciousness,* Assoc. Res. Nerv. Ment. Dis. Monographs, No. 45. Baltimore: Williams & Wilkins, 1967.

3. Feinberg, I., Braun, M., Koresko, R. L., and Gottlieb, F. Stage 4 sleep in schizophrenia. *Arch. Gen. Psychiat.* (Chicago) 21:262, 1969.
4. Feinberg, I., Braun, M., and Shulman, E. EEG sleep patterns in mental retardation. *Electroenceph. Clin. Neurophysiol.* 27:128, 1969.
5. Feinberg, I., Koresko, R. L., and Heller, N. EEG sleep patterns as a function of normal and pathological aging in man. *J. Psychiat. Res.* 5:107, 1967.
6. Gresham, S. C., Agnew, H. W., Jr., and Williams, R. L. The sleep of depressed patients. *Arch. Gen. Psychiat.* (Chicago) 10:503, 1965.
7. Hartmann, E. Longitudinal studies of sleep and dream patterns in manic depressive patients. *Arch. Gen. Psychiat.* (Chicago) 19:312, 1968.
8. Hawkins, D. R., and Mendels, J. Sleep disturbance in depressive syndromes. *Amer. J. Psychiat.* 123:682, 1966.
9. Hawkins, D. R., Mendels, J., Scott, J., Bensch, G., and Teachey, W. The psychophysiology of sleep in psychotic depression: A longitudinal study. *Psychosom. Med.* 29:329, 1967.
10. Kales, A., Beall, G. N., Bajor, G., Jacobson, A., Kales, J. D., Sly, R. M., and Wilson, T. E. Sleep studies of adult and child asthmatics. *Psychophysiology* 4:397, 1968.
11. Kales, A., Jacobson, A., Kales, J. D., Marusak, C., and Hanley, J. Effects of drugs on sleep (Noludar, Doriden, Nembutal, Chloral Hydrate, Benadryl). *Psychophysiology* 4:391, 1968.
12. Mendels, J., and Hawkins, D. R. Sleep and depression: A controlled EEG study. *Arch. Gen. Psychiat.* (Chicago) 16:344, 1967.
13. Mendels, J., and Hawkins, D. R. Sleep and depression: Further considerations. *Arch. Gen. Psychiat.* (Chicago) 19:445, 1968.
14. Nowlin, J. B., Troyer, W. G., Jr., Collins, W. S., Silverman, G., Nichols, C. R., McIntosh, H. D., Estes, E. H., Jr., and Bogdonoff, M. D. The association of nocturnal angina pectoris with dreaming. *Ann. Intern. Med.* 63:1040, 1965.
15. Ross, J. J., Johnson, L. C., and Walter, R. D. Spike and wave discharges during stages of sleep. *Arch. Neurol.* (Chicago) 14:399, 1966.
16. Stein, M., Fram, D. H., Wyatt, R., Grinspoon, L., and Tursky, B. All-night sleep studies of acute schizophrenics. *Arch. Gen. Psychiat.* (Chicago) 20:470, 1969.

The Relationship of Sleep Disturbances to Psychopathology

ISMET KARACAN AND ROBERT L. WILLIAMS

Since the beginning of time man has wondered about the importance of sleep and dreams to his health, happiness, and well-being. For most of his history his inquiries have been limited to idle speculation, parables, poems, and omens. Man has roamed the earth and the space beyond the earth. He has learned to build and to destroy whole civilizations. He has created works of art, music, and literature which have outlived these civilizations. He has developed complex systems of law and social order to enhance human interaction. Yet throughout this odyssey of inquiry and achievement, man has learned remarkably little about sleep—a state in which he spends one-third of his life.

During this century, man has made considerable progress in his study of sleep and dreams. He has crossed a Rubicon of scientific achievement, and he has begun to replace idle speculation with empirical investigations. Throughout this paper we attempt to chart the progress of this empirical investigation. We begin by discussing the theoretical framework which provided a foundation for later experimental studies. We then cite the early rapid eye movement sleep experiments which tested the theoretical notions concerning sleep, dreaming, and their relationship to psychopathology. We discuss the controversy which has surrounded these initial REM sleep studies and the studies of NREM sleep which followed. Finally we discuss pregnancy and postpartum psychosis as a suitable paradigm for investigating the relationship of sleep disturbances to psychopathology.

THEORETICAL FRAMEWORK

Allusions to the etiological importance of sleep disturbances in psychopathology are common in the early psychiatric literature.

Tuke [53] in 1892 stated that "loss of sleep may frequently be a cause, or one of several causes, of mental disorders." In the early twentieth century Bleuler [7] distinguished himself by literally living with schizophrenic patients for several years to observe their behavior. He is considered one of the most knowledgable in the field of schizophrenia. He discussed the similarities between the schizophrenic process and dreaming:

> In dreams, a similar dissociation of thinking occurs; symbolism, condensations, predominance of emotions which often remain hidden, hallucinations—all these can be found in both states and in the same way, and in spite of the difference in genesis and in spite of the minor differences, it may well be possible to show the secondary symptomatology of schizophrenia as wholly identical with that of dreams.

In addition, Bleuler noted that other deliria had also been compared with dreams. He cited the classification by French psychiatrists of "oneiro deliria" and suggested that alcoholic delirium and the various types of fever deliria bear a resemblance to the dreaming process. Similar notions relating dreams to psychopathology have been advanced by others [16, 19, 28, 32].

REM SLEEP EXPERIMENTS

These authorities lacked the technological means with which to investigate their hypotheses concerning sleep, dreaming, and psychopathology. However, their theoretical formulations were based on a wealth of insightful clinical experience and provided the impetus for latter-day investigations of the functional significance of REM sleep in psychopathology. Aserinsky and Kleitman's discovery [2] in 1953 of the cyclical occurrence of REM periods provided the first major breakthrough for measurement of biological indices of the dreaming state. A new technique which could be utilized in testing the previous theoretical notions was already overdue. REM sleep in normal subjects as well as schizophrenic patients became the target of experimentation.

In 1960 Dement [12] published the findings of his historic REM deprivation experiment and opened a new frontier in experimental psychiatry. Dement found that during REM deprivation there was a steady increase in the number of awakenings required to suppress REM sleep. On the recovery nights there was a substantial increase in the total amount of REM sleep from previously established baseline levels. In addition he reported that "distinct personality changes" occurred in the 2 subjects who had been deprived the longest. Dement's findings have been interpreted as demonstrating a need for REM sleep. Because of the great impact of Dement's results on the scientific community, many young investigators were attracted to the field of sleep research. His work was replicated by other established sleep laboratories. Most investigators confirmed the findings of a greater number of awakenings required to maintain REM deprivation and an increase in REM time from baseline to recovery-night levels. His suggestion that prolonged REM deprivation might produce severe psychological alterations has not, however, been substantiated [34, 44, 48, 54]. More recently Cartwright et al. [9] reported finding marked differences in physiological response between individuals on REM recovery nights and finding some subjects who apparently had no rebound recovery.

Because a positive correlation between dreaming periods and REM periods had been shown [3, 13], researchers hypothesized that REM frequency in psychotics—particularly in schizophrenics—would differ from the REM frequency of normal subjects. Paradoxically, however, a difference in opinion as to the underlying mechanism of the hallucinatory process and its relationship to REM resulted in the polarization of investigators into two schools of thought. One group assumed that since schizophrenia is accompanied by a higher level of arousal, and REM is a physiological expression of instinctual drive, then REM time should be greater in schizophrenic patients than in normal subjects. Dement [11] was the first to study the sleep patterns of schizophrenic patients and found that they did not differ from a control population. Feinberg [15] also found that there was no significant difference in amount of REM time between schizophrenic and nonschizophrenic subjects. Similar findings were reported by Onheiber et al. [42] and Vogel and Traub [55].

The other group assumed that since the hallucinatory process is similar to the dreaming process, schizophrenics should evidence less REM time than normal persons (since these subjects "dream" during the day). Rechtschaffen [45] studied the waking electroencephalogram, electro-oculogram (EOG) and electromyogram (EMG) of 5 acute schizophrenic subjects in order to determine whether there were indications of an "intrusion" of REM into wakefulness. He reported that the waking EEG failed to show any patterns resembling those obtained during the REM period.

The failure of the investigators to find outstanding differences in the REM activity of schizophrenics when compared to controls was unexpected. Soon, however, positive but controversial findings began to be reported. Fisher and Dement [17] studied one patient before, during, and after the onset of acute paranoid psychosis and reported finding an "unusually high" base-line REM time. A later reevaluation suggested that the report was in error. It should also be noted that the treatment of this patient with high doses of Stelazine contaminated the results. Gulevich [23] reported that chronic schizophrenics in remission exhibit a greater amount of REM time than do normal individuals. Snyder [50] reported finding a reduction of REM time in schizophrenic patients who were studied during the early stage of the illness.

Other investigators performed experimental REM deprivation studies with the expectancy that schizophrenic subjects would react adversely to deprivation of the REM stage. Azumi [4] found no exacerbation of psychotic symptoms after REM deprivation, but he found that psychotics show less compensatory REM time on recovery nights than do normal persons. It should be mentioned, however, that the control group was not age-matched. Zarcone [59] reported that REM compensation is greater in remission than in the acute phase. In contrast to these findings, Vogel and Traub [55] reported observing a normal rebound in schizophrenic patients. In a total sleep deprivation study, Koranyi [39] found that schizophrenic subjects react more adversely to deprivation than do normal subjects. Freedman et al. [18] studied the manifest dream content of acute schizophrenic patients during REM sleep and found that it contained more hallucinatory experiences than that obtained during the remission phase.

Thus far the results of studies of schizophrenic populations have been contradictory and controversial. Most of these studies have been cross-sectional, and there are several disadvantages to this type of study. Differences in symptomatology exhibited by the patients tend to mask the diagnostic picture. These phenomenological differences may indicate different stages of the same disease process, or they may indicate different forms of the same psychosis. On the whole there is a need for a more universally accepted and more precisely defined set of criteria for diagnosis. Generally the effects of somatic and psychological treatment have been disregarded. Most of the studies have focused on small and heterogeneous groups.

Laboratory settings differ somewhat from each other, yet the individual differences in patients' reactions to the experimental setting have not been considered. It is known, for instance, that there is a "first-night" effect on sleep patterns of normal subjects. For this reason, the first night's recording is generally disregarded in normal subjects. It is important that we determine whether schizophrenic patients respond to environmental effects in the same way as normal persons. If this is the case, the duration of this response to environmental effects should be determined. In addition, measures of anxiety level of each subject and of differential effects of environment on anxiety level in a particular laboratory might provide a basis for comparison of sleep responses produced in separate laboratory settings.

The fact that environmental effects may intrude has been illustrated by Baekeland [5], who investigated the effects on sleep of two films, one psychologically stressful, the other neutral. He found that the stress film significantly increased the number of awakenings and the REM density.

Another complication encountered in the study of schizophrenics can, paradoxically, be attributed to modern medical and technological advances. Presently most patients seek psychiatric attention only after unsuccessful drug treatment. The validity of using these patients as subjects for sleep research is doubtful. The effects of psychotropic drugs on the clinical conditions and the sleep pattern must be taken into account.

STUDIES OF NREM SLEEP

Because of the historical and theoretical impact of the discovery of REM sleep, most sleep research—and justly so—has been directed toward the study of REM sleep. Some investigators do not even report their findings on the other stages of sleep. Consequently only a few studies have focused on the significance of the other stages.

There are no doubt several other variables which should be investigated and reported. With the exception of Caldwell's work [8], most studies of schizophrenics have neglected the NREM stages of sleep (stages 1, 2, 3, 4). In the process of collecting data on REM, investigators have acquired an abundance of NREM data, but these data have for the most part been neglected.

Theories about dreaming, and the evidence which linked dreaming to REM, caused this area of sleep to be placed high on the scale of experimental priorities. Yet it is interesting to note that stage 4 suppression in depressed patients was discovered long before the REM stage was recognized [14]. Thus far in sleep research, sleep has been equated with EEG activity, and dreaming has been equated with REM. In fact, however, EEG and eye movement activity are but a small part of the total process of sleep and dreaming.

In a study of sleep deprivation, it was found [6] that REM sleep was somewhat suppressed on the night immediately following sleep deprivation, but that it rebounded to high levels on the second and subsequent recovery nights. On the other hand, stage 4 significantly increased on the first recovery night. These investigators suggested that the restitution of stage 4 might be more important to the organism than the restitution of REM sleep.

In a study of stage 4 deprivation, Agnew, Webb, and Williams [1] found that there is a significant increase in stage 4 sleep on the night following stage 4 deprivation, when compared with pre-deprivation base-line nights, demonstrating a compensation or rebound phenomenon. In a later study [57] these investigators used psychological tests to compare the psychological effects of REM-deprivation and stage 4 deprivation on two matched groups. It was found that those subjects who were REM deprived manifested, on testing, anxiety, confusion, insecurity, and withdrawal, while those who were stage 4 deprived showed, on testing, symptoms of depression and hypochondriasis. A study by Webb [56] indicates that subjects who have been partially deprived tend to sleep as if they were going to obtain a full night's sleep. In other words, they begin with a large amount of stage 4 rather than "compressing" their sleep patterns to obtain a proportionately shortened amount of each of the EEG sleep stages. This indicates the importance of stage 4 sleep for the organism.

In another recent study [8], a marked suppression of stage 4 sleep was observed in 40 percent of schizophrenic patients as compared to normal subjects. Reduced stage 4 activity in psychotic depressive patients has been reported by several other investigators (14, 22, 25, 50, 61). Stage 4 suppression has also been found in certain metabolic disorders, such as hypothyroidism (26, 33, 36). It has also been shown [22, 60] that stage 4 sleep returned to normal levels in depressed patients after successful treatment of their clinical condition. These reports have produced consistent evidence demonstrating the importance of stage 4 sleep in certain pathological conditions. In addition, recent experiments have shown a link between stage 4 sleep and certain growth processes. It has been shown that stage 4 decreases with age, and Honda et al. [27] found increased human growth hormone (HGH) levels during stage 4 sleep.

The results of the cross-sectional schizophrenia studies do not necessarily rule out sleep disturbances as an etiological factor in the development of acute psychosis. Sleep changes may have occurred prior to the onset of clinical symptoms. The only manner in which such a relationship could be investigated would be to carry out a longitudinal study of the entire illness—from a time prior to the onset of clinical symptoms, through remission. Longitudinal studies might help clarify the conflicting results produced by cross-sectional studies. However, many complications would be encountered in a longitudinal study of most types of psychopathological conditions: It is extremely difficult to select "normal" subjects in whom clinical symptoms will develop during the course of the study. Moreover, the lack of a refined, universally accepted set of criteria for selecting patients, the many months and years of continuous investigation required, and the attrition of subjects during the course of the study usually render a longitudinal study impractical. Furthermore, the investigator is hampered by the moral and social complications inherent in prolonged experimental study of psychotic patients where some treatment modalities must be eliminated or held constant. There are also problems in collecting and analyzing the large amount of data produced by such a study, and in obtaining the necessary financial resources. Through an intramural research program, the National Institute of Mental Health (NIMH) provides facilities for overcoming some of these problems. Unfortunately, however, this program is available only to a select few. In addition, young investigators are often discouraged from applying for long-range extramural NIMH support because they are usually not yet distinguished enough to qualify and because the fruits of their endeavors may not be forthcoming for several years. At the same time, this type of research requires more commitment than most senior investigators are willing to give to a new area.

One practical paradigm with which to study the relationship between sleep disturbances and psychopathology would be a regularly recurring acute schizophrenia, in which a rapid progression occurs from the acute stage through remission. Periodic catatonia is an example of such a paradigm. Unfortunately, however, this condition is described far less frequently in the modern literature than was the case a few decades ago, and it is doubtful that adequate patient populations could be selected within a reasonable period of time. On the other hand, the manic-depressive psychosis might well serve as the basis of such a cyclical study. Diaz-Guerrero et al. [14] found that profound sleep disturbances accompany the depressed type of manic-depressive psychosis. Subsequent studies have substantiated these findings. However, it remains to be shown when in the illness these sleep disturbances begin to occur and whether sleep disturbances precede or follow the depression. Again, the answers to these questions must come from longitudinal studies which need to be carried out before depression becomes clinically obvious.

SLEEP STUDIES OF PREGNANCY AND POSTPARTUM PSYCHOSIS

In the past several years, sleep investigators have attempted without success to show a causal relationship between stages of sleep and various illnesses. Part of their problem has been the difficulty of obtaining symptom-free subjects in whom clinical symptoms develop during the course of the research.

Pregnancy in the complicated as well as the uncomplicated state provides the necessary and sufficient conditions for a longitudinal investigation of the relationship between psychopathology and sleep disturbances. The pregnancy experience is time-limited with a clearly defined beginning (conception) and definitely marked end (parturition, return of the menses). These events take long enough for study of the ongoing processes, but not so long that an investigator cannot complete a project in his lifetime. Pregnant subjects are available at all times throughout the year. Furthermore, it is quite easy to obtain control subjects who are matched for age, social and economic background, and parity.

Perhaps the most attractive inducement for studying pregnancy is that it is now possible to predict with appropriate testing during early pregnancy which pregnant women will be most likely to develop postpartum emotional disturbances [20, 40, 46]. The view that sleep disturbances are one of the most common symptoms accompanying postpartum depression has been expressed by several authors [10, 24, 29, 58]. It has also been observed that insomnia starts before the onset of the psychosis, and clinical symptoms first appear during this period of sleep disturbance. The colorful term *miserable sleeplessness* [49] has become a classic description of this insomnia. It was suggested [31] that sleeplessness receive early attention in puerperal cases in order to prevent mental breakdowns. Jelly [30] reported that patients with puerperal psychosis were described as follows: "Nearly all showed early loss of appetite and inability to sleep."

Therefore pregnancy and the postpartum period provide a natural paradigm through which the relationship of sleep and dreaming to psychopathology may be examined and through which the chronological appearance of clinical symptoms may be charted.

After several years of clinical involvement with postpartum psychosis, our laboratory at the University of Florida became involved in investigating the etiological importance of sleep disturbances in psychopathology. A thorough review of the literature revealed to our surprise that there was not a single published study in which modern EEG and EOG techniques were used to investigate sleep in postpartum psychosis, which is a psychobiological complication of pregnancy.

Over the past four years we have been carrying on an intensive investigation of sleep and dreaming during pregnancy and the postpartum period. It has been shown that the onset of clinical symptoms of postpartum psychosis occurs most frequently in the early postpartum period [43, 46, 47, 51, 52]. We were interested in charting the sleep patterns from a time prior to the onset of clinical symptoms. Therefore our preliminary investigation [36, 38] focused on sleep patterns during late pregnancy and the early postpartum period.* Seven white females of middle socioeconomic class, ranging in age from 22 to 30 years (mean 24.5), were studied for three consecutive nights during the last month of pregnancy,

* At the 1967 meeting of the Association for the Psychophysiological Study of Sleep, Santa Monica, Cal., where our first results were reported, another investigator, Mme. Olga Petre-Quaden, also presented data on sleep patterns during pregnancy.

for three consecutive nights immediately following delivery, and for one night between the second and third week of the postpartum period. An eight-channel EEG and a two-channel EOG were used to monitor sleep throughout the night. In order to assess the nature of sleep pattern changes during pregnancy and the immediate postpartum period, each pregnant woman was age-matched with a control subject who had slept in the laboratory for three consecutive nights. The overall sleep pattern observed during gestation seemed similar in some respects to insomnia and was characterized by a longer sleep latency, frequent awakenings, shorter sleep time, and a marked reduction of deep sleep (stage 4). In addition, immediately after delivery there was a suppression of 1-REM sleep. By the second postpartum week, these profound sleep changes tended to normalize.

Our data indicate that in normal pregnancy, sleep disturbances are of greater intensity than had been generally suspected and presumably can profoundly affect the woman's physiological disposition, perhaps to the point of inducing disease. The observation of a marked reduction in stage 4 sleep during the last trimester of pregnancy in these subjects is indeed significant, because it had not been reported in normal subjects of the childbearing age group. When coupled with recent reports of reduced stage 4 sleep in psychotically depressed and schizophrenic patients [8, 14, 22, 25, 50, 61], it gives considerable credence to the hypothesis that there might be a relationship between sleep disturbances and postpartum psychosis.

In order to determine exactly when in pregnancy these changes begin to take place, we followed our preliminary study with a more extensive investigation of the entire pregnancy and postpartum periods [37]. A group of subjects whose ages ranged from 20 to 30 years (mean 24.0) were selected during the first month of pregnancy. Their sleep was monitored after they had been pregnant four to six weeks, and thereafter once every two weeks until delivery. They were again monitored for three consecutive nights immediately following delivery, and then every two weeks until the first week after the return of the menses. Records were compared with those obtained from age-matched control subjects.

Data from this study will continue to be analyzed as the subjects complete the postpartum periods. Analysis of the 3 subjects whose records are complete produced the following preliminary findings. Subjects' greatest total sleep time occurred during the first trimester. (All subjects reported more frequent naps during early pregnancy.) Their sleep time approached normal in the second trimester, and decreased to below normal in the third trimester. Immediately after delivery, sleep time increased to above-normal levels, decreasing to normal levels during the control period, i.e., the period from 2½ to 4 months after the first postpartum menses. The average total sleep time for the experimental subjects during the control period was 328.7 minutes, and the average total sleep time for nonpregnant controls was 448.4 minutes. This striking difference emphasizes the possibility that the return of the menses does not necessarily indicate a return to the same psychobiological stage exhibited before pregnancy. There were differences in amount of stage 4 between and within individual patterns. As a group, the subjects exhibited significantly increased stage 4 after the first menses. This level was greater than that of nonpregnant control subjects. The report of increased sleepiness and an increased number of naps during the first trimester demonstrated that changes in the sleep pattern had already taken place at this early stage of pregnancy. In fact, 3 subjects mentioned that they had consulted their physicians about being tired and sleepy, and the resulting examination revealed that they were pregnant.

Because of the need to determine the time at which sleep changes begin to occur, we have recently begun a study of subjects who intend to become pregnant, but who are not yet pregnant. Subjects for this study are being screened to determine risk of possibly developing postpartum psychological complications. Criteria for prediction and classification of risk are given in the Gordon Stress Questionnaire [21] and the Larsen Stress Scale [40]. It has become obvious that there is a highly complex interaction between psychophysiological systems throughout pregnancy and the postpartum period. There is a highly integrated, delicately balanced network of the life processes which is at no time static during this period of reproduction. It is of fundamental importance that we investigate all the relevant variables in pregnancy: the social environmental system; the psychological system, including the personality structure and the emotional response to physiological change; the hormonal system; and the sleep system, including dreams. An investigation of all these relevant systems will provide increased knowledge about each system, about the interaction among the systems in a normal pregnancy, and about the relationship between dynamic alterations of these systems and the development of abnormal complications—in particular, postpartum psychosis.

Stage 4 suppression thus far has been associated with psychopathological conditions such as depression and schizophrenia, and with hormonal dysfunction such as hypothyroidism. However, in the age group represented by our pregnancy subjects, during late pregnancy and the postpartum period we have found stage 4 suppression without any clinically recognizable pathology. While there are individual differences in the duration, amount, and time of supression, once we have established the normal parameters for all these variables, it will be possible to distinguish critical deviations from these values. Stage 4 suppression, then, will have predictive value for the early detection of postpartum emotional disturbance.

The results of our study are expected to show the heuristic value of examining sleep disturbances as predictors of psychopathology. Thus the approach taken using pregnancy as a paradigm may serve as a model for the investigation of other types of psychosis.

IMPLICATIONS OF SLEEP RESEARCH FOR THE FUTURE

The theoretical conceptions of men like Freud, Bleuler, and Jackson—the patriarchs and mentors of modern day psychiatrists—engendered a curiosity about the essence of sleep and dreaming in the human organism. It is this curiosity which has compelled, and which will continue to compel their successors to probe further and to utilize the appropriate technological tools for fruitful inquiry. Scientific research is one of the most dynamic of human endeavors. Therefore it is crucial that the scientist and the inquiring student retain a constant awareness that today's knowledge is but a glimpse of tomorrow's knowledge—and that present-day technological advances merely provide the spark with which to ignite the fires of tomorrow's inquiry.

During the past few decades we have been content to describe sleep in terms of a very limited amount of neurophysiological data as measured by electrical activity. We have observed, through use of the electroencephalograph, that several distinct patterns of amplitude and frequency occur during sleep. We have labeled these patterns as stages, and we have observed that these stages can be used to identify various types of sleep such as deep and dreaming sleep. We have learned that there is some relationship between the relative frequency and proportion of these stages and other life processes—such as somatic or psychopathological conditions. But there is a great deal more to learn about sleep, and some of this information can be revealed with present-day technological tools.

Thus far we have not studied the frequency of the stages of sleep in periods less than one-third of a night. One of the observations from our laboratory is that many changes in sleep patterns occur within the first hour of sleep. The analysis of data on an hour-by-hour basis, for instance, would reveal the temporal distribution as well as the frequency distribution of sleep parameters throughout the night. It has been observed that in infants REM sleep occurs immediately after falling asleep. Yet in adults this would be very unusual. It would be appropriate to determine the manner in which REM latency changes with age and with various clinical conditions.

The EEG description of the various sleep stages has yet to be refined. For instance, it is not uncommon to observe spindle activity* during REM periods. In our laboratory we have observed that

* See Glossary.

several schizophrenic and depressed patients, and one patient with uremic syndrome, exhibited abundant alpha activity* during stage 4. All these patients had complained of sleep disturbances. Poor spindle activity has been observed in cardiac patients and prominent K-complexes* have been observed in pregnant subjects.

The electrical impulses, as described by EEG, measure one set of variables in the sleep process. Autonomic variables should also be investigated. It has been observed [35], for instance, that during REM deprivation, penile erection—an autonomic variable which has been shown to be associated with REM—continues to occur in the NREM time when REM would have occurred.

A more meaningful tool for monitoring sleep response would be one which would directly measure the actual level of arousal. Such a technological advance is within our realm and may provide a new frontier for scientific inquiry into the nature of sleep and pathology. In the meantime, it would be well for us to scrutinize everything we are obtaining with our present technology so that, regardless of the directions dictated by our theoretical convictions, we will not overlook the information presented to us by our data.

REFERENCES

1. Agnew, H. W., Jr., Webb, W. B., and Williams, R. L. The effects of stage 4 sleep deprivation. *Electroenceph. Clin. Neurophysiol.* 17:68, 1964.
2. Aserinsky, E., and Kleitman, N. Regularly occurring periods of eye motility, and concomitant phenomena during sleep. *Science* 118:273, 1953.
3. Aserinsky, E., and Kleitman, N. Two types of ocular motility occurring in sleep. *J. Appl. Physiol.* 8:1, 1955.
4. Azumi, K., Takahashi, S., Takahashi, K., Maruyama, N., and Kikuti, S. The effects of dream deprivation on chronic schizophrenics and normal adults: A comparative study. *Folia Psychiat. Neurol. Jap.* 21:205, 1967.
5. Baekeland, F., Koulack, D., and Lasky, R. Effects of a stressful

* See Glossary.

presleep experience on electroencephalograph-recorded sleep. *Psychophysiology.* In press.

6. Berger, R. J., and Oswald, I. Effects of sleep deprivation on behaviour, subsequent sleep, and dreaming. *J. Ment. Sci.* 108: 457, 1962.
7. Bleuler, E. *Dementia Praecox* (1908). Translated by J. Zinkin. New York: International Universities Press, 1950. Pp. 439, 441.
8. Caldwell, D. F., and Domino, E. F. Electroencephalographic and eye movement patterns during sleep in chronic schizophrenic patients. *Electroenceph. Clin. Neurophysiol.* 22:414, 1967.
9. Cartwright, R. D., Monroe, L. J., and Palmer, C. Individual differences in response to REM deprivation. *Arch. Gen. Psychiat.* (Chicago) 16:297, 1967.
10. Davidson, G. M. Concerning schizophrenia and manic-depressive psychosis associated with pregnancy and childbirth. *Amer. J. Psychiat.* 92:1332, 1936.
11. Dement, W. Dream recall and eye movements during sleep in schizophrenics and normals. *J. Nerv. Ment. Dis.* 122:263, 1955.
12. Dement, W. The effect of dream deprivation. *Science* 131: 1705, 1960.
13. Dement, W., and Kleitman, N. Cyclic variations in EEG during sleep and their relation to eye movements, body motility and dreaming. *Electroenceph. Clin. Neurophysiol.* 9: 673, 1957.
14. Diaz-Guerrero, R., Gottlieb, J. S., and Knott, J. R. The sleep of patients with manic-depressive psychosis, depressive type. *Psychosom. Med.* 8:399, 1946.
15. Feinberg, I., Koresko, R. L., Gottlieb, F., and Wender, P. H. Sleep electroencephalographic and eye movement patterns in schizophrenic patients. *Compr. Psychiat.* 5:44, 1964.
16. Ferenczi, S. *The Theory and Technique of Psychoanalysis,* Vol. VII. New York: Basic Books, 1960. Pp. 96–98.
17. Fisher, C., and Dement, W. Studies on the psychopathology of sleep and dreams. *Amer. J. Psychiat.* 119:1160, 1963.
18. Freedman, N., Grand, S., and Karacan, I. An approach to the study of dreaming and changes in psychopathological states. *J. Nerv. Ment. Dis.* 143:339, 1966.
19. Freud, S. *The Standard Edition of the Complete Psychological Works of Sigmund Freud,* tr. and ed. by J. Strachey with others. London: Hogarth and the Institute of Psycho-Analysis, 1964. Vol. XII, pp. 15–16, 221, 244–245.

20. Gordon, R. E. *Prevention of Postpartum Emotional Difficulties* (monograph). Ann Arbor, Mich.: University Microfilms, 1961.
21. Gordon, R. E., Kapostins, E. E., and Gordon, K. K. Factors in postpartum emotional adjustment. *Obstet. Gynec.* 25:158, 1965.
22. Gresham, S. C., Agnew, H. W., Jr., and Williams, R. L. The sleep of depressed patients. *Arch. Gen. Psychiat.* (Chicago) 13: 503, 1965.
23. Gulevich, G., and Dement, W. All Night Sleep Recordings in a Group of Schizophrenic Patients in Remission. Paper read at the Association for Psychophysiological Study of Sleep (APSS), Palo Alto, Cal., 1964.
24. Hamilton, J. A. *Postpartum Psychiatric Illness.* St. Louis: Mosby, 1962.
25. Hawkins, D. R., and Mendels, J. The psychophysiologic investigation of sleep in patients with depression. *Amer. J. Psychiat.* 123:1893, 1966.
26. Heuser, G., Kales, A., Jacobson, A., Paulson, M. J., Zweizig, J. R., Walter, R. D., and Kales, J. D. Sleep patterns in hypothyroid patients. *Physiologist* Vol. 9, No. 3, 1966.
27. Honda, Y., Takahashi, K., Takahashi, S., Azumi, K., Irie, M., Sakuma, M., Tsushima, T., and Shizume, K. Growth hormone secretion during nocturnal sleep in normal subjects. *J. Clin. Endocr.* 29:20, 1969.
28. Jackson, H., quoted by E. Jones. In *Papers on Psychoanalysis.* Boston: Beacon Press, 1948. Pp. 251–272.
29. Jansson, B. Psychic insufficiencies associated with childbearing. *Acta Psychiat. Scand.* 38:172, Suppl. 5–164, 1964.
30. Jelly, A. C. Puerperal insanity. *Boston Med. Surg. J.* 144:271, 1901.
31. Jones, R. Puerperal insanity. *Brit. Med. J.* 1:579, 1902.
32. Jung, C. G. *The Practice of Psychotherapy,* tr. by R. F. C. Hull. New York: Pantheon Books, 1954. Pp. 139–143.
33. Kales, A., Beall, G. N., Berger, R. J., Heuser, G., Jacobson, A., Kales, J. D., Parmelee, A. H., and Walter, R. D. Sleep and dreams: Recent research on clinical aspects. *Ann. Intern. Med.* 65:1078, 1968.
34. Kales, A., Hoedemaker, F., Jacobson, A., and Lichtenstein, E. Dream deprivation: An experimental reappraisal. *Nature* 204: 1337, 1964.
35. Karacan, I., Goodenough, D. R., Shapiro, A., and Starker, S.

Erection cycle during sleep in relation to dream anxiety. *Arch. Gen. Psychiat.* (Chicago) 15:183, 1966.

36. Karacan, I., Heine, M., Agnew, H. W., Jr., Williams, R. L., Webb, W. B., and Ross, J. J. Characteristics of sleep patterns during late pregnancy and the postpartum periods. *Amer. J. Obstet. Gynec.* 101:579, 1968.
37. Karacan, I., Williams, R. L., Hursch, C. J., Heine, M., and McCaulley, M. Some implications of the sleep patterns of pregnancy for postpartum emotional disturbances. *Brit. J. Psychiat.* 115:929, 1969.
38. Karacan, I., Williams, R. L., Webb, W. B., Agnew, H. W., Jr., and Ross, J. J. Sleep and dreaming during late pregnancy and postpartum. *Psychophysiology* 4:378, 1968.
39. Koranyi, E. K., and Lehmann, H. E. Experimental sleep deprivation in schizophrenic patients. *Arch. Gen. Psychiat.* (Chicago) 2:76, 1960.
40. Larsen, V. L. Stresses of the childbearing year. *Amer. J. Public Health* 56:32, 1966.
41. Larsen, V. L., Evans, T., Brodsack, J., Dungey, L., Elliott, J., Harmon, J., Kaess, S., Karman, I., Main, D., Martin, L., and Ramer, J. Attitudes and stresses affecting perinatal adjustment. Final Report, NIMH Grant No. MH-01381-01-02, 1966.
42. Onheiber, P., White, P. T., DeMyer, M. K., and Ottinger, D. R. Sleep and dream patterns of child schizophrenics. *Arch. Gen. Psychiat.* (Chicago) 12:568, 1965.
43. Pugh, T. F., Jerath, B. K., Schmidt, W. M., and Reed, R. B. Rates of mental disease related to childbearing. *New Eng. J. Med.* 268:1224, 1963.
44. Rechtschaffen, A., and Maron, L. The effect of amphetamine on the sleep cycle. *Electroenceph. Clin. Neurophysiol.* 16:438, 1964.
45. Rechtschaffen, A., Schulsinger, F., and Mednick, S. A. Schizophrenia and physiological indices of dreaming. *Arch. Gen. Psychiat.* (Chicago) 10:89, 1964.
46. Richardson, S., and Guttmacher, A. F. *Childbearing: Its Social and Psychological Aspects.* Baltimore: Williams & Wilkins, 1967. P. 72.
47. Ryle, A. The psychological disturbances associated with 345 pregnancies in 137 women. *J. Ment. Sci.* 107:279, 1961.
48. Sampson, H. Deprivation of dreaming sleep by two methods. *Arch. Gen. Psychiat.* (Chicago) 13:79, 1965.
49. Savage, G. H. Prevention and treatment of insanity of pregnancy and the puerperal period. *Lancet* 1:164, 1896.

50. Snyder, F., Anderson, D., Bunney, W., Jr., Kupfer, D., Scott, J., and Wyatt, R. Longitudinal variation in the sleep of severely depressed and acutely schizophrenic patients with changing clinical status. *Psychophysiology* 5:235, 1968.
51. Strecker, E. A., and Ebaugh, F. G. Psychoses occurring during the puerperium. *Arch. Neurol. Psychiat.* 15:239, 1926.
52. Tobin, S. M. Emotional depression during pregnancy. *Obstet. Gynec.* 10:677, 1957.
53. Tuke, D. H. Sleep; Dreaming. In *Dictionary of Psychological Medicine,* 1892.
54. Vogel, G. W. REM deprivation. III. Dreaming and psychosis. *Arch. Gen. Psychiat.* (Chicago) 18:312, 1968.
55. Vogel, G. W., and Traub, A. C. REM deprivation. I. The effect on schizophrenic patients. *Arch. Gen. Psychiat.* (Chicago) 18:287, 1968.
56. Webb, W. B., Agnew, H. W., Jr. Sleep: Effects of a restricted regime. *Science* 150:1745, 1965.
57. Williams, R. L., Agnew, H. W., Jr., and Webb, W. B. *Effects of Prolonged Stage Four and 1-REM Sleep Deprivation (EEG, Task Performance, and Psychologic Responses).* Brooks Air Force Base, Texas: USAF School of Aerospace Medicine, Aerospace Med. Div. (AFSC), 1967.
58. Wolff, H. G., and Curran, D. Nature of delirium and allied states: The dysergastic reaction. *Arch. Neurol. Psychiat.* 33:1175, 1935.
59. Zarcone, V., Gulevich, G., Pivik, T., and Dement, W. C. Partial REM phase deprivation and schizophrenia. *Arch. Gen. Psychiat.* (Chicago) 18:194, 1968.
60. Zung, W. W. K. *Effect of antidepressant drugs on sleeping and dreaming. II. On the adult male.* Excerpta Medica International Congress Series, No. 150. Proceedings of the Fourth World Congress of Psychiatry, Madrid, 1966.
61. Zung, W. W. K., Wilson, W. P., and Dodson, W. E. Effect of depressive disorders on sleep EEG responses. *Arch. Gen. Psychiat.* (Chicago) 10:439, 1964.

REM Sleep and the Autistic Child

EDWARD M. ORNITZ

Our interest in the interrelationships between sleep research and mental illness has focused on certain parallels between the neurophysiological organization of REM sleep (D-state) and the behavior of autistic children [4].

The syndrome of early infantile autism, which may be the earliest manifestation of schizophrenia in childhood, is characterized by profound disturbances of relating, language, motility, developmental rate, and perception beginning in the first year of life [5]. The disturbance of relating is primarily a pervasive disregard of all social and pleasurable aspects of the environment that are ordinarily meaningful to normal children. The disturbances of language encompass both complete muteness and the development of echolalic speech accompanied by a peculiar tendency to speak of the self in the second or third person. Speech is also hollow-sounding, atonal, and arrhythmic. Disturbances of motility include dramatic fluctuations between states of frenetic overactivity and brief episodes of posturing characteristic of catatonic immobility. During the hyperactivity, a number of particular behaviors recur: these include toe-walking, hand flapping, and body whirling. The disturbances of developmental sequence involve such extreme irregularities in the normal schedule of psychomotor development as to suggest a basic disturbance of the maturational rate. The disturbances of perception appear to be basic to the entire disease process and can present striking contradictions between apparent obliviousness to environmental stimulation, easily mistaken for a sensory loss, and acute states of agitation, panic, or overexcitement in response to sensory input. These perceptual disturbances affect all sensory modalities, involve hyposensitivity and hypersensitivity to the basic elements of sensation—e.g., pitch, loudness, brightness, alteration of visual field, pattern, and texture—and occur as early as the neonatal period [5]. The same type of basic failure to regulate the impact of sensory input has been observed during the prodromal and incipient stages of acute schizophrenic psychoses in adulthood [2].

The pathological behaviors of the autistic child, particularly the disturbances of motility and perception, occur as rapidly fluctuating states of overexcitation and extreme inhibition [4]. In addition, some of the behaviors suggest an abnormal reaction to vestibular input in these children. On the one hand the autistic child seems to seek out vestibular stimulation by whirling himself, engaging in perseverative body-rocking and head-rolling and paying undue attention to spinning objects. On the other hand the same child may have a history of marked agitation when thrown up into the air or whirled around, as in ordinary roughhouse, or when taken into an elevator. In the latter case, in the very young autistic child, specific reactions to the acceleration and deceleration of the elevator have been observed. In the laboratory depressed postrotational and calorically induced nystagmus has been observed in both schizophrenic children [3] and adults [1]. Recently we have found that the reduced duration of postrotational nystagmus in autistic children is dependent on a free visual field. This suggests that there is an interaction between the vestibular and visual input which determines the abnormal finding in the autistic child [14].

While dreaming has been thought since ancient times to be related to mental illness, recent neurophysiological understanding of the REM sleep state, during which dreaming occurs, has suggested some relationships to the hyperexcitation and inhibition, and the vestibular dysfunction, found in autistic children [4]. The REM state has been shown to consist of a tonic inhibitory state, manifested by diminished muscle tone and generally decreased amplitude of sensory evoked responses. This inhibitory state, which coincides roughly with the period of relatively low voltage mixed frequency stage 1 EEG, is punctuated by coexisting states of more profound phasic inhibition and phasic excitation coinciding with the bursts of rapid eye movements occurring during REM sleep. Both the phasic excitatory and inhibitory phenomena, as well as the eye movement activity itself, have been shown to be dependent upon integrity of the vestibular nuclei [13]. Thus we have, during

REM sleep, neurophysiological states of excitation and inhibition which exert an effect on sensory input and which involve the normal functioning of central vestibular mechanisms. In the autistic child's behavior we see dissociated states of excitation and inhibition, with extreme hyporeactivity and paradoxical hyperreactivity to sensory input, and suggestions of central vestibular dysfunction.

Earlier attempts to demonstrate abnormalities of REM sleep in autistic children began with a study of REM sleep time. The percentage of time spent in REM sleep, as well as the patterning of the REM sleep cycle throughout the night, was not unusual in autistic children [9, 10]. Against this background of a normal REM sleep cycle, we have looked for abnormalities within the REM state itself. When auditory responses to repetitive clicks were summated, it was found that the relative amplitude of the auditory evoked response was increased during REM sleep in young autistic children, as compared to normal controls. When these responses were summated during the eye movement bursts and compared to those obtained during NREM sleep, a significant inhibition of the response to sound was found in the normal controls. In contrast, there was a marked overriding of this inhibition in the young autistic children [8]. A significant difference between autistic children and controls could not, however, be demonstrated in autistic children over 5 years of age. This suggested that maturational factors might be involved. Therefore we studied a group of 6- to 12-month-old normal babies. They also showed a lack of inhibition of auditory evoked response amplitude during the eye movement bursts of REM sleep [7]. Thus the development of phasic inhibition of sensory input during the ocular activity of REM sleep seems to be a maturational phenomenon; the autistic children are late in this development. This finding parallels the tendency for hypersensitivity to sensory stimuli to occur during the early years in autistic children, and to become less disturbing after the children are 5 to 6 years of age.

In a smaller group of autistic children under 4 years of age, EEG activity in the range of spindle frequencies was observed during REM sleep [6]. This was rarely noted during the REM sleep of normal controls. In an age-matched group of 8 autistic and 6 normal children, the amount of this spindle-like activity was found to be significantly increased during the REM sleep of the autistic children. The occurrence of this activity was reduced in those autistic children who were reexamined at an older age. Again a maturational factor seems to be at play, in this instance influencing the organization of the EEG pattern in autistic children. Studies of prematures and neonates suggest that the occurrence of activity in the spindle frequency range during REM sleep is characteristic of a more immature organization [11].

In the autistic children under 4 years old the duration of the eye movement bursts during REM sleep was significantly reduced. This decrease in the eye movement activity also attenuated as the autistic children matured [6]. The ocular activity during REM sleep has been shown to be dependent upon the integrity of the vestibular system [12]. Thus in very young autistic children we have found a depression of ocular activity during the spontaneous vestibular discharges of REM sleep analogous to the depression of oculomotor responses (nystagmus) to externally applied vestibular stimulation in the waking autistic child.

In summary, preliminary studies on small groups of young autistic children have suggested a relationship between the clinical findings in this earliest form of schizophrenia and disruption of the normal homeostatic balance between excitation and inhibition during the oculomotor activity of REM sleep. This disruption is manifest by an overriding of the normal inhibition of the auditory evoked response and a reduced duration of the oculomotor activity itself. As both the oculomotor activity and the normal phasic inhibition of sensory input are dependent upon the vestibular system, a basic disturbance of central vestibular mechanisms is suggested in early infantile autism. Since these findings tend to be mitigated with increasing age and are characteristic of the less mature organism, and since EEG patterns characteristic of earlier development are found during REM sleep in young autistic children, these findings taken together suggest the possibility of a basic dysmaturation of vestibular mechanisms in autistic children. These vestibular mechanisms mediate the phasic excitatory and inhibitory events of REM sleep, including the modulation of sensory input. It is suggested that the symptoms of early infantile autism, particularly the perceptual changes, are manifestations of a breaking into waking life of the disordered phasic activity of REM sleep. On the psychological level, this postulated pathophysiology of REM sleep may be reflected in the disruption of normal mental functioning by the hallucinatory phenomena of dreaming. This, then, may be the nature of schizophrenia.

REFERENCES

1. Angyal, A., and Blackman, N. Vestibular reactivity in schizophrenia. *Arch. Neurol. Psychiat.* 44:611, 1940.
2. Chapman, J. The early symptoms of schizophrenia. *Brit. J. Psychiat.* 112:225, 1966.
3. Colbert, E. G., Koegler, R. R., and Markham, C. H. Vestibular dysfunction in childhood schizophrenia. *Arch. Gen. Psychiat.* (Chicago) 1:600, 1959.
4. Ornitz, E. M., and Ritvo, E. R. Neurophysiologic mechanisms underlying perceptual inconstancy in autistic and schizophrenic children. *Arch. Gen. Psychiat.* (Chicago) 19:22, 1968.
5. Ornitz, E. M., and Ritvo, E. R. Perceptual inconstancy in early infantile autism. *Arch. Gen. Psychiat.* (Chicago) 18:76, 1968.
6. Ornitz, E. M., Ritvo, E. R., Brown, M. B., La Franchi, S., Parmelee, T., and Walter, R. D. The EEG and rapid eye movements during REM sleep in normal and autistic children. *Electroenceph. Clin. Neurophysiol.* 26:167, 1969.
7. Ornitz, E. M., Ritvo, E. R., Lee, Y. H., Panman, L. M., Walter, R. D., and Mason, A. The auditory evoked response in babies during REM sleep. *Electroenceph. Clin. Neurophysiol.* 27:195, 1969.
8. Ornitz, E. M., Ritvo, E. R., Panman, L. M., Lee, Y. H., Carr, E. M., and Walter, R. D. The auditory evoked response in normal and autistic children during sleep. *Electroenceph. Clin. Neurophysiol.* 25:221, 1968.
9. Ornitz, E. M., Ritvo, E. R., and Walter, R. D. Dreaming

sleep in autistic and schizophrenic children. *Amer. J. Psychiat.* 122:419, 1965.
10. Ornitz, E. M., Ritvo, E. R., and Walter, R. D. Dreaming sleep in autistic twins. *Arch. Gen. Psychiat.* (Chicago) 12:77, 1965.
11. Parmelee, A. H., Jr., Schulte, F. J., Akiyama, Y., Wenner, W. H., Schultz, M. A., and Stern, E. Maturation of EEG activity during sleep in premature infants. *Electroenceph. Clin. Neurophysiol.* 24:319, 1968.
12. Pompeiano, O., and Morrison, A. R. Vestibular influences during sleep. I. Abolition of the rapid eye movements of desynchronized sleep following vestibular lesions. *Arch. Ital. Biol.* 103:569, 1965.
13. Pompeiano, O., and Morrison, A. R. Vestibular influences during sleep. III. Dissociation of the tonic and phasic inhibition of spinal reflexes during desynchronized sleep following vestibular lesions. *Arch. Ital. Biol.* 104:231, 1966.
14. Ritvo, E. R., Ornitz, E. M., Eviatar, A., Markham, C., Brown, M., and Mason, A. Decreased postrotatory nystagmus in early infantile autism. *Neurology* 19:653, 1969.

*Contributions of Sleep Research to the Understanding and Treatment of Enuresis**

EDWARD R. RITVO

The vast majority of children evaluated for nocturnal enuresis show no evidence of organic pathology to explain their wetting. Such cases are usually labeled primary, idiopathic, or essential. Many theories have been put forward to explain why such children wet the bed—and they are exceeded by an even larger number of recommended therapeutic procedures. Indeed, this is the state of

* The research on which this paper is based was supported by a grant from the McGregor Fund, Detroit, Mich.

our medical art today: On the advice of doctors, enuretic children are scolded, ignored, dehydrated, bladder stretched, drugged with energizers or hypnotics, shocked by electrodes attached to their penises, blinded by flashing lights, deafened by buzzers, and sent for psychoanalysis.

The latest insult some of these poor victims of enuresis had to endure was an all-night EEG study [1]. Here they were wired up to strange machines and made to slumber while we monitored signals from their scalp and jockey shorts. We perpetrated these insults in order to understand during which stages of sleep wetting actually occurred and what EEG activity accompanied wetting. We also wished to learn if there were different types of wetting and, if so, what personality characteristics accompanied them. We hoped such data might put our knowledge of enuresis on a more scientific footing and lead to more rational approaches to therapy.

THE EXPERIMENT

Seven 8- to 10-year-old boys were selected as representing a typical cross section of primary enuretic patients. They were all in excellent physical health with negative medical and neurological examinations. Urinalysis was normal. Psychiatric interviews were used to assess their emotional development and to detect any major neurotic constellations. A total of 62 nights of EEG monitoring were obtained. Each all-night recording was scored for EEG stages and minutely analyzed during the 10 minutes before and after each wet. Furthermore, certain background phenomena were defined* as evidence of cortical arousal and scored separately. A total of 48 wets were observed. If one defines the 60- to 30-second interval

* The criteria for arousal phenomena were (1) flattening from slow wave sleep to low voltage fast activity with prompt return to slow wave pattern, (2) transient appearance of alpha rhythm, (3) clear-cut emergence of monorhythmic theta (3–8 cps hypersynchronous slow waves) over background slow activity, (4) "V" waves and K-complexes occurring in series over a background of stage 1,2 or 3,4 sleep, (5) gross muscle movement obscuring the record combined with clinical evidence of transient awakening.

before wetting as the stage of sleep during which a wet occurred, the distribution of wets was as follows:

Awake: 5 episodes (10 percent)
REM sleep: 3 episodes (6 percent)
Stage 2 sleep: 19 episodes (40 percent)
Stage 3 and stage 4: 21 episodes (44 percent)

Close examination of the records revealed that each patient had at least one wet that was preceded by evidence of arousal during the 60 to 30 seconds prior to micturition and at least one that was not. Of the 48 total wets observed, 65 percent were preceded by arousal signals and 35 percent were not. All the boys wet in each stage of sleep except stage 1-REM (3 episodes from 3 subjects). Most non-arousal wets took place during the first half of the night and thus would have been most likely to occur during stage 3 or 4 sleep which predominates during this part of the night. Stage 1-REM, awake, and arousal wets occurred mainly during the last quarter of the night and almost exclusively in children with frank neurotic conflicts.

CONCLUSIONS

It appears from our data that a child with primary nocturnal enuresis can have several different types of enuretic events. This fact no doubt underlies the difficulty that certain investigators have had explaining enuresis from a single point of view and the failure of any specific therapeutic regimen to yield consistent results in a large population. Three distinct types of enuretic events were noted: (1) awake enuresis, (2) arousal enuresis, and (3) nonarousal enuresis. In this last type we can make the assumption that no evidence of bladder activity reached cortical levels with sufficient intensity to arouse the boy and thus allow for a choice to take place as to whether he should get up, inhibit the reflex while remaining asleep, or wet the bed.

The observation of these various types of enuretic events suggests a somatopsychic model for the etiology of nocturnal enuresis. Since all our subjects on at least one occasion showed a failure to register arousal signals prior to micturition (a nonarousal enuretic event) it appears that they all had a pathophysiological substrate for their symptoms. When this type of enuresis persists past the age of expected night training (ages 3 to 4 years) it provides a core about which neurotic constellations can gather. Reactions from parents and peers and the child's own awareness of his inability to control his urination can lead to a neurotic basis for the symptom. In this way a child with nonarousal enuretic events is predisposed to have this symptom continue on a psychogenic basis. Wetting on a neurotic basis, we believe, accounts for waking and arousal enuresis.

TREATMENT APPROACHES

Once we have established a diagnosis of primary nocturnal enuresis, a careful assessment as to the proportion of arousal and nonarousal events is the first step in designing a therapeutic program. All-night EEG observations are not necessary, as we have found that those children with predominantly arousal and awake enuresis are characterized as follows:

1. Presence of several neurotic symptoms, e.g., fire setting, compulsions, poor peer relationships, poor school adjustment, day wetting
2. History of sporadic wetting
3. Anxiety and discomfort about the bed wetting may indicate that the symptoms are ego dystonic
4. Much parental concern, overinvolvement, and infantilization of the patient
5. Wets usually occur in the early morning just prior to arising
6. Family histories usually negative for enuresis

Characteristics typical of those boys with predominantly nonarousal enuresis are these:

1. Minimal evidence of maladjustment or neurotic symptomatology
2. History of having wet regularly
3. Nonchalant attitude toward the wetting on the part of patients and families usually noted
4. Reportedly deep sleepers
5. Wets occur early in the night
6. Frequent positive family histories of enuresis

In a child with predominantly arousal and awake enuresis, psychiatric consultation is indicated if the severity of the symptom or the patient's general condition warrants. If psychotherapy is recommended, conditioning or drug treatment, or both, aimed at the nonarousal wets can be concurrently administered by the pediatrician if proper preparation is undertaken in discussions with the patient.

In cases where little psychopathology is present and the history indicates that the episodes are predominantly of the nonarousal type, medication and conditioning therapy can be of great help when administered within the context of a continuing supportive relationship with the doctor.

In both instances it is necessary to explain to the child that the medication or conditioning device will not stop all the enuresis or magically allow him to awaken. Rather these aids can help him master his symptom over a period of months and thus increase his feelings of self-esteem. We further encourage a child to gain control of his symptom by recommending that he take care of his own bed sheets, take his own medication, plug in and manage his own conditioning device, and in general be responsible for the consequences of his wetting. We have found that imipramine has the most predictably beneficial response among those medications we have tested and that other measures, such as fluid restriction or increasing fluid intake to stretch the bladder, are not helpful.

REFERENCES

1. Ritvo, E. R., Ornitz, E. M., Gottlieb, F., Poussaint, A. F., Maron, B., Ditman, K. S., and Blinn, K. A. Arousal and nonarousal types of enuretic events. *Amer. J. Psychiat.* 126:1, 1969.

Insomnia and Disordered Sleep

*What has recent research taught us about insomnia and disordered sleep? What about its pharmacological treatment?**

The Pharmacology of Disordered Sleep: A Laboratory Approach†

WILLIAM W. K. ZUNG

The following presentation is a synthesis based upon general knowledge and hypotheses taken from several areas including clinical psychiatry, electroencephalography, neurophysiology, and pharmacology in an attempt to understand the possible relationship between drugs and disordered sleep. It is hoped that this heuristic approach may suggest and eventually lead us to a rational basis for the treatment of the various states of sleep disturbance, present either as a symptom or as part of a disease process. In view of the

* The reader interested in these questions may wish to refer also to papers by Baekeland and Hartmann (p. 33), Hartmann (p. 59 and p. 192), Hawkins (p. 85), and Stoyva (p. 355).

† This work was in part supported by Research Scientist Development Grant MH 35232 National Institute of Mental Health.

state of the art as it is today, the achievement of this goal will be some time in coming and the present discussion will be at times walking on untested soil. However, as new grounds are broken and new findings reaped by investigators in the various fields, the tentative assumptions made in this paper on the pharmacology of disordered sleep as a laboratory approach will be rejected, accepted, or modified. With this caveat, we proceed by posing the following questions:

1. What do we know about sleep disturbance in the various clinical disorders?
2. What are the possible relationships between these disturbances and the neurophysiology of the brain?
3. What are the effects on the brain of the drugs used in the treatment of clinical disorders?
4. What are the effects of these same drugs on sleep?

CHARACTERISTICS OF THE ALL-NIGHT SLEEP OF VARIOUS SUBJECT GROUPS

The Sleep of Normal Subjects

Onset of sleep. The onset of sleep is defined as the time from saying "good night" to the subject to the onset of stage 1, using EEG criteria. Some authors [45] define this parameter as from "good night" to the onset of sleep spindles, which is the characteristic EEG pattern of stage 2. As for the duration of this period, in a questionnaire survey of the sleep habits of 2446 normal subjects, the authors stated that the reported upper limit for normal onset of sleep was 1½ hours [38] and defined initial or early insomnia as requiring over 1½ hours before the subject was able to get to sleep [37]. Perusal of values reported from laboratory studies indicates that 15 minutes, plus or minus 5 minutes, is representative for this parameter (see Table 1).

TABLE 1. *Characteristics of all-night sleep of various subject groups.* + = Increased, − = Decreased, 0 = No change, × = No data available.

Conditions Studied	Onset of Sleep (min.)	Percent Time in Sleep Stage						Shifts to Wakefulness & Between Stages of Sleep
		A	1	2	3	4	REM	
Normal subjects	15 ± 5	<1	10 ± 5	35 ± 10	10 ± 5	20 ± 5	20 ± 5	10 ± 5
"Insomnia"		These values cannot be determined except individually by laboratory studies using all-night sleep recordings						
Anxiety	+++	×	×	×	×	−	0	×
Schizophrenia	+	0	0	0	0	−	−	+
Depression	+	+	+	0	0	−	−	+++

TOTAL SLEEP TIME. Total sleep time can be defined as time from the first minute of EEG evidence of sleep to the last minute of sleep just before the final awakening. Although statistical data on the duration of sleep in adults is fairly consistent (mean = 8 hours), the range of the number of hours slept for any individual may vary considerably. In the McGhie and Russell study [38] 6 percent of the subjects reported that they slept less than 5 hours per night, 15 percent for 5 to 6 hours, 62 percent for 7 to 8 hours, 13 percent for 9 to 10 hours, and 2 percent slept over 10 hours. In a survey [37] of sleep patterns in psychiatric patients, a sleep period of 5 hours or less was considered abnormal. Jones and Oswald [31] reported 2 normal healthy subjects who had a mean total sleep time of less than 3 hours per 24 hours. Mean percentage time in stage 4 and REM indicated no loss in these states which were 24 percent and 23 percent, respectively. The concept of total sleep time, therefore, can only be relevant in terms of any given individual's own base-line sleep time. Unfortunately it is difficult in laboratory studies to obtain premorbid all-night sleep studies on patients, a problem not uncommon in clinical medicine.

DISTRIBUTION OF PERCENTAGE OF TIME IN THE VARIOUS STAGES OF SLEEP-REM. Although the original classification of sleep into stages [8] was first published in 1937, and the description of rapid eye movements measured by electrooculographic (EOG) recordings 20 years later [10], the actual "scoring" of an all-night sleep record still poses methodological problems. There does not exist common agreement among sleep researchers on the actual quantitative distribution of the various EEG frequencies which occur during sleep and on the criteria for defining a particular stage of sleep.

Attempts to define criteria based upon the various rhythms (alpha, beta, delta, and sigma or spindles*) present in the stages of sleep have been made by several authors [10, 24, 49, 56], but their values vary considerably. Because of this, reported values for percentage of time spent in the stages of sleep during an all-night recording cannot be compared from laboratory to laboratory. An-

* See Glossary.

other difficulty encountered when studies from different laboratories are to be compared is that because of differences in focus and interest between investigators, percentages of time in the various stages of sleep are "lumped together" in different ways. For example, as a result of the recent interest in REM sleep or D-state, it is common to find the other stages of sleep (A, 1, 2, 3, and 4) reported together as NREM sleep or S-state. For these reasons, comparisons in this paper are restricted to stating whether there is an increase, decrease, or no change of the various sleep parameters as reported by each laboratory, using its own control data. In general, the many reported values for the distribution of percent time in the various stages of sleep for normal control subjects in the young and middle-age adult will be in range of the data in Table 1.

TRANSITIONS. The transitions between stages of sleep during sleep can be described as follows: The normal subject during an all-night sleep will have 5 to 6 periods of NREM sleep and 4 to 5 periods of REM sleep. These occur in cycles approximately every 90 minutes and have been described [20] to be basic to the mammalian body. Hartmann proposed that the 90-minute cycle may be related to the id and is associated with the primary process of dreaming. Alternatively, we propose that these cycles are part of the primitive defenses of man against hostile environment, just as arousal mechanisms from sleep to wakefulness are part of this same primitive mechanism [51]. In addition, the 8-hour period of a total night's sleep may itself be a basic cycle of man. Thus once a subject reaches the deepest stage of sleep which occurs during the first third of the night [49], he spends the rest of the night slowly "waking up," as indicated by the slope of the all-night sleep pattern (see Fig. 1). This concept becomes important when we later consider the disturbance of sleep in depression, and the effect that certain drugs have on sleep patterns.

During an all-night sleep, a subject at any given moment of time will be in one of the six operationally defined stages of sleep (A, 1, 2, 3, 4, or REM). Preceding this moment and following it, he must still be in one of those six stages. From this "closed system" one can

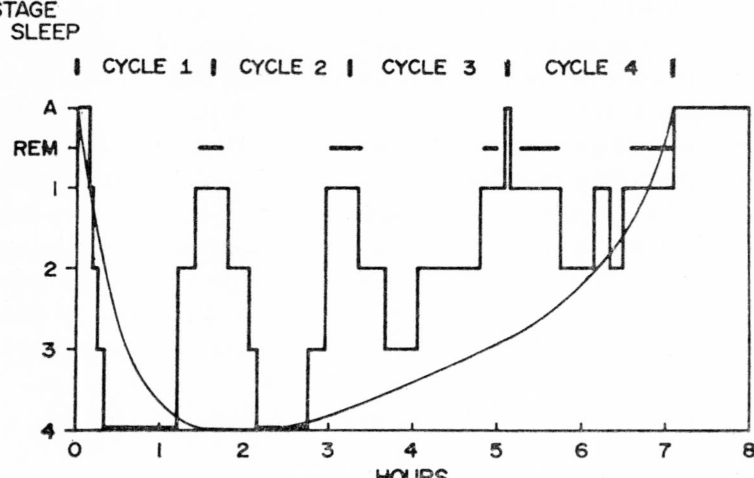

FIGURE 1. *A typical all-night sleep pattern of a normal adult, illustrating the presence of NREM and REM cycles. The bottom curve illustrates that the all-night sleep itself is also a cycle.*

construct a contingency table so as to study this continuous process [49]. Taking the mathematical model one step further, it is possible to study the transitional probabilities of sleep as a time dependent matrix by using a Markov chain [57]. Transitions from one stage of sleep to another (in any number of steps) and the duration and number of cycles occurring during an all-night sleep are all parameters which reflect the neurophysiological status of the sleep-arousal system (to be discussed in the section on the neurophysiology of sleep). Suffice it to say here that alterations of these characteristics may be just as important, if not more so, than changes in percent time spent in any stage of sleep-REM.

The Sleep of Insomniacs

Insomnia is defined in the fifth edition of Dorland's *Medical Dictionary* as the inability to sleep and abnormal wakefulness. Inasmuch as insomnia is a symptomatic complaint, all the values in

Table 1 on the characteristics of the all-night sleep EEG and EOG must be determined individually by actual laboratory studies.

One general conclusion about the sleep of insomniacs from laboratory studies is that almost without exception, these individuals underestimate the amount of sleep obtained and overestimate their sleep disturbance [19, 55]. In a study we reported [55], a patient with a 25-year history of insomnia was found to have (1) no difficulty in falling asleep; (2) mean total sleep time of 484 minutes; and (3) a mean distribution of total sleep time as follows: stage A, 19 percent; 1, 26 percent; 2, 7 percent; 3, 14 percent; 4, 23 percent; and REM, 10 percent. However, according to the patient, she "didn't sleep a wink" on those 4 nights of investigation. We also found that the subject had an increase in the number of shifts from one sleep stage to another, and that this was reflected in the increase in the number of cycles during an all-night recording to a mean of 9 per night.

Sleep and Anxiety

The main characteristic finding associated with anxiety states clinically and in the laboratory is the difficulty in falling asleep [19, 44]. A sleep study on medical students during the period of their comprehensive examination, as a chronic stress related to anxiety, has been reported [35]. They observed some decrease in stage 4 as daytime stress increased, while percent time in REM was unaffected.

Sleep and Schizophrenia

A review of disorders of sleep in schizophrenia by Bliss [5] concluded that most schizophrenic subjects do not have sleep problems. Analyses of data available reveal the following:

1. Onset of sleep: varied from normal [7] to prolonged onset [33, 34].

2. NREM sleep: varied from no difference [9] to decreases in stages 3 and 4 [33, 34].
3. REM sleep: varied from no change [9, 15, 33] to a decrease [34].
4. Spontaneous interruptions: reported both present [34] and absent [7].

It is most likely that the variations in the reported studies on the sleep patterns of "schizophrenics" reflect more the disparate nature of the illness and its varied types rather than a fundamental defect.

Sleep and Depression

Of all the clinical entities, depression has been the most thoroughly studied in terms of its disordered sleep. This is because sleep disturbance is one of the most, if not the most important physiological sign in depressive disorders. Further, the restoration of sleep may be the first sign of approaching recovery, and improvement in sleep is often used as a measure of response to treatment. Witness the use of "sleep charts" kept on many psychiatric wards on depressed patients by night nurses and aides, and the morning rounds of the doctor whose first question to the staff is, "How much did the patient sleep last night?"

A summary of the most frequently found characteristics from laboratory studies [11, 17, 23, 40–43, 45, 56, 58] are as follows:

1. There is more wakefulness or stage A present after the onset of sleep.
2. There is an increase in stage 1 sleep.
3. There is a decrease of stage 4.
4. There is decreased REM time.
5. There is an increase in the activity of the arousal system.

As a result of these disturbances, there is a marked change in the normal 90-minute cycle. The number of cycles in the sleep of depressives may increase to 10 or more per night, and the cycle length may decrease to 30 minutes (Fig. 2).

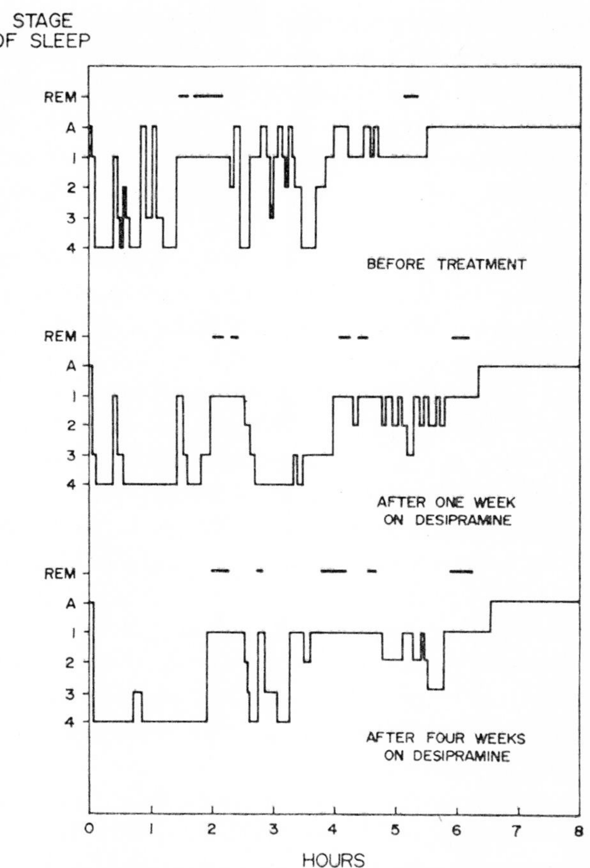

FIGURE 2. *All-night sleep patterns of a depressed patient treated with desipramine (25 mg. q.i.d.), comparing data obtained before treatment and after one and four weeks on drug.*

Sleep disturbance in depressive disorders has been described clinically and by laboratory studies as frequent waking and early awakenings. It is most likely that these two characteristics are interrelated and based upon the following three factors: (1) The disturbances in sleep indicate a pathophysiology of the arousal system which accounts for the frequent wakings. (2) The repeated awakenings together with the light sleep during the early morning hours leave the patient with the subjective feeling of having been "more awake than asleep." (3) The approaching daylight hours bring increased ambient light and noise levels, which lead the depressed patient to stay up on that "last" awakening. In most instances this is an earlier awakening time than is usual for the patient. Thus the report of depressed patients that they sleep all night but don't feel rested may be based on physiological, psychological, and environmental factors.

Although both stage 4 and REM sleep are decreased in this disorder, it is likely that it is the loss of stage 4 sleep which is primary. In one longitudinal study [56] of the sleep of depressives during treatment, stage 4 was increased or made up first, and the increase in REM time appeared much later. Studies [1] on totally sleep-deprived subjects indicate that the first compensation is for stage 4, and then later for lost REM time. Furthermore it has been found [2] that stage 4 deprivation in normal subjects resulted psychologically in depression and reduced functioning, while REM deprivation psychologically resulted in a state of higher irritability and lability.

Several studies have attempted to compare the sleep of "reactive" and "endogenous" depressives on a basis of observer rating of behavioral sleep, or questionnaires. Results of these have been generally negative, with no significant difference. Thus one author [28] reported no difference in insomnia or motility between the two groups. Another author [18] reported that, while there were no differences in the number of hours slept, the quality of sleep, or the number of interruptions present during a night's sleep (disturbed in both), the reactive group had more difficulty in falling asleep while the endogenous group had early morning awakening.

NEUROPHYSIOLOGY OF SLEEP

Anatomical Substrate of Sleep

Sleep as a normal physiological process is an end product of both active and passive mechanisms which in turn produce decreased activity of an arousal system. Akert [3] summarized our present knowledge about the anatomical substrate of sleep and localizes the arousal system in the rostral portion of the brain stem, including areas of the mesencephalon, posterior hypothalamus, and the anterior third of the pons in a network of interconnecting neurons called the reticular formation. Functionally, the reticular formation has been shown to have facilitory or activating influence on the cerebral cortex, hence the name *reticular activating system* (RAS).

Localization of the sleep system, which actively inhibits the arousal system, includes anatomical pathways which are both ascending and descending. These pathways originate from the frontal lobes, limbic system, intralaminary nuclei of the thalamus, caudate nucleus, preoptic area, and medullary areas around the nucleus solitarius. Passive mechanisms which contribute to the inhibition of the arousal system include decreased stimuli from the external environment which are transmitted through the exteroceptive systems. These sensory pathways include the skin (tactile and thermal), muscles and joints, auditory and visual modalities. Passive mechanisms also include decreased stimuli from the internal environment or enteroceptive systems, an example of which would be the diurnal hormonal levels and their fluctuating effects on the central nervous system.

Jouvet [32] summarized the results of his work since 1958 in REM sleep and its anatomical substrate as follows: Lesions of the pontine reticular formation (dorsal and lateral part of the nucleus reticularis pontis oralis et caudalis) suppressed REM sleep without producing any change in slow wave sleep, while stimulation of this area in an intact animal induced REM sleep.

The anatomical substrate of the normal EEG rhythms observed during sleep has been described [25]: (1) alpha rhythm, from the parieto-occipital region; (2) beta rhythm, from the frontocentral region (motor cortex); (3) delta rhythm, from the frontal lobe; (4) theta rhythm, from the parietotemporal region; and (5) sleep spindles, from the thalamocortical regions.

Disturbance in Onset of Sleep

Disturbance in onset of sleep is thought to be an inability of the normal sleep mechanism to inhibit sufficiently a hyperactive waking system, which is being bombarded primarily by cortical excitatory impulses. Thus a person in a state of anxiety is unable to fall asleep at his usual bedtime as a result of continued psychic activity. In addition there is increased stimulation of the cortex through the exteroceptive sensory pathways as a result of the increased muscular tension so often found in anxiety states (Table 2).

TABLE 2. *The neurophysiology of sleep*

Phenomenon	Cerebral Cortex	Thalamus	Hypothalamus	Limbic System	Reticular Formation
Disturbance in onset of sleep	X	—	—	—	—
Origin of sleep-arousal system	X	X	X	X	X
Origin of REM sleep	—	—	—	—	X
Origin of EEG rhythms occurring during sleep	X	X	—	—	—
Increased number of shifts to wakefulness & between stages of sleep	—	—	—	—	X

Disturbance in the Arousal System

The increased number of shifts from one sleep stage to another, shifts to wakefulness, and the inability to obtain adequate amounts of deep sleep as manifested by a marked decrease in stage 4 sleep, all found in depression, indicate a disturbance of the arousal system. A study [17] on the effect of depressive disorders on EEG responses to auditory stimulation during all-night sleep demonstrated that depressed patients when compared to a group of normal control subjects did respond significantly more often in all the stages. Further, after completion of treatment of their illness, there were no differences when compared to normal subjects of their arousal responses to auditory stimulation in any stage of sleep. Further evidence [46, 50] for the presence of a disturbed arousal system in depressed patients has been presented by investigators using the duration of the EEG arousal response elicited by photic stimulation as a measure of the level of the activity of the RAS. Both studies reported increased duration of the arousal response in depressed patients and postulated that the longer response represented increased activity of the RAS. This increase in responsitivity of the arousal system may be based upon several postulated mechanisms: (1) an increase in neuronal activity of the RAS, (2) a release of inhibitory mechanism of the RAS without increased RAS activity, or (3) a combination of both. The evidence [12, 39, 52] to date tends to support the first hypothesis—that it is the increased activity of the neurons of the RAS.

One study [15] on the sleep of schizophrenics postulated the presence of an increased level of arousal as a possible defect in this disorder based upon the abnormalities found in their investigation.

Insomnia may be a disturbance of the arousal system involving the mechanisms discussed above, or it may be a disturbance of the sleep or inhibitory system. It has been postulated [14] that the decrease in stage 4 noted in the sleep patterns of the geriatric population may be based upon a degenerative process of the inhibitory system involving both cortical and subcortical areas of the brain.

EFFECT OF PSYCHOTROPIC DRUGS ON THE BRAIN

In "picking the right drug for the right patient" in the treatment of clinical disorders, the practicing physician often chooses on the basis of "potency" of a given drug to match the "severity" of the diagnosis. Little or no attention has been paid to the manner in which the specific drugs might affect specific areas of the brain, and what this effect means in terms of the total patient. Experiments on some of the basic actions of different psychotropic drugs on key areas of the brain have been demonstrated using doses comparable with clinical usage by Himwich [26, 27]. The author points out that it is true that all drugs affect every organ of the body to a greater or lesser extent, and that systems and areas of the central nervous system are not independent but interconnected and act in integrated units. The focus of these studies was the areas of the brain most susceptible to a given drug.

Using after-discharges evoked by direct stimulation of various areas of the brain as a measure of reactivity, neurophysiological studies were performed of the following drugs: barbiturates; meprobamate; phenothiazines: chlorpromazine (Thorazine), prochlorperazine (Compazine); and tricyclic antidepressants: amitriptyline (Elavil), desipramine (Norpramin), desmethylamitriptyline (Nortriptyline) and imipramine (Tofrānil).

CORTEX. The cortex is the site of the discriminative aspect of consciousness (vision, hearing, speech, and fine motor activities). Barbiturates depress the cortex so as to produce a sedative action.

TABLE 3. *Action of psychotropic drugs on the brain.* + = Stimulates, — = Inhibits, 0 = No effect.

Region of the Brain	Function	Barbiturates	Meprobamate	Phenothiazines	Tricyclic Antidepressants
Cerebral Cortex	Discriminative aspects of consciousness	—	0	0	0
Thalamus	Relay station to cortex	+	—	+	
Hypothalamus	Regulation of vegetative & emotional functions	—	0	—	+
Limbic system	Regulation of emotions	—	—	+	+
Reticular formation	Arousal system	—	0	—	—
Neurohumoral depots	Regulation of emotions	0	0	—	+

Meprobamate, phenothiazines, and the antidepressants have no effect on this region (see Table 3).

THALAMUS. The thalamus is a relay station which transmits alerting impulses from the reticular formation to the cortex. The response to slow (7 per second) repetitive stimulation is sleep, while high frequency stimulation produces arousal. Barbiturates and phenothiazines enhance the sleep pattern mediated through this system and thus further diminish alertness, while meprobamate attenuates the response.

HYPOTHALAMUS. The hypothalamus is the center for the regulation of autonomic and vegetative functions (temperature, appetite, sex). Barbiturates and phenothiazines both decrease its function, while meprobamate has no effect. In contrast to this, the group of tricyclic antidepressant compounds increase the sensitivity of the hypothalamus to stimulation.

LIMBIC SYSTEM. The limbic system regulates the emotions, including preservation of the organism as in satisfying hunger for food, and the preservation of the species through sexual activities. Barbiturates and meprobamate inhibit this system and diminish its functions. Thus stimuli traversing this system after administration of either drug will be decreased with subsequent attenuation of the emotional behavior. The phenothiazines stimulate and evoke seizure-like patterns and it is suggested that as a result of this, there is loss of normal function of this system, which could account for the cessation of pathological thinking in schizophrenia. The antidepressant compounds increase the sensitivity of this system to stimulation and increase its various functions.

RETICULAR FORMATION. Among other functions, stimulation of the reticular formation produces alerting and arousing, both behavioral and EEG. Barbiturates, phenothiazines, and antidepressants all block the alerting response to a stimuli such as external sound. The decreased activity of the RAS results in a diminished behavioral alertness, or sleepiness. Meprobamate on the other hand neither stimulates nor inhibits the RAS. It should be noted that the descending component of the RAS also plays a role in the extrapyramidal regulation of posture and movement, so that phenothiazine-induced parkinsonism is via this system.

NEUROHUMORAL DEPOTS. Only the effects of norepinephrine (NE) and serotonin on neurohumoral depots are considered here. They are present in considerable amounts in the limbic system and reticular formation, and lowest in the cerebral cortex. A recent hypothesis concerning depression is that it is a state associated with the relative deficiency of NE. Treatment of depression with tricyclic antidepressant drugs may be related to NE metabolism, since these drugs have been shown [6] to increase biologically active NE in the central nervous system by blocking re-uptake of NE by axonal membranes.

Neither barbiturates nor meprobamate affect NE or serotonin levels. Phenothiazines block the action of the neurohormones, and their blocking of the hypothalamus may be based on this mechanism. The tricyclic antidepressants increase the concentration of these biogenic amines in the special parts of the brain where they occur.

Choosing a Therapeutic Drug

A study of Table 3 reveals some very fundamental differences among drugs which, when correlated with descriptive psychopathology of the various disorders, give some insight into the proper use of drugs in specific disorders. For example, symptoms of depressive disorders can be divided into (1) disturbance in mood with a pervasive affect of depression, (2) disturbance in biological functions, including those of sleep, appetite, sex, and autonomic dysfunctions, and (3) psychological disturbances. If we look at the drug action of barbiturates, meprobamate, phenothiazines, and tricyclic antidepressants, we can discern very rapidly that, if we were going to pick a priori the right drug for the treatment of depression, it would be the tricyclic compounds. The data speaks for itself: (1) This drug stimulates the limbic system and therefore improves mood. (2) It stimulates the hypothalamus and therefore improves the various biological dysfunctions present in depression such as decreased appetite, sleep, and libido. (3) It inhibits the reticular formation, which further improves the sleep disturbance. (4) It increases the neurohumoral depots, which are deficient in depressive disorders. None of the other drugs have these combined properties.

One other observation of note: If sleep disturbance is one of the cardinal signs of depression, why haven't "sleep-inducing" drugs helped this disorder? Again, perusal of Table 3 reveals some relevant facts which may help to answer this question. It can be seen that although barbiturates and phenothiazines both inhibit the reticular formation, they both also inhibit the hypothalamus. Further, they have opposite effects on the limbic system: While barbiturates have no effect on neurohumoral depots, phenothiazines inhibit their activity.

It is upon these complex anatomic and functional relationships that psychotropic drugs presumably produce therapeutic actions. To ameliorate or correct the pathophysiology of any disorder, one must alter the functioning of the cerebral substrate at the molecular level, which after all is where drugs act.

EFFECT OF PSYCHOTROPIC DRUGS ON SLEEP

The specific effects of the following drugs on the sleep of normal and psychiatric subjects have been reported and the results summarized in Table 4.

Barbiturates. Barbiturates are reported [45] to decrease percent time in stages A, 1, and REM. They also reduce frequency of movements and shifts of depth of sleep, both from one stage to another and to stage A. Effect on stage 4 is conflicting, with reports of decreases [4, 45] and increases [36].

TABLE 4. *Effect of psychotropic drugs on all-night sleep of normal adults.* + = Increased, — = Decreased, 0 = No change, × = Not known

Psychotropic Drugs	Percent Time in Sleep Stage						Shifts to Wakefulness & Between Stages of Sleep
	A	1	2	3	4	REM	
Barbiturates	—	—	+	0	±	—	—
Meprobamate	0	—	+	0	0	—	—
Phenothiazines	—	—	×	×	±	—	—
Tricyclic antidepressants	—	—	0	0	+	—	—

MEPROBAMATE. Meprobamate is reported [16] to decrease stages 1 and REM, with no effect on stages A, 3, and 4, and to increase stage 2 sleep. In another study [29] using motility as a sleep index (measured by an electronic recording device attached to the bed), results indicated that this drug significantly reduced motility and restlessness.

PHENOTHIAZINES. Several studies on the effect of chlorpromazine on the sleep of subjects have been conflicting. Stage 4 or slow wave sleep has been reported to be decreased by one author [47] and increased by another [36]. Percent time in REM has been reported [36, 47] to be decreased [13, 22] and increased in both normal and psychiatric subjects.

Percent time in the arousal stage was reported [47] to be unchanged in normal subjects, but decreased in psychiatric patients.

TRICYCLIC ANTIDEPRESSANTS. Sleep studies on the following compounds have been reported: amitriptyline [21, 47], desipramine [30, 47, 54, 56], and imipramine [30, 47]. These psychotropic agents have been shown to have the following effects on all-night sleep: (1) decrease in number of awakenings [30, 54, 56], (2) increase in stage 4 sleep [47, 54, 56], (3) decrease in REM time [21, 30, 47, 54, 56], (4) depression of RAS [58], and (5) increase in duration of the normal 90-minute cycle [54, 56].

From these observations, a mechanism for the therapeutic effects of antidepressant drugs may be postulated: that they ameliorate the very same disturbances of sleep which investigators have reported as characteristically present in depressed patients. This was illustrated by the results of a longitudinal investigation [56] on the effect of desipramine on the sleep of depressed patients. The all-night sleep of 6 patients was studied before drug treatment and during the first and fourth weeks of desipramine, 25 mg. 4 times a day. Concurrent with the laboratory study, ratings of the patient's depression were obtained using the Self-rating Depression Scale (SDS), the results of which are expressed as an index [53]. High indices (> 50) on the scale indicate the presence of significant depressive symptomatology while low scores (< 50) indicate the absence of psychopathology. Data obtained from this study are summarized in Table 5.

TABLE 5. *Longitudinal effects of desipramine on sleep of depressed patients*

Nights	Distribution of All-Night Sleep as Mean % Time in Stages						SDS Index
	A	B	C	D	E	REM	
Before treatment	6.4	32.7	18.7	10.7	15.2	16.3	65
Week 1, desipramine	1.2	22.6	23.1	18.2	20.4	14.5	57
Week 4, desipramine	0.2	23.1	20.0	14.6	24.0	18.1	42

It can be seen that the pretreatment sleep of the depressed patients as it is distributed as mean percent sleep time spent in the various stages of sleep fits the previously described characteristics for the sleep of depressives (see section Characteristics of All-Night Sleep).

The distribution of the mean percent sleep time in the various stages of sleep-REM after treatment indicated a reversal of these values so that there were decreases of stages A and 1, and increases of stages 2, 3, and 4. Percent time in REM was decreased further after one week of desipramine, but by the fourth week it had increased to above the pretreatment level. Lastly, shifts during the night to wakefulness and between stages of sleep were abnormal prior to treatment and decreased with treatment. In addition the clinical status of the patients' depressive illnesses was reflected by the mean SDS indices. Thus it was 65 (equivalent of moderate to severe depression) before treatment, decreased to 57 at the end of one week, and was 42 (within normal range) by the end of the fourth week.

Data from one subject will illustrate the effect on all-night sleep pattern of treatment with desipramine (see Fig. 2). The patient's sleep before treatment showed the characteristic disturbances with numerous awakenings present after the onset of sleep, decreased stage 4 sleep which was of short duration when present, decreased REM time, and alternating periods of light-deep-light sleep, most of which occurred in durations shorter than 30 minutes. During drug treatment, the number of shifts of sleep stages decreased, while shifts to stage A or awakening were abolished. The overall effect of these changes was to increase the short pretreatment periodicity (of about 30 minutes) to longer periods (from 1 to 2 hours).

Thus the antidepressants seem to have a normalizing effect on the all-night pattern and its cyclic nature. This mechanism may be very important therapeutically to the depressed patient, in view of his increased number of awakenings. There is evidence that sleep does not normally simply "recycle" with sleep onset. Instead, the sleep of subjects who returned to sleep in the morning hours resembled more the sleep characteristics which occur late in a full night's sleep [48].

The decrease in percent REM time found in the sleep of depressives and in sleep after antidepressant drug intake may be based upon a mechanism common to both, which is the alteration of the normal biological rhythm of sleep. In the sleep of depressives the cyclic pattern is disturbed by the frequent wakings, present probably as a result of the increased activity of the RAS. In the sleep with antidepressant drugs, there is an inhibitory action on the arousal system by the drugs, decreasing the number of awakenings and of shifts in stages of sleep and thereby changing the cycles in this manner. The result in both instances is an altered sleep-arousal mechanism, which in turn affects the REM phenomenon by decreasing its occurrence in number or duration or both.

REFERENCES

1. Agnew, H., Webb, W., and Williams, R. The effect of stage 4 sleep deprivation. *Electroenceph. Clin. Neurophysiol.* 17:68, 1964.
2. Agnew, H., Webb, W., and Williams, R. L. Comparison of stage 4 and 1-REM sleep deprivation. *Percept. Motor Skills* 24: 851, 1967.
3. Akert, K. The anatomical substrate of sleep. *Progr. Brain Res.* 18:9, 1965.
4. Baekeland, F. Pentobarbital and dextroamphetamine sulfate: Effects on the sleep cycle in man. *Psychopharmacologia* (Berlin) 11:388, 1967.
5. Bliss, E. Sleep in schizophrenia and depression: Studies of sleep loss in man and animals. *Res. Publ. Ass. Nerv. Ment. Dis.* 45:195, 1967.
6. Bunney, W. E., Jr., and Davis, J. M. Norepinephrine in depressive reactions. *Arch. Gen. Psychiat.* (Chicago) 13:483, 1965.
7. Caldwell, D. F., and Domino, E. F. Electroencephalographic and eye movement patterns during sleep in chronic schizophrenic patients. *Electroenceph. Clin. Neurophysiol.* 22:414, 1967.
8. Davis, H., Davis, P. A., Loomis, A. L., and Harvey, E. N. Changes in human brain potentials during the onset of sleep. *Science* 86:448, 1937.
9. Dement, W. Dream recall and eye movements during sleep in schizophrenics and normals. *J. Nerv. Ment. Dis.* 122:263, 1955.
10. Dement, W., and Kleitman, N. Cyclic variations in EEG during sleep and their relation to eye movements, body motility, and dreaming. *Electroenceph. Clin. Neurophysiol.* 9:673, 1957.
11. Diaz-Guerrero, R., Gottlieb, J. S., and Knott, J. R. The sleep

of patients with manic-depressive psychosis, depressive type. *Psychosom. Med.* 8:399, 1946.

12. Evarts, E. V. Effects of Sleep and Waking on Activity of Single Units in the Unrestrained Cat. In G. W. Wolstenholme and M. O'Conner (Eds.), *Ciba Symposium on the Nature of Sleep*. London: Churchill, 1961. P. 171.
13. Feinberg, I. Current Studies of Sleep and Dreaming in Psychiatric Patients. Paper read at Association for the Psychophysiological Study of Sleep (APSS), Palo Alto, Cal., 1964.
14. Feinberg, I. Sleep electroencephalographic and eye-movement patterns in patients with schizophrenia and with chronic brain syndrome. *Res. Publ. Ass. Res. Nerv. Ment. Dis.* 45:211, 1967.
15. Feinberg, I., Koresko, R. L., and Gottlieb, F. Further observations on electrophysiological sleep patterns in schizophrenia. *Compr. Psychiat.* 6:21, 1965.
16. Freeman, F., Agnew, H. W., Jr., and Williams, R. An EEG study of the effects of meprobamate on human sleep. *Clin. Pharmacol. Ther.* 6:172, 1965.
17. Gresham, S. C., Agnew, H. W., Jr., and Williams, R. L. The sleep of depressed patients. *Arch. Gen. Psychiat.* (Chicago) 13:503, 1965.
18. Haider, I. Patterns of insomnia in depressive illness: A subjective evaluation. *Brit. J. Psychiat.* 114:1127, 1968.
19. Hartmann, E. *The Biology of Dreaming*. Springfield, Ill.: Thomas, 1967.
20. Hartmann, E. The 90-minute sleep-dream cycle. *Arch. Gen. Psychiat.* (Chicago) 18:280, 1968.
21. Hartmann, E. The effect of four drugs on sleep patterns in man. *Psychopharmacologia* (Berlin) 12:346, 1969.
22. Hartmann, E., and Verdone, P. Sleep and Dream Patterns of a Pair of Identical Twins Discordant for Schizophrenia. Paper read at APSS, Gainesville, Fla., 1966.
23. Hawkins, D. R., and Mendels, J. Sleep disturbance in depressive syndromes. *Amer. J. Psychiat.* 123:682, 1966.
24. Hess, R. The electroencephalogram in sleep. *Electroenceph. Clin. Neurophysiol.* 16:44, 1964.
25. Hill, D., and Paar, G. *Electroencephalography*. New York: Macmillan, 1963.
26. Himwich, H. E. Tranquilizers, barbiturates, and the brain. *J. Neuropsychiat.* 3:279, 1962.
27. Himwich, H. E., Morillo, A., and Steiner, W. C. Drugs affecting rhinencephalic structures. *J. Neuropsychiat.* 3:S15, 1962.

28. Hinton, J. M. Patterns of insomnia in depressive states. *J. Neurol. Neurosurg. Psychiat.* 26:184, 1963.
29. Hinton, J., and Marley, E. The effects of meprobamate and pentobarbitone sodium on sleep and motility during sleep. *J. Neurol. Neurosurg. Psychiat.* 22:137, 1959.
30. Hishikawa, Y., Nakai, K., Ida, H., and Kaneko, Z. The effect of imipramine, desmethylimipramine and chlorpromazine on the sleep-wakefulness cycle of the cat. *Electroenceph. Clin. Neurophysiol.* 19:518, 1965.
31. Jones, H. S., and Oswald, I. Two cases of healthy insomnia. *Electroenceph. Clin. Neurophysiol.* 24:378, 1968.
32. Jouvet, M. Paradoxical sleep: A study of its nature and mechanisms. *Progr. Brain Res.* 18:20, 1965.
33. Kleitman, N. *Sleep and Wakefulness.* Chicago: University of Chicago Press, 1963.
34. Koresko, R. L., Snyder, F., and Feinberg, I. Dream time in hallucinating and non-hallucinating schizophrenic patients. *Nature* (London) 199:1118, 1963.
35. Lester, B., Burch, N., and Dossett, R. Nocturnal EEG-GSR profiles: The influence of presleep states. *Psychophysiol.* 3:238, 1967.
36. Lester, B., and Guerrero-Figueroa, R. Effects of some drugs on EEG fast activity and dream time. *Psychophysiol.* 2:224, 1966.
37. McGhie, A. The subjective assessment of sleep patterns in psychiatric illness. *Brit. J. Med. Psychol.* 39:221, 1966.
38. McGhie, A., and Russell, S. M. The subjective assessment of normal sleep patterns. *J. Ment. Sci.* 108:642, 1962.
39. Machne, X., Calma, I., and Magoun, H. W. Unit activity of central cephalic brain stem in electroencephalogram arousal. *J. Neurophysiol.* 18:547, 1966.
40. Mendels, J., and Hawkins, D. R. Sleep and depression: A controlled EEG study. *Arch. Gen. Psychiat.* (Chicago) 16:344, 1967.
41. Mendels, J., and Hawkins, D. R. Sleep and depression: A follow-up study. *Arch. Gen. Psychiat.* (Chicago) 16:536, 1967.
42. Mendels, J., and Hawkins, D. R. Sleep and depression. *Arch. Gen. Psychiat.* (Chicago) 19:445, 1968.
43. Muratorio, A., Maggini, C., and Murri, L. Il sonno notturno nelle sindromi depressive studio poligrafico di 35 casi. *Estratto da Neopsichiatria* 33:1, 1967.
44. Oswald, I. *Sleeping and Waking.* Amsterdam: Elsevier, 1962.
45. Oswald, I., Berger, R. J., Jaramillo, R. A., Keddie, K. M. G.,

Olley, P. C., and Plunkett, G. B. Melancholia and barbiturates: A controlled EEG, body and eye movement study of sleep. *Brit. J. Psychiat.* 109:66, 1963.

46. Paulson, G., and Gottlieb, G. A longitudinal study of the electroencephalographic arousal response in depressed patients. *J. Nerv. Ment. Dis.* 133:524, 1961.
47. Toyoda, J. The effects of chlorpromazine and imipramine on the human nocturnal sleep electroencephalogram. *Folia Psychiat. Neurol. Jap.* 18:198, 1964.
48. Webb, W. B., Agnew, H. W., Jr., and Sternthal, H. Sleep during the early morning. *Psychonomic Science* 6:277, 1966.
49. Williams, R. L., Agnew, H. W., Jr., and Webb, W. B. Sleep patterns in young adults: An EEG study. *Electroenceph. Clin. Neurophysiol.* 17:376, 1964.
50. Wilson, W. P., and Wilson, N. J. Observations on the duration of photically elicited arousal responses in depressive psychoses. *J. Nerv. Ment. Dis.* 133: 438, 1961.
51. Wilson, W. P., and Zung, W. W. K. Attention, discrimination, and arousal during sleep. *Arch. Gen. Psychiat.* (Chicago) 15: 523, 1966.
52. Winters, W. D. Neuropharmacological studies and postulates on excitation and depression in the central nervous system. *Recent Advances Biol. Psychiat.* 9:313, 1961.
53. Zung, W. W. K. A self-rating depression scale. *Arch. Gen. Psychiat.* (Chicago) 12:63, 1965.
54. Zung, W. W. K. Effect of antidepressant drugs on sleeping and dreaming. Part II. On the adult male. *Excerpta Med. Int. Congress Series* No. 150:1824, 1968.
55. Zung, W. W. K. The treatment of insomnia with antidepressant drugs. *Psychophysiology* 5:234, 1968.
56. Zung, W. W. K. Effect of antidepressant drugs on sleeping and dreaming. Part III. On the depressed patient. *Biol. Psychiat.* In press.
57. Zung, W. W. K., Naylor, T. H., Gianturco, D. T., and Wilson, W. P. Computer simulation of sleep EEG patterns with a Markov chain model. *Recent Advances Biol. Psychiat.* 8:335, 1966.
58. Zung, W. W. K., Wilson, W. P., and Dodson, W. E. Effect of depressive disorders on sleep EEG responses. *Arch. Gen. Psychiat.* (Chicago) 10:439, 1964.

Personality, Sleep, and Dreaming

*How is personality related to sleep and dreaming? Do personality variables affect amount of sleep, amount of dreaming, type of dream, or recollection of dreams?**

Personality and Dreams†

DAVID FOULKES

Despite demonstrations that reports of having dreamed can be elicited upon awakenings from all varieties of electroencephalographically recorded sleep [6], it has become apparent that the most vivid and dreamlike dreams are generally reported from EEG stage REM ("ascending" EEG sleep stage 1, a low-voltage, mixed frequency tracing associated with intermittent rapid eye movement) [2, 22]. The question of the relationship of personality variables to frequency of dreaming, then, is most often conceptualized in terms of the association of personality with the frequency of stage REM

* The reader interested in these questions may wish to refer also to papers by Baekeland and Hartmann (p. 33), Webb (p. 44), Hauri (p. 70), Lewis (p. 199), Jones (p. 221), Cartwright (p. 227), and Hawkins (p. 233) and to another paper by Foulkes (p. 165).

† Supported by National Science Foundation Grant GS-2123.

sleep periods or the proportion of total sleep time spent in stage REM (REM percent).

Limited variability across persons in REM percent [26] makes it unlikely that many significant personality correlates of the proportion of sleep spent in stage REM will be found within the normal range. One report [26] has indicated a positive relationship between an inventory measure of manifest anxiety and REM percent, but this finding was not replicated in another study [21]. Shading into the realm of psychopathology, however, it has been observed that self-described poor sleepers averaged markedly less REM sleep (REM percent = 16.93) than did self-described good sleepers (REM percent = 24.34). The poor-sleep group also showed greater peripheral physiological activation (e.g., heart rate, phasic vasoconstrictions) during sleep, more awakenings during the night, reduced total sleep time, and greater psychological disturbance as assessed by the Cornell Medical Index and the Minnesota Multiphasic Personality Inventory (MMPI) [21].

Studies of psychiatric patients have been extensive, many having been conducted in the hope of demonstrating either that a derangement of the anatomical-physiological mechanisms of REM sleep underlies psychosis or that chronic deprivation of stage REM induces the appearance of REM-like phenomena in wakefulness (the psychotic as a "waking dreamer"). Findings to date have been inconclusive but mostly negative [13]. Although there have been occasional reports to the contrary [e.g., 4], schizophrenics seem to have neither strikingly more nor strikingly less REM sleep than normals. Depressive disorders, and exacerbations of symptoms in both schizophrenics and depressives, seem to be associated with some reduction in REM percent [18, 19, 31, 32]. It seems likely, however, that these effects are produced by generally disturbed sleep rather than being indicative of any direct link between clinical symptomatology and stage REM mechanisms. Attempts to demonstrate the role of stage REM in psychotic disorders have recently taken another direction: the assessment of variability of response to stage REM deprivation in relation to clinical diagnosis or state. It has been reported that actively ill schizophrenics fail to compensate (i.e., to show increased REM percent) following selective stage REM deprivation [38], but this finding has not been confirmed by others [36]. Furthermore, adequate evidence is still lacking of any consistent deleterious behavioral consequences, much less of psychotic breakthroughs, following stage REM deprivation in either normal subjects or psychiatric patients [35].

Questionnaire studies of dream recall frequency have consistently, if weakly, associated repression or defensiveness with the relative failure to be aware of the many dreams each person presumably experiences every night [3, 28, 29, 30, 34]. Questionnaire nonrecallers do become more aware of their dreams when awakened during stage REM in the laboratory [12], although variability in daytime impressions of dreaming is positively correlated with variability in nocturnal recall upon stage REM arousals [10]. Conscious, deliberate interest in dreams may well both underlie this last correlation and be a generally good predictor of daytime variability in dream recall [3].

Dream recall under laboratory conditions (awakening from electroencephalographically defined sleep phases for immediate dream retrieval) is much more variable in NREM sleep stages than in stage REM [7]. It is not known whether variability in NREM recall reflects individual differences in the actual occurrence of NREM mentation or differential success in its retrieval. The nature of those NREM experiences that are reported, however, suggests that NREM mentation is generally less memorable in many of its features (e.g., length, intensity) than is REM mentation [5, 27]. Dreams reported during the night in the laboratory are most likely to be recalled the next morning if, as originally reported, they were long and intense [17]. These same factors are probably operative at the point of the original report as well: there is likely to be a close relationship between what is dreamed and how often one is aware of having dreamed. Memory is apparently less adequate during NREM sleep than during REM sleep [16, 20, 25], and cognitive-skill factors may also play some role in individual variability in NREM recall.

Relationships between dream content variables and waking behavioral variables have generally been considered within the framework of two alternative possibilities: complementarity or continuity [1, 15]. Evidence collected on the association of personality with laboratory dream reports is overwhelmingly in favor of the latter alternative. For both REM and NREM sleep, nocturnal mental experiences are reported to be more vivid and bizarre for subjects with greater evidence of pathological response on standard personality inventories such as the MMPI [9, 23, 24]. Similarly, disturbed male adolescents were found to have more vivid and unpleasant REM dreams than their controls, and male adolescents high in a test measure of social dominance were found to play a more active role in their dreams than those low in the test measure [8]. In still another investigation [1] MMPI and behavioral rating measures of hostile and sexual impulse expression in wakefulness were found to be positively correlated with like measures derived from laboratory-reported REM dreams.

The continuity hypothesis is also consistent with a number of findings relating experimentally induced or naturally occurring variations in daytime behavior with variations in nocturnal dream content. In one study [33], for instance, college girls' REM dreams were most unpleasant during that phase of the menstrual cycle in which they felt most depressed. With respect to drive-related experiences, it appears that if a drive is subject to presleep satiation, it has less of an influence than otherwise upon nocturnal mentation; whereas if it is subject to frustration or arousal without satisfaction, it has more of an influence than otherwise. Illustrative of the former effect is the finding [14] that subjects had REM dreams less concerned with thinking and problem-solving following 6 presleep hours of concentrated studying, and REM dreams containing less physical activity after 6 presleep hours of strenuous physical exercise. Consistent with the latter effect are findings that subjects who experienced social isolation in the presleep period had increased social dream content [37] and that college girls' dreams were most manifestly sexual during that phase of the menstrual cycle associated with low waking sexual interest [33].

The period of sleep onset does not appear to be an exception to the continuity hypothesis of personality–dream relations, but the nature of the continuity is somewhat different than for either REM or other NREM sleep. Sleep-onset fantasy seems to be much more closely related to voluntary waking fantasy than is either REM or NREM fantasy [10]. At sleep onset, voluntary control of the course taken by mental activity is still possible to a degree unknown during sleep proper. Subjects with constricted waking fantasy and rigid waking defenses against impulse life thus are still able to defend themselves against the intrusion of vivid mentation during the decathexis of reality that occurs at sleep onset [10, 11]. During this period, then, it may be psychologically healthier persons who have more vivid and intense mental activity, apparently because regressive mental content is less threatening to them.

REFERENCES

1. Ben-Horin, P. The Manifestation of Some Basic Personality Dimensions in Wakefulness, Fantasy, and Dreams. University of Chicago Ph.D. Dissertation, 1967.
2. Bosinelli, M., Bagnaresi, G., Molinari, S., and Salzarulo, P. Caratteristiche dell' attivita psichofisiologica durante il sonno: Un contributo alle tecniche di valutazione. *Riv. Sper. Freniat.* 92:128, 1968.
3. Domhoff, B., and Gerson, A. Replication and critique of three studies on personality correlates of dream recall. *J. Consult. Psychol.* 31:431, 1967.
4. Feinberg, I., Koresko, R. L., Heller, N., and Steinberg, H. R. Unusually high dream time in an hallucinating patient. *Amer. J. Psychiat.* 121:1018, 1965.
5. Foulkes, D. Dream reports from different stages of sleep. *J. Abnorm. Soc. Psychol.* 65:14, 1962.
6. Foulkes, D. *The Psychology of Sleep.* New York: Scribner's, 1966.
7. Foulkes, D. Nonrapid eye movement mentation. *Exp. Neurol.* [Suppl.] 4:28, 1967.
8. Foulkes, D., Larson, J. D., Swanson, E. M., and Rardin, M. Two studies of childhood dreaming. *Amer. J. Orthopsychiat.* 39:627, 1969.

9. Foulkes, D., and Rechtschaffen, A. Presleep determinants of dream content: Effects of two films. *Percept. Motor Skills* 19: 983, 1964.
10. Foulkes, D., Spear, P. S., and Symonds, J. D. Individual differences in mental activity at sleep onset. *J. Abnorm. Psychol.* 71:280, 1966.
11. Foulkes, D., and Vogel, G. Mental activity at sleep onset. *J. Abnorm. Psychol.* 70:231, 1965.
12. Goodenough, D. R., Shapiro, A., Holden, M., and Steinschriber, L. A comparison of "dreamers" and "nondreamers": Eye movements, electroencephalograms, and the recall of dreams. *J. Abnorm. Soc. Psychol.* 59:295, 1959.
13. Hartmann, E. *The Biology of Dreaming*. Springfield, Ill.: Thomas, 1967.
14. Hauri, P. Effects of Evening Activity on Subsequent Sleep and Dreams. University of Chicago Ph.D. Dissertation, 1966.
15. Kirsch, T. B. The relationship of the REM state to analytical psychology. *Amer. J. Psychiat.* 124:1459, 1968.
16. Mandell, M. P., Mandell, A. J., and Jacobson, A. Biochemical and neurophysiological studies of paradoxical sleep. *Recent Advances Biol. Psychiat.* 7:115, 1964.
17. Meier, C. A., Ruef, H., Ziegler, A., and Hall, C. S. Forgetting of dreams in the laboratory. *Percept. Motor Skills* 26:551, 1968.
18. Mendels, J., and Hawkins, D. R. Sleep and depression: A controlled EEG study. *Arch. Gen. Psychiat.* (Chicago) 16:344, 1967.
19. Mendels, J., and Hawkins, D. R. Sleep and depression: A follow-up study. *Arch. Gen. Psychiat.* (Chicago) 16:536, 1967.
20. Molinari, S., Foulkes, D., and Weisz, R. The Phenomenology of Different Sleep Periods: Psychological Correlates of Phasic and Tonic Events. Paper read at Association for the Psychophysiological Study of Sleep, Boston, 1969.
21. Monroe, L. J. Psychological and physiological differences between good and poor sleepers. *J. Abnorm. Psychol.* 72:255, 1967.
22. Monroe, L. J., Rechtschaffen, A., Foulkes, D., and Jensen, J. Discriminability of REM and NREM reports. *J. Personality Soc. Psychol.* 2:456, 1965.
23. Pivik, T., and Foulkes, D. "Dream deprivation": Effects on dream content. *Science* 153:1282, 1966.
24. Pivik, T., and Foulkes, D. NREM mentation: Relation to personality, orientation time, and time of night. *J. Consult. Clin. Psychol.* 32:144, 1968.

25. Portnoff, G., Baekeland, F., Goodenough, D. R., Karacan, I., and Shapiro, A. Retention of verbal materials perceived immediately prior to onset of non-REM sleep. *Percept. Motor Skills* 22:751, 1966.
26. Rechtschaffen, A., and Verdone, P. Amount of dreaming: Effect of incentive, adaptation to laboratory, and individual differences. *Percept. Motor Skills* 19:947, 1964.
27. Rechtschaffen, A., Verdone, P., and Wheaton, J. Reports of mental activity during sleep. *Canad. Psychiat. Ass. J.* 8:409, 1963.
28. Schonbar, R. A. Some manifest characteristics of recallers and nonrecallers of dreams. *J. Consult. Psychol.* 23:414, 1959.
29. Schonbar, R. A. Differential dream recall frequency as a component of "life style." *J. Consult. Psychol.* 29:468, 1965.
30. Singer, J. L., and Schonbar, R. A. Correlates of daydreaming: A dimension of self-awareness. *J. Consult. Psychol.* 25:1, 1961.
31. Snyder, F., Anderson, D., Bunney, W., Kupfer, D., Scott, J., and Wyatt, R. Longitudinal variation in the sleep of severely depressed and acutely schizophrenic patients with changing clinical status. *Psychophysiology* 5:235, 1968.
32. Snyder, F., Scott, J., Karacan, I., and Anderson, D. Presumptive evidence of REMS deprivation in depressive illness. *Psychophysiology* 4:382, 1968.
33. Swanson, E. M., and Foulkes, D. Dream content and the menstrual cycle. *J. Nerv. Ment. Dis.* 145:358, 1968.
34. Tart, C. T. Frequency of dream recall and some personality measures. *J. Consult. Psychol.* 26:467, 1962.
35. Vogel, G. W. REM deprivation. III. Dreaming and psychosis. *Arch. Gen. Psychiat.* (Chicago) 18:312, 1968.
36. Vogel, G. W., and Traub, A. C. REM deprivation. I. The effect on schizophrenic patients. *Arch. Gen. Psychiat.* (Chicago) 18:287, 1968.
37. Wood, P. Dreaming and Social Isolation. University of North Carolina Ph.D. Dissertation, 1962.
38. Zarcone, V., Pivik, T., Gulevich, G., Azumi, K., and Dement, W. Partial deprivation of the REM state in schizophrenics with active symptomatology. *Psychophysiology* 5:239, 1968.

Individual Differences in Dreaming

HERMAN A. WITKIN

Psychological individuality is a central concern of the clinician in both his practical and theoretical work. Yet the writings of clinicians on dreaming show little attention to individual differences in characteristic mode of dreaming and typical dream content (i.e., stylistic differences in dreaming) or in dream recall. Research with the laboratory monitoring method has begun to identify such individual differences and to contribute to our understanding of them.

INDIVIDUAL DIFFERENCES IN DREAM RECALL

Work with the monitoring method has shown that everyone dreams a good deal each night, and though individual differences may exist in time spent in REM sleep, the period of "dreamy" dreams [1, 9], these differences are small compared to the differences in amount of dream experience people are able to report in the morning. The real difference is between persons who remember their dreams and those who do not—or *reporters* and *nonreporters*, as they have come to be designated.

Two recent reports by Goodenough [15, 16] have reviewed the evidence, coming mainly from the extensive research by Goodenough and his collaborators, on differences between home reporters and nonreporters in a variety of characteristics of sleeping and dreaming in the laboratory. Of particular relevance here is the evidence that the category of nonreporters consists of subgroups identifiably different in their laboratory behavior and therefore possibly nonreporters for qualitatively different reasons [20]. Some home nonreporters characteristically fail to remember any dream content on awakening from REM periods. Others, when awakened, characteristically report that they were awake and thinking. Still others become reporters in the laboratory and in fact seem indistinguishable from home reporters in most characteristics of laboratory behavior. This breakup of the nonreporter category, originally considered homogenous, may make possible a more fruitful approach to exploring the personality characteristics of persons who forget their dreams and the processes mediating such forgetting.

Studies that have sought distinguishing personality correlates of a tendency to forget dreams have used subjects classified as reporters or nonreporters on the basis of frequency of home dream recall and have considered nonreporters (and reporters, for that matter) as a unitary group.

Some of these studies have identified specific personality attributes of nonreporters. Considering results of studies which have been replicated, nonreporters, as compared to reporters, appear more prone to use repression as a defense, to experience less anxiety, to be lower in ego strength, and to have less self-awareness [11, 12, 23, 28, 31]. Other studies, not yet replicated, have shown that nonreporters experience the locus of control outside themselves [30], are more common among engineers than among artists (considered the more creative group) [27], and on the Rorschach are low on indices of fantasy predominance and associative productivity and tend to respond to form determinants only [23]. Conflicting results have been obtained on need-achievement [12, 28, 31], psychological maladjustment [6, 11, 22, 32], and extroversion [6, 31, 32]. Some of these discrepancies may be due to failure to take account of sex differences in personality variables associated with dream recall [6]. Other characteristics have been looked at but failed to discriminate reporters from nonreporters [5, 27, 29].

Field Dependence and Independence

Another group of studies compared reporters and nonreporters with regard to a broader characterological dimension—extent of psychological differentiation as reflected particularly in a more field-dependent or field-independent cognitive style.* Field dependence

* Lachman, Lapkin, and Handelman [19] examined another cognitive style, leveling-sharpening, in relation to home dream recall.

represents a relatively global way of perceiving world and self and field independence, an articulated mode of perception. Persons who are field independent tend to have a relatively articulated body concept and developed sense of separate identity (together signifying a differentiated self), and they are likely to have a developed defensive structure and to use such specialized defenses as intellectualization and isolation, in contrast to the more global defenses of repression and denial typically used by field-dependent persons [34, 36]. These attributes, which tend to cluster together in the same person, reflect developed psychological differentiation; the contrasting cluster found in more field-dependent persons reflects limited differentiation. In this conception field dependence or field independence signifies less developed or more developed differentiation.

Studies have repeatedly shown that home dream nonreporters, both adults and children, are significantly more field-dependent than reporters [13, 20,* 21, 30]. If we consider the cluster of characteristics for which field-dependence stands, this well-confirmed result is congruent with the findings on the more specific personality attributes, previously described, which have recurrently distinguished reporters from nonreporters. Thus repression, one of these specific attributes, is also a characteristic of field-dependent persons; and the relatively low level of experienced anxiety, another of the specific attributes, may, as Schonbar has suggested, reflect the use of denial, a defense typical of field-dependent persons. Low level of ego strength, still another of the specific attributes of nonreporters, has also been linked to field dependence. Finally, the six Rorschach measures found by Orlinsky [36] to distinguish reporters from nonreporters are very similar to those which distinguish field-dependent from field-independent persons.

This picture of home nonreporters as limitedly differentiated persons cannot be assumed to fit all nonreporters. Separate personality study of the subgroups of nonreporters identified by Lewis et al.

* Evidence on the relation between field dependence and dream characteristics obtained in this study, and referred to at several points in the present paper, was not included in the published report.

[20] may be one route to identification of the psychological variety that very likely exists among them.

Granting that many or most nonreporters are limitedly differentiated, there remains the important question of the mechanism by which such persons come to forget their dreams. One mechanism may be their ready exercise of repression over their dream experiences, in keeping with their easy use of this defense in other areas of experience. A study in our laboratory, in which my collaborators are Goodenough, Lewis, Shapiro, and Koulack [33], is attempting to check this possibility by determining whether dreams made emotionally charged by arousing presleep experiences will more often fail to be recalled by less differentiated than more differentiated persons. A recent study by Baekeland and Lasky [3] suggests that repression may also work in the field-dependent person to cause loss of morning recall of content given at the time of awakening from the dream. A check on whether repression is a factor in memory loss from on-the-spot to postsleep reporting is being made in a study we are now conducting by determining whether the particular elements lost are emotionally more charged than the recalled elements; this is being done for groups of more differentiated and less differentiated subjects. Baekeland's findings help explain the behavior of the subgroups in the Lewis et al. study who were nonreporters at home but became reporters in the laboratory, when it is noted that these subjects were quite field-dependent. In light of Baekeland's results we may consider that an important factor in the tendency for at least some limitedly differentiated persons to be home nonreporters is their loss of the dream experience between the time it takes place and morning recall, even when they are able to reproduce the experience immediately upon awakening.

Baekeland's observation that less differentiated persons suffer greater memory loss from on-the-spot to morning reporting may reflect the operation of other psychological mechanisms, in addition to repression. One possibility is that, as with their waking experiences [34], the dream experiences of these people lack clear cognitive structure, and their dream loss reflects the typical fate of vaguely organized material in memory. Another mechanism may be their less effective consolidation of the dream experience. It has been shown [25] that an "alert" state of the nervous system, achieved by a period of wakefulness, may be needed to consolidate the trace of the antecedent dream experience and make it available to subsequent recall. The evidence that limitedly differentiated persons may characteristically function at a lower level of arousal [37] lends credence to the possibility that, among them, restoration of the nervous system to an "alert" state on awakening does not proceed as rapidly or go as far as in differentiated persons, thereby making consolidation of the dream experience, and its subsequent recall, less effective. Consistent with the consolidation hypothesis is the finding [20] of a positive but not quite significant correlation between field-dependence and REM period arousal threshold.

INDIVIDUAL DIFFERENCES IN THE EFFECTS OF REM SLEEP DEPRIVATION

Results of studies of the effects of REM sleep deprivation have frequently been inconsistent. Though this is surely due in part to differences in methodology, it may also reflect differences in kinds of subjects used. The kind-of-subject factor can be a particularly important contributor to inconsistent results when, as is so often true in monitored sleep research, the number of cases used is small. The importance of individual differences in the effects of REM sleep deprivation lies, however, not so much in their methodological nuisance value as in the route they open to more complete understanding of the function of REM sleep and the consequences of its loss.

Published reports on REM sleep deprivation, in which data for individual subjects have been included, provide evidence of striking individual differences in some of the most salient deprivation effects. Repeatedly, subjects have been found to differ in the persistence of their attempt to remain in REM sleep, reflected in number of awakenings required to maintain REM sleep deprivation, and in the extent of their indulgence in REM sleep during recovery, reflected in amount of compensatory REM time [e.g., 9, 10, 14]. Such individual differences were in fact to be found in the report on the very first study of deprivation by Dement. In Dement's group of 8 subjects, 1—in fact the very one who required the largest number of awakening to maintain REM deprivation—showed no increase in REM time during recovery. The prevalence of the individual differences noted leads inevitably to the question of whether people differ in drive toward REM sleep, contributing to differences in the effects of REM sleep reduction.

Pivik and Foulkes [24]* have found that deprivation effects may show themselves not only in increased compensatory REM time, but in more intense dreaming (and greater eye movement activity) afterward as well. Similarly there has been observed some tendency for dreams from REM period deprivation awakenings to be more elaborate and more vivid [17, 18, 26]. These observations raise the possibility that the person's characteristic way of dreaming, to begin with (as more intense or less intense), may be a factor in determining the consequences of deprivation for him. That individual difference in usual quality of dreaming may in fact contribute to individual differences in the effects of deprivation is suggested by a recent study of Cartwright et al. [9].

Within the small group of subjects used, 3 subgroups were identified with regard to patterns of response to deprivation. One subgroup ("compensators") consisted of subjects who were field-independent and "good dreamers" (reflected in imaginative dreams and high base-night REM percent) and who were found in another study [7] to be well controlled under a hallucinatory drug (reflected in the absence of both hallucinatory experiences and deterioration of intellectual performance). In the deprivation period these subjects did not show insistent need for REM sleep, and in the recovery period they showed increased REM compensatory time with no EEG disturbance. These relatively differentiated persons, who make more effective use of the normal REM period for imaginative

* This study investigated deprivation effects within a single night. The effects observed were not found, however, in a later study using a cross-night design [14]. The difference in results may be a function of differences in methods used.

dreaming, seem better able to tolerate REM deprivation and to delay fantasy gratifications without ill effects, until the opportunity next arises.*†

A second subgroup ("disrupters") gave evidence of an insistent need for REM sleep during deprivation, and on recovery nights showed EEG disruption with no increase in REM time. Subjects in this group reacted to a hallucinatory drug with bizarre imagery and loss of intellectual competence; they were "poor dreamers" and likely to be field-dependent. These are then less differentiated persons, with poor controls, who seem to have a greater need for their ordinary REM sleep dreaming, are disturbed by its reduction, and do not seem able to "make up for it" effectively afterwards.

A third group ("substitutors") showed considerable fantasy content in dream reports given on REM awakenings during deprivation, with no increase in REM time on recovery nights. In this pattern, which may be typical of some field-independent persons, deprivation seems to be dealt with by more intense dreaming "on the spot."

These first findings on individual differences in the effects of REM sleep deprivation suggest that the question, "What are the effects of REM sleep deprivation?" may be profitably amended to read, "What are the effects for which kinds of persons?"

INDIVIDUAL DIFFERENCES IN DREAM CONTENT

Some of the very sparse evidence available on individual differences in dream content has already been cited. The review of additional evidence that follows is limited to studies which specifically related personality attributes or personality structure to features of dream content. A body of evidence on individual differences in

* A study by Cartwright and Monroe [8] provides additional evidence that field-independent persons who are "compensators," when blocked from fantasy expression, will "make up for it" at a later time.

† Fitting in with the Cartwright et al. finding that field-independent persons tend to have more imaginative dreams is the observation [4] that the dream reports of field-independent subjects contain a larger number of elements.

dream content has accumulated around the differentiation dimension.

Reflecting their developed sense of separate identity, more differentiated persons are likely to represent the self as an active participant in their dreams [13]. In this connection Lewis et al. [20] have observed that reporters are likely to represent the self as a protagonist of the action in their dreams, and they suggest that this contributes to better organization of the dream experience, thereby facilitating its recall. It may be that the more frequent presence of an active self in the dreams of differentiated persons provides still another basis for their better dream recall. The observed tendency of limitedly differentiated persons to dream more often about the experimenter [2, 35] may also be understood to reflect their limited sense of separate identity. In the presleep period, these persons are likely to be "caught up" by their relation with the experimenter, and this experience, so important to them, is carried over into the dream. Less differentiated persons are likely to dream about the experimenter openly, in his own proper person [2, 35]. This finding, taken together with the observation of Baekeland et al. [4] that relatively undifferentiated persons tend to represent elements from a presleep association period in their dreams as direct incorporations and differentiated persons in transformed fashion, suggests that openness or disguise of representation of waking experiences in dreams may be an important stylistic difference in dreaming between these two kinds of people.

Probably as a function of differences in structure of controls, more differentiated and less differentiated persons seem to differ in extent of anxiety in their dreams. Lewis et al. [20] found significantly higher REM density among their limitedly differentiated subjects, a characteristic frequently associated with intense, aroused dream content. The tendency of undifferentiated persons to dream more about the laboratory [20] may also reflect anxious concern about the experimental procedure. If proneness to anxious dreams is also a feature of the home dreams of less differentiated persons, it should make their home dreams more subject to repression; this lends credence to the possibility that repression is one factor in their being home nonreporters. Also relevant here is the observation [7, 9] that more differentiated persons are better able to tolerate delay in REM sleep dreaming, without disruptive effects, and to prevent fantasy intrusions and loss of reality contact under drugs, as they have been found able to prevent these during sensory isolation. Differentiated persons give evidence of more effectively operating controls in both these altered ego states as they do in the normal waking state.

REFERENCES

1. Antrobus, J. S., Dement, W. C., and Fisher, C. Patterns of dreaming and dream recall: An EEG study. *J. Abnorm. Soc. Psychol.* 69:341, 1964.
2. Baekeland, F. Personal communication.
3. Baekeland, F., and Lasky, R. The morning recall of REM-period reports given earlier in the night. *J. Nerv. Ment. Dis.* 147:570, 1968.
4. Baekeland, F., Resch, R., and Katz, D. Presleep mentation and dream reports. *Arch. Gen. Psychiat.* (Chicago) 19:300, 1968.
5. Berrien, F. K. A statistical study of dreams in relation to emotional stability. *J. Abnorm. Soc. Psychol.* 28:194, 1933.
6. Bone, R. N. Extroversion, neuroticism and dream recall. *Psychol. Rep.* 23:922, 1968.
7. Cartwright, R. D. Dream and drug-induced fantasy behavior. *Arch. Gen. Psychiat.* (Chicago) 15:7, 1966.
8. Cartwright, R. D., and Monroe, L. Personal communication.
9. Cartwright, R. D., Monroe, L., and Palmer, C. Individual differences in response to REM deprivation. *Arch. Gen. Psychiat.* 16:297, 1967.
10. Dement, W. C. The effect of dream deprivation. *Science* 131: 1705, 1960.
11. Desroches, H. F., and Kalman, B. D. The relationship between dream recall and symptoms of emotional instability. *J. Consult. Psychol.* 20:350, 1967.
12. Domhoff, B., and Gerson, A. Replication and critique of three studies on personality correlates of dream recall. *J. Consult. Psychol.* 31:431, 1967.
13. Eagle, C. Personal communication.

14. Foulkes, D., Pivik, T., Ahrens, J. B., and Swanson, E. M. Effects of "dream deprivation" on dream content: An attempted cross-night replication. *J. Abnorm. Psychol.* 73:403, 1968.
15. Goodenough, D. R. Some Recent Studies of Dream Recall. In H. A. Witkin and H. B. Lewis (Eds.), *Experimental Studies of Dreaming.* New York: Random House, 1967. Pp. 128–147.
16. Goodenough, D. R. The Phenomena of Dream Recall. In *Progress in Clinical Psychology.* New York: Grune & Stratton, 1969. Pp. 136–153.
17. Kales, A., Hoedemaker, F. S., Jacobson, A., and Lichtenstein E. L. Dream deprivation: An experimental approach. *Nature* (London) 204:1337, 1964.
18. Kales, A., and Jacobson, A. Mental Activity During Sleep: Recall Studies, Somnambulism and Effects of Rapid Eye Movement Deprivation and Drugs. In C. D. Clemente (Ed.), Physiological Correlates of Dreaming. *Exp. Neurol.* [Suppl. 4], Dec., 1967. Pp. 81–91.
19. Lachmann, F. M., Lapkin, B., and Handelman, N. S. The recall of dreams: Its relation to repression and cognitive control. *J. Abnorm. Soc. Psychol.* 64:160, 1962.
20. Lewis, H. B., Goodenough, D. R., Shapiro, A., and Sleser, I. Individual differences in dream recall. *J. Abnorm. Psychol.* 71: 52, 1966.
21. Linton, H. B. Personal communication.
22. McElroy, W. A. The frequency of dreams. *Bull. Brit. Psychol. Soc.* 3:91, 1952.
23. Orlinsky, D. E. Rorschach test correlates of dreaming and dream recall. *J. Project. Techn.* 30:250, 1966.
24. Pivik, T., and Foulkes, D. Dream deprivation: Effects on dream content. *Science* 153:1282, 1966.
25. Portnoff, G., Baekeland, F., Goodenough, D. R., Karacan, I., and Shapiro, A. Retention of verbal materials perceived immediately prior to onset of non-REM sleep. *Percept. Motor Skills* 22:751, 1966.
26. Sampson, H. Psychological effects of deprivation of dreaming sleep. *J. Nerv. Ment. Dis.* 143:305, 1966.
27. Schechter, N., Schmiedler, G. R., and Staal, M. Dream reports and creative tendencies in students of the arts, sciences, and engineering. *J. Consult. Psychol.* 29:415, 1965.
28. Schonbar, R. A. Some manifest characteristics of recallers and nonrecallers of dreams. *J. Consult. Psychol.* 23:414, 1959.
29. Schonbar, R. A. Some Dimensions of Sensitivity of Recallers

and Nonrecallers of Dreams. Paper read at Symposium on Dream Recall and Theory, Post Graduate Center for Mental Health, New York, 1964.

30. Schonbar, R. A. Differential dream recall frequency as a component of "life style." *J. Consult. Psychol.* 29:468, 1965.
31. Singer, J. L., and Schonbar, R. A. Correlates of daydreaming: A dimension of self-awareness. *J. Consult. Psychol.* 25:1, 1961.
32. Tart, C. T. Frequency of dream recall and some personality measures. *J. Consult. Psychol.* 26:467, 1962.
33. Witkin, H. A. Influencing Dream Content. In M. Kramer and R. M. Whitman (Eds.), *Dream Psychology and the New Biology of Dreaming*. New York: Thomas, 1969. Pp. 285–359.
34. Witkin, H. A., Dyk, R. B., Faterson, H. F., Goodenough, D. R., and Karp, S. A. *Psychological Differentiation*. New York: Wiley, 1962.
35. Witkin, H. A., and Lewis, H. B. The relation of experimentally induced presleep experiences to dreams: A report on method and preliminary findings. *J. Amer. Psychoanal. Ass.* 13:819, 1965.
36. Witkin, H. A., Lewis, H. B., Hertzman, M., Machover, K., Meissner, P. B., and Wapner, S. *Personality Through Perception*. New York: Harper, 1954.
37. Witkin, H. A., and Oltman, P. K. Cognitive style. *Int. J. Neurol.* 6:119, 1967.

Changes in Dream Content during a D-Period and during a Night

*Is there a discernible regular pattern of change in dream content during the course of a single D-period (REM period)? During the course of a single night? Across several nights?**

Stage REM Variability and Dreaming†

DAVID FOULKES

A number of experimental studies have attempted to relate preawakening REM period differences with differences in dreams subsequently retrieved upon arousals from such periods. At least three general lines of approach have been followed.

1. Variable lengths of preawakening stage REM have been correlated with dream report variables. Longer prearousal REM pe-

* The reader interested in this question may wish to refer also to a paper by Hartmann (p. 192).

† Supported by National Science Foundation Grant GS-2123.

riods, even with time of night held constant, appear to be associated with clearer and more vivid, active, and emotional dream reports, but the plausibility or sensibleness of dream content in relation to the dreamer's daily life is apparently unaffected by the length of the REM period [8, 25]. It is not clear from these findings whether dream experience during, for example, the twenty-fourth minute of the REM period differs systematically from that in the first, or whether the report on awakening from a long REM period simply encompasses a larger time span of material than does the report on awakening from a short REM period.

2. Dreams reported from different periods of stage REM during the night have been compared. Dreams from the first REM period of the night have generally been found to be less vivid than those reported from later REM periods [4, 8], but differences among subsequent REM periods are slight. Similar findings have been reported for successive periods of NREM sleep, the first such period being associated with less vivid mentation than all subsequent ones, and the latter differing little among themselves [17]. Studies of sequential dreams have suggested waxing and waning relative strengths of motives for drive expression and motives of drive defense across the night, leading to the absence of any simple time-of-night trends in dream content [15, 24].

3. In general, even where findings have been consistent across studies on either the length or ordinal position of an REM period in relation to dream content, effects have been small. A possible reason for this may be that short-term variability within a stage REM period is more significant than stage REM length per se or differences among successive periods of stage REM. A third experimental approach, therefore, has attempted to correlate momentary changes in stage REM physiology with dream content variables.

Studies of dream content in association with autonomic activity during stage REM have not always met with success [12], but some positive results have been reported. These include observations that penile detumescence is associated with anxiety-provoking dream content [7], that respiratory variability is correlated with dream intensity [11] and with goodness of dream recall [23], and that increased variability of heart rate and vasoconstriction is related to relatively emotional dream content [10].

Several investigations have been concerned with demonstrating that eye movement presence or direction is correlated with specific visual parameters of dream content (the so-called scanning hypothesis). Statistically significant correlations were observed between preawakening eye movement density and the active quality of reported dream experiences, and between eye movement direction and the directionality of visualization in such reports [2, 3, 22]. Doubts have been cast on the generality of these relationships, however, in view of the presence of REMs in neonates [21] and in the congenitally blind [9].

Perhaps the most exciting recent conceptualization in the psychophysiology of sleep is Moruzzi's [14] distinction between tonic and phasic aspects of stage REM. This distinction has focused attention upon the fact that there are relatively stable background characteristics of stage REM (e.g., its typical electroencephalograph pattern) upon which are intermittently superimposed momentary bursts of correlated physiological activation of a number of different structures and systems. The rapid eye movements that give stage REM its name are the most conspicuous phasic events in the intact human; in animal preparations, pontine-geniculo-occipital (PGO) spikes are a favored index of phasic activation. But the phasic activation of stage REM is not seen merely in the visual system: it has been reported [1], for instance, that reduced respiratory amplitude accompanies REM bursts during stage REM.

Moruzzi [14] suggested that phasic events during stage REM would be of particular interest to psychologists studying the dream. Aserinsky [1] developed the idea that ocularly motile segments of stage REM may be associated with a different "level" of dreaming than are ocularly quiet segments, but he seemingly despaired of obtaining precise data on the phenomenal accompaniments of phasic and nonphasic moments in stage REM.

Molinari et al. [13], however, have reported an investigation of the subjective correlates of brief periods of REM bursts or of ocular quiescence within stage REM. In contrast to earlier studies of specifically visual experiences that might be related to REMs, these authors interpreted REMs as a sign of overall phasic activation and were interested in nonvisual as well as visual correlates of the presence and absence of such activation. Their results indicated that REM bursts were accompanied by "primary visual experience," i.e., visual imagery experienced in an intellectually passive fashion and unaccompanied by cognitive elaboration, while periods of ocular quiescence within stage REM either were lacking in reported visual experience or produced reports of visual imagery that was being reflected upon or reacted to in a more intellectually active manner ("secondary cognitive elaboration").

From these results it appears that the phasic REM bursts in stage REM may provide the vivid, visual elements of the dream, while a more secondary-process activity in the interburst lulls links these elements together in a reasonably coherent dramatic unity. Observations by Ferguson et al. [5] of the behavior of cats showing drug-induced PGO spikes during wakefulness support the hypothesis that phasic activation is associated with a preemptory kind of internally generated visual experience.

The Molinari [13] findings suggest, then, that the major experiential correlate of REM sleep—the vivid, perceptual dream—may owe many of its most distinctive features to the phasic, rather than the tonic, aspects of stage REM. In parallel fashion, Ferguson et al. [6] had earlier proposed that it is phasic PGO spiking that is actually interfered with and compensated for in the apparent deprivation and recovery of tonic stage REM electroencephalograph patterns.

It thus seems likely that the phasic-tonic dichotomy will become a powerful tool for the interpretation of variations in dream content within stage REM. At the same time, this dichotomy can be useful in understanding earlier but more conceptually limited observations of stage REM dream variability—such as, for instance, that moment-to-moment (phasic) variability in autonomic functioning is apparently better related to dream intensity than is overall mean (tonic) level, that the frequency of REM bursts is related to the amount of activity in dream reports, and that the first REM period of the night, which Aserinsky [1] reports to contain only half as much time on a percentage basis actually occupied by REM, is associated with more conceptual and less visual dreaming than are subsequent episodes of stage REM.

Focusing upon phasic events in stage REM also promises a reconciliation with results [8, 20] indicating the occasional reporting of quite vivid dreams from NREM sleep. Neurophysiological phasic activity, as represented, for example, by the PGO spike, occurs in the cat during NREM sleep as well as during stage REM, albeit relatively less frequently. It may prove difficult to associate NREM phasic events with reports of mental activity, however, since the REM bursts used to index such events in stage REM are, by definition, absent. Nevertheless, Pivik and Dement [16] have reported momentary suppressions of submental electromyogram tracings during NREM sleep that may provide an externally recordable index of NREM phasic activity. Pompeiano [19] noted that momentarily augmented electromyogram suppressions in the cat are temporally related to other phasic events, including REMs. Pivik et al. [18] also have reported preliminary attempts at correlating possible NREM phasic indicators with variations in NREM dream reports, and this line of investigation seems to be a most promising approach to the "problem" of NREM dreaming.

REFERENCES

1. Aserinsky, E. Physiological Activity Associated with Segments of the Rapid Eye Movement Period. In S. S. Kety, E. V. Evarts, and H. L. Williams (Eds.), *Sleep and Altered States of Consciousness.* Baltimore: Williams & Wilkins, 1967.
2. Berger, R. J., and Oswald, I. Eye movements during active and passive dreams. *Science* 137:601, 1962.
3. Dement, W., and Wolpert, E. A. The relation of eye movements, body motility, and external stimuli to dream content. *J. Exp. Psychol.* 55:543, 1958.
4. Domhoff, B., and Kamiya, J. Problems in dream content study with objective indicators. III. Changes in dream content

throughout the night. *Arch. Gen. Psychiat.* (Chicago) 11:529, 1964.

5. Ferguson, J., Henriksen, S., Cohen, H., Hoyt, G., Mitchell, G., McGarr, K., Rubenson, D., Ryan, L., and Dement, W. The Effect of Chronic Administration of PCPA on the Behavior of Cats and Monkeys. Paper read at Association for the Psychophysiological Study of Sleep (APSS), Boston, 1969.
6. Ferguson, J., Henriksen, S., McGarr, K., Belenky, G., Mitchell, G., Gonda, W., Cohen, H., and Dement, W. Phasic event deprivation in the cat. *Psychophysiology* 5:238, 1968.
7. Fisher, C., Gross, J., and Zuch, J. Cycle of penile erection synchronous with dreaming (REM) sleep. *Arch. Gen. Psychiat.* (Chicago) 12:29, 1965.
8. Foulkes, D. Dream Reports from Different Stages of Sleep. University of Chicago Ph.D. Dissertation, 1960.
9. Gross, J., Byrne, J., and Fisher, C. Eye movements during emergent stage 1 EEG in subjects with lifelong blindness. *J. Nerv. Ment. Dis.* 141:365, 1965.
10. Hauri, P., and Van de Castle, R. L. Some Relationships Between Dream Content and Autonomic Functioning. Paper read at APSS, Boston, 1969.
11. Hobson, J. A., Goldfrank, F., and Snyder, F. Respiration and mental activity in sleep. *J. Psychiat. Res.* 3:79, 1965.
12. Knopf, N. A Study of Heart and Respiration Rates During Dreaming. University of Chicago M.A. Thesis, 1962.
13. Molinari, S., Foulkes, D., and Weisz, R. The Phenomenology of Different Sleep Periods: Psychological Correlates of Phasic and Tonic Events. Paper read at APSS, Boston, 1969.
14. Moruzzi, G. Discussion. In M. Jouvet (Ed.), *Aspects Anatomo-Fonctionnels de la Physiologie du Sommeil.* Paris: Centre National de la Recherche Scientifique, 1965.
15. Offenkrantz, W., and Rechtschaffen, A. Clinical studies of sequential dreams. I. A patient in psychotherapy. *Arch. Gen. Psychiat.* (Chicago) 8:497, 1963.
16. Pivik, T., and Dement, W. Amphetamine, REM deprivation, and K-complexes. *Psychophysiology* 5:241, 1968.
17. Pivik, T., and Foulkes, D. NREM mentation: Relation to personality, orientation time, and time of night. *J. Consult. Clin. Psychol.* 32:144, 1968.
18. Pivik, T., Halper, C., and Dement, W. Phasic Events and Mentation During Sleep. Paper read at APSS, Boston, 1969.
19. Pompeiano, O. The Neurophysiological Mechanisms of the

Postural and Motor Events During Desynchronized Sleep. In S. S. Kety, E. V. Evarts, and H. L. Williams (Eds.), *Sleep and Altered States of Consciousness.* Baltimore: Williams & Wilkins, 1967.
20. Rechtschaffen, A., Verdone, P., and Wheaton, J. Reports of mental activity during sleep. *Canad. Psychiat. Ass. J.* 8:409, 1963.
21. Roffwarg, H. P., Dement, W., and Fisher, C. Preliminary Observations of the Sleep-Dream Pattern in Neonates, Infants, Children and Adults. In E. Harms (Ed.), *Problems of Sleep and Dream in Children.* New York: Pergamon, 1964.
22. Roffwarg, H. P., Dement, W., Muzio, J., and Fisher, C. Dream imagery: Relationship to rapid eye movements of sleep. *Arch. Gen. Psychiat.* (Chicago) 7:235, 1962.
23. Shapiro, A., Goodenough, D. R., Biederman, I., and Sleser, I. Dream recall and the physiology of sleep. *J. Appl. Physiol.* 19: 778, 1964.
24. Trosman, H., Rechtschaffen, A., Offenkrantz, W., and Wolpert, E. Studies in psychophysiology of dreams. IV. Relations among dreams in sequence. *Arch. Gen. Psychiat.* (Chicago) 3:602, 1960.
25. Verdone, P. Variables Related to the Temporal Reference of Manifest Dream Content. University of Chicago Ph.D. Dissertation, 1963.

Temporal Patterns of Dreams

R. L. VAN DE CASTLE

Do dreams contain some recognizable temporal patternings or interrelationships? Before attempting to answer this frequently asked question, a review will be made of various studies that have investigated patterns of dream content occurring within two different temporal units: the individual dream and the multiple dreams of a single night.

TEMPORAL PATTERNS WITHIN A DREAM

Several definitional problems face the dream investigator when he attempts to study the organizational pattern of a single dream. How long does an individual dream last? If one accepts a simplistic equation that each separate REM period (D-period) indicates an individual dream, then a dream can last from a minute to over an hour. However, there is some evidence [3] that several dreams may occur within a separate REM period and that their termination is signalled by a gross body movement. How is the termination of a dream indicated psychologically? What are the appropriate criteria to be used to mark the point when the dreamer seems to have achieved cognitive closure on a topic? Is a dream limited to a description of events that occur within a single setting, e.g., a forest, or can a single dream encompass several changes of settings? There has not even been a start made toward reaching agreement on these slippery issues.

No studies have reported any statistical data about the patterns of organization that appear *within* a given dream such as whether the frequencies of characters, affects, colors, and so on, are greater at the beginning than at the conclusion of the same dream. There is some data showing differences *between* dream reports when the dreamer is awakened shortly after the REM period begins, when the REM period has lasted several minutes, and when it has just terminated.

The differences between "short REM" (1 minute or less of REM sleep) and "long REM" (9 minutes or more of REM sleep) awakenings indicated that dreamers rated long REM dreams as containing many more clearly visualized scenes and felt that long REM dreams were more active, dramatic, and emotional [9]. Dreams obtained after very brief REM periods during an REM deprivation study [7] were described as showing that day residue material appears in relatively undistorted form at REM period onset and that the content then gradually becomes transformed and distorted by primary process mechanisms as the REM periods increase in length. A very detailed analysis of the progression of imagery found in a single long REM dream has been provided by Foulkes [9]. Other studies [8] have suggested that when dreamers are frequently awakened so that REM periods never exceed 11 minutes in duration, these interrupted dreams were longer and more vivid with more drive and sensual themes present than in dreams obtained from REM periods which were allowed to continue until they were judged to be just coming to an end.

TEMPORAL PATTERNS WITHIN A NIGHT

Before the advent of electrophysiological dream studies, various speculations about the temporal patterning of dreams had been offered. Freud [11] had made the following general remarks:

> In interpreting . . . dreams occurring during the same night, the possibility should not be overlooked that separate and successive dreams of this kind may have the same meaning, and may be giving expression to the same impulses in different material. If so, the first of these homologous dreams to occur is often the more distorted and timid, while the succeeding one will be more confident and distinct.

French [10] felt that the organization of dreams depended upon the consequences of attempted solutions to conflicts in previous dreams. The sequential pattern may thus be one of alternating gratification and disturbance. This *focal conflict* theory would predict a continually changing motivational hierarchy as the result of the shifts caused by disturbing wishes versus the reactive wishes. Alexander [1], in discussing pairs of dreams, advanced the idea that the gratification of a wish might be obtained in a two-stage process to escape the notice of the censor. If the dreamer had a wish for forbidden behavior toward a particular person, the person could appear in the first dream along with the behavior disguised, while in the second dream the behavior would be represented, but the person disguised.

Since it is possible to obtain four or five dream reports per night by awakening subjects from REM periods, several investigators have sought to examine the relationships among multiple dreams of the same night. Dement and Wolpert [4] obtained 38 nights of sequential dreams from 8 subjects and reported that on only 7 of the 38 nights did they seem united by a common theme. Linkage "varied from single seemingly trivial details to occasions of similarity in plot." No formal classification was attempted to find continuity. The authors concluded that "for the most part, each dream seemed to be a self-contained drama relatively independent of the preceding or following drama."

Trosman et al. [19] utilized 2 subjects for a total of 32 nights of sequential dreams and observed that only once in these 32 nights was it possible to identify a readily apparent sequential relationship. Ratings on twelve dream dimensions were made by judges to assess whether these ratings varied with dream position during the night. No relationships were found, although it was pointed out that a few instances of "lateral homology" occurred. This term refers to between-night serial correspondences, e.g., on 2 nights some type of athletic event was mentioned in the first dream, a rejection by a friend occurred in the second dream, and a buried object was freed from the ground in the third dream. In the authors' opinion, more concrete imagery and primitive thinking emerged as the night progressed.

One psychotherapy patient who participated for 15 nights of mutiple awakenings was studied by Offenkrantz and Rechtschaffen [16]. The dreams of 2 nights were discussed in detail to support their notion that all of the dreams of a night were concerned either with the same conflict or with a limited number of conflicts. They interpreted their data in accordance with French's approach and as supporting the hypothesis of a parallel between the sequence of waking behavior and the defensive-adaptive ego activities in the dream sequence. They noted that earlier dreams of the night often dealt with the experimental situation and that on the 9 occasions when a geographical setting of childhood or adolescence was reported, such dreams occurred after 4:30 A.M. Verdone [20] has also reported that his 4 subjects rated their later dreams of the night as dealing with earlier time periods of the dreamer's life. Later dreams were also rated as more vivid and emotional by Verdone's dreamers.

Kramer et al. [15] obtained a total of 29 nights of multiple awakenings from 2 subjects. Only the 18 nights on which three or more dreams had been reported were used for classification. They divided dream series into three patterns. A sequential pattern was one showing an alternating ascendancy of disturbing and reactive motives and concomitant tension accumulation, discharge and regression pattern. This pattern occurred on 9 nights. A repetitive pattern, in which the conflict is restated in each of the dreams of the night, sometimes in different settings or with different degrees of concreteness, occurred on 6 nights. On 1 night, an intermediate pattern combining both sequential and repetitive aspects was reported. The other 2 nights were not classified.

In this same paper, some figures were given on the frequency with which multiple dreams were reported to one of the authors during analytic sessions. Material concerning dreams was available for 8 patients who had been in analysis an average of 343 hours (range 86–749 hours). At least one dream had been reported in 58 percent of the 2744 sessions. A single dream had been reported in 1092 sessions, two dreams in 291 sessions and three dreams in 201 sessions. Thus, on 31 percent of the occasions when patients reported dreams, their reports involved two or more dreams.

Domhoff and Kamiya [5] examined 219 dreams to discover whether there were any changes in objective dream scores that were related to REM position. An equal number of dreams (73) from each of the first 3 REM periods of the night had been obtained from 22 college students. REM periods 2 and 3 were very similar, although there were more room settings in REM period 2. The dreams of REM period 1 had fewer characters and fewer elements of an aggression-misfortune nature. Food and drink as well as building elements increased during the night and terrain settings decreased. Foulkes [9] also reports some data on the first 3 REM periods of 22 college students. These dreamers rated their own dreams on nine different dimensions. None of the ratings for the 3 REM periods differed very noticeably except that REM period 1 had less sensory imagery. There were some trends toward the dreamer's becoming more active and the dreams becoming more emotional and dramatic during the later REM periods.

Differences in REM period dream scores were also investigated by Hall and Van de Castle [13]. After several adjustment nights, 15 male college students were awakened once per night until 16 dreams had been obtained, four dreams from each of the first 4 REM periods. After this single series, subjects were also awakened for a multiple series. During the multiple series, subjects were awakened after every REM period for several nights. The total of 196 single and 273 multiple dreams were analyzed on several of the Hall–Van de Castle scales. These latter scales have been shown to possess high reliability, and normative material based upon their use with 1000 dreams is available [12]. In addition to laboratory dreams, 264 home dreams from these same subjects were also analyzed. Fewer differences between late dreams (REM periods 4–8) and home dreams were found than there were between early dreams (REM periods 1–3) and home dreams. Several differences were still present, however, as home dreams were shorter and had more aggressions and other types of outcomes while late REM period dreams had more single human characters and references to the experimental situation.

When dreams from the single series were compared against each other, no systematic differences were found among dreams collected from different REM periods. When the late REM periods (4–8) of the multiple series were compared with the early REM periods (1–3), it was found that later REM periods were longer, had more single female characters, and contained more misfortunes. Because of the large number of comparisons made, it is possible that some of these were only chance differences. A 12-item questionnaire about various dream properties had also been answered by subjects after each awakening. No differences were found among single dreams, but later REM periods for the multiple series were judged by the subjects to have more clarity and were easier to recall, and they were also rated as being more bizarre and containing more color elements. Herman et al. [14] also reported that color references increased as the night progressed.

When all single dreams were compared to all multiple dreams, utilizing the Hall–Van de Castle scales as well as the questionnaire replies, the multiple dreams were found to be very similar to single dreams. Experimenters may find some solace in these latter findings, because it appears that marked systematic bias in the direction of increased scores for hostility, misfortunes, and so on, is not introduced when a subject is repeatedly awakened throughout the night.

One of the factors which can contribute to the similarity of the dream scores from multiple awakenings is that some subjects experience rather enduring waking interests which are subsequently reflected in their dreams. Hall and Van de Castle [13] reported that 30 percent of the 50 lab dreams of a subject who was a sports car buff contained references to sports cars, 36 percent of the 36 dreams of an avid football fan dealt with football activities, another subject had airplanes in 32 percent of his 34 dreams, while 23 percent of the lab dreams of another subject dealt with situations involving the color guard to which he belonged.

With the increasing attention that has been paid to stages 2, 3, and 4 (NREM) mentation, some investigators have looked for linkages between REM and NREM content during the same night. Rechtschaffen et al. [17] report on two series they carried out to investigate the possible interrelatedness of mental activity during sleep. Their first series involved 2 subjects, known to be good NREM recallers, who were each studied for 3 nights and awakened from several REM and NREM periods. Their second series involved reexamining the reports from a previous study where REM and NREM awakenings had been made. They summarized their findings by stating that "the structure of sleep mentation, at least on the manifest level, is marked both by an apparent lack of observable connections between different episodes of mental activity on some nights and by the repetition of elements in varying contexts on other nights." These authors hypothesized that manifest elements tend to exert a "press" for repetition when recent preoccupations are particularly intense. Fisher et al. [6], in examining nightmares, offered the observation that "in some instances, the NREM nightmare and REM dreams of the same night appear to deal with the same content."

Before concluding this section, mention should also be made of efforts to study successive dreams through hypnotic suggestions. A leading proponent of the technique, Sacerdote [18], attempts to have patients produce a series of several hypnotic dreams within a single therapy session. If one is willing to assume an equivalence between hypnotic and nocturnal dreams, this approach could be a useful one to study changes in imagery and affect as a patient is instructed to experience a series of dreams about a selected topic.

SUMMARY

Our understanding of the time phasing as a dream unfolds is very incomplete. When some acceptable criteria for setting the temporal limits of a dream can be established, it will be possible to investigate the pattern of organization that exists among the various subunits within the overall dream. About all we know, so far, is that different types of dream reports are obtained from short and long REM period awakenings. The best guess regarding dream chronology is that the dream begins with a reexperiencing of the imagery that accompanied some recent significant emotional event. The dreamer then moves on to express related imagery that is sequentially triggered off in a fashion that corresponds to the associated conceptual hierarchy that has been developed by the dreamer in response to his unique life experiences.

Although more research attention has been devoted to studying the interrelationships of multiple dreams within the night, our current knowledge is still meager. It is apparent that there are no special characteristics necessarily associated with any specific REM period. The initial dream of the night is generally short, deals with situations from the preceding day, and is rather impoverished in content. As the night progresses, dreams become longer, more vivid and emotional, and they are easier to recall. There are some suggestions that more oral components and earlier time references appear during later dreams in a context where dream occurrences are more bizarre and visualized in greater chromatic detail. It could thus be said that psychological intensity builds up during the night as the dreamer continues to grapple with incompletely solved emotional problems that were highlighted during the recent past.

If the focus is placed upon manifest content, there are seldom any observable links between separate dreams of the night. Unless considerable information is available about the individual dreamer and his conceptual schemata, the continuity of successive manifest dreams is difficult to find. Once the dreams are available for post hoc interpretative speculations, it is generally possible to arrive at a synthesis that is satisfying for the speculating investigator, but conviction will not be forthcoming until advance predictions can be made and subsequently confirmed. Perhaps predictions of the sequence to be expected in REM period series can be offered on the basis of how an individual subject proceeds when he constructs a series of daytime hypnotic dreams.

It is probable that significant insights will be derived about the manner in which waking thoughts are transformed into nocturnal mentation when more detailed scrutiny is made of the interrelationships between NREM and REM reports. It may be that NREM elements, with their more apparent secondary process form of thinking, arise from preconscious processes, while REM elements are more traceable to unconscious determinants. The final fabric of dreams may be woven from the warp and woof interplay of these different forms of thinking.

REFERENCES

1. Alexander, F. Dreams in Pairs. In R. Fliess (Ed.), *The Psychoanalytic Reader,* Vol. I. New York: International Universities Press, 1948.

2. Dement, W., Kahn, E., and Roffwarg, H. The influence of the laboratory situation on the dreams of the experimental subject. *J. Nerv. Ment. Dis.* 140:119, 1965.
3. Dement, W., and Wolpert, E. The relation of eye movements, body motility, and external stimuli to dream content. *J. Exp. Psychology* 55:543, 1958.
4. Dement, W., and Wolpert, E. Relationships in manifest content of dreams occurring on the same night. *J. Nerv. Ment. Dis.* 126:568, 1958.
5. Domhoff, B., and Kamiya, J. Problems in dream content study with objective indicators. III. Changes in dream content throughout the night. *Arch. Gen. Psychiat.* (Chicago) 11:529, 1964.
6. Fisher, C., Byrne, J., and Edwards, A. NREM and REM nightmares. *Psychophysiology* 5:221, 1968.
7. Fisher, C., and Dement, W. Dream Development in Relation to NREM and REM Stages of Sleep. Paper read at the Association for the Psychophysiological Study of Sleep, Brooklyn, N.Y., 1963.
8. Fiss, H. The Need to Complete One's Dream. In J. Fisher and L. Breger (Eds.), *The Meaning of Dreams: Recent Insights from the Laboratory.* Research Symposium No. 3, California Department of Mental Hygiene, 1969.
9. Foulkes, D. *The Psychology of Sleep.* New York: Scribner's, 1966.
10. French, T. M. *The Integration of Behavior. I. Basic Postulates.* Chicago: University of Chicago Press, 1952.
11. Freud, S. *The Interpretation of Dreams.* New York: Science Editions, Wiley, 1961.
12. Hall, C., and Van de Castle, R. *The Content Analysis of Dreams.* New York: Appleton-Century-Crofts, 1966.
13. Hall, C., and Van de Castle, R. Studies of Dreams Reported in the Laboratory and at Home. Institute of Dream Research Monograph Series, No. 1. Santa Cruz, Cal., 1966.
14. Herman, J., Roffwarg, H., and Tauber, E. S. Color and other perceptual qualities of REM and NREM sleep. *Psychophysiology* 5:223, 1968.
15. Kramer, R., Whitman, R. M., Baldridge, B. J., and Lansky, L. M. Patterns of dreaming: The interrelationship of the dreams of a night. *J. Nerv. Ment. Dis.* 139:426, 1964.
16. Offenkrantz, W., and Rechtschaffen, A. Clinical studies of sequential dreams. I. A patient in psychotherapy. *Arch. Gen. Psychiat.* (Chicago) 8:497, 1963.

17. Rechtschaffen, A., Vogel, G., and Shaikun, G. Interrelatedness of mental activity during sleep. *Arch. Gen. Psychiat.* 9:536, 1963.
18. Sacerdote, P. *Induced Dreams.* New York: Vantage, 1967.
19. Trosman, H., Rechtschaffen, A., Offenkrantz, W., and Wolpert, E. Studies in psychophysiology of dreams. IV. Relations among dreams in sequence. *Arch. Gen. Psychiat.* (Chicago) 3:602, 1960.
20. Verdone, P. Temporal reference of manifest dream content. *Percept. Motor Skills* 20:1253, 1965.

The Nightmare

What have we learned about the nightmare?

REM and NREM Nightmares

CHARLES FISHER, JOSEPH V. BYRNE,
ADELE EDWARDS, AND EDWIN KAHN

Thirty-seven subjects (14 male, 23 female) with a history of nightmares were studied for 150 nights with continuous all-night EEG, EOG, heart and respiratory rates, and tape recordings. The subjects were allowed to sleep undisturbed until they spontaneously had a nightmare, when they were interviewed.

Spontaneous awakenings with some degree of anxiety from mild to severe panic occurred during all stages of sleep. Nightmares can be classified into three varieties: (1) The stage 4 arousal reaction nightmare is the most severe observed. It includes the night terror (pavor nocturnus) of children and adults, the latter often of lifelong duration and related to traumatic fixations of childhood. It also includes the nightmare of the traumatic neurosis that has its onset in adult life. (2) The REM anxiety dream which may be of all degrees of intensity and is frequently characterized by subjects as a nightmare. (3) Stage 2 arousals appear to be related to stage 4, but the degree of anxiety involved is much less.

STAGE 4 AROUSAL REACTION NIGHTMARE OR "INCUBUS ATTACK"

We confirm and extend the findings of Broughton [1] and Gastaut and Broughton [2]. Six subjects had 50 severe nightmares of this type, characterized by sudden cataclysmic breakthrough of panic with intense vocalization or bloodcurdling screams. This type of nightmare arises out of stage 4 sleep, mostly during the first two NREM periods, 70 percent occurring during the first NREM. With the scream, the subject passes into an arousal reaction: alpha rhythm, dissociated, confused, unresponsive, hallucinating, hypermotile, and somnambulistic with intense autonomic discharge, heart rate more than doubling, with increases up to 90–100 beats per minute—e.g., one subject showed an increase from 64 to 152 per minute. There is increased rate and amplitude of respiration. Note that there is no increase in heart and respiratory rate in the minutes just prior to the onset of the nightmare.

Broughton [1] suggested that subjects with nightmare show heightened physiological responses all through sleep, e.g., increased heart rate during stage 4 prior to the attack. We have not been able to confirm this. On the contrary, average heart rate during stage 4 sleep in our nightmare subjects was considerably lower than normal, around 54 per minute as opposed to the normal rate of 60 [3, 4]. Several subjects ran heart rates as low as 44 or 48 per minute.

Other findings indicate decreased physiological activation during stage 4 prior to onset of the nightmare. For example, the length of time in stage 4 prior to outbreak of the nightmare and the quality of stage 4 sleep (higher percentage of delta waves) was found to correlate significantly with intensity of the nightmare: The longer the period of stage 4 preceding outbreak of the nightmare, the greater the postarousal increase in heart rate, the latter representing a measure of the intensity of the nightmare. For several subjects, respiratory rate and variability tended to decrease slightly during stage 4 just prior to the outbreak of the nightmare. Thus longer and better quality stage 4 sleep and slightly slower and less variable respiration were associated with the more intense nightmares. These findings suggest that the more severe the nightmare the deeper the sleep, but we are aware of the ambiguities of the concept of sleep depth.

The stage 4 arousal nightmare is not really a dream but a pathological formation that occurs in a postarousal stage in which the subject may be hallucinating and somnambulistic. Its severity is determined by certain physiological conditions, e.g., deeper stage 4 sleep promoting ego regression, dissolution of controls and defenses, and eruption of intense traumatic anxiety. Contrary to Broughton [1], who reported nearly complete amnesia for stage 4 nightmare content, we recovered some content in 83 percent of 50 stage 4 nightmares. We believe that this content plays a role in instigating the nightmare.

In several subjects, however, severe nightmares were produced simply by sounding a buzzer during stage 4 sleep. As with the spontaneous nightmare, we discovered that the more severe the buzzer arousal nightmare, the deeper the sleep preceding its onset, as indicated by longer periods of good delta. Thus a factor of external stimulation may be involved in the onset of the stage 4 nightmare; this finding can be brought into relation with Broughton's formulation about the arousal reaction. This matter needs further investigation.

REM ANXIETY DREAMS AND NIGHTMARES

Eleven subjects had 22 spontaneous awakenings (with dream content) from REM sleep in which mild to moderate anxiety was manifest. For each subject, heart and respiratory rates for intervals prior to these anxious REM awakenings were compared with similar control intervals during REM sleep on a different night when no spontaneous awakenings occurred. Much to our surprise, in 18 of the 22 REM anxiety awakenings, heart and respiratory rates did not differ from the same subjects' control rates. In the remaining 4 instances, in which considerable fright was associated with dream content, there were physiological changes during the REM period. For example, one subject reported a very frightening dream in which she was being attacked by large cats; heart rate increased from 76 to 92 and respiration became shallow and rapid, increasing from 15 to 30 per minute. Thus in a few instances, when anxiety passed a certain threshold, the REM dream was associated with cardiorespiratory increase. For the vast majority of the anxiety dreams reported there appeared to be a dissociation between the subjectively experienced anxiety and autonomic discharge.

The REM anxiety dream is mostly desomatized; that is, there is an absence of or decrease in autonomic discharge that mutes anxiety. This may constitute a regulating mechanism blunting affect and guarding the subject's REM sleep. The REM dream, we have found, can deal with the same conflict material as the stage 4 nightmare but without anxiety or disruptive arousal. Even when heart rate changes occur during the REM anxiety dream, they are minimal compared to the great increases during the stage 4 nightmare. In the former, mild increases of 16–20 beats per minute occur after awakening, but these appear for the most part to be caused by body movement rather than anxiety, while in the stage 4 nightmare, increases of 90–100 per minute may develop. In short, while the stage 4 nightmare is characterized by full resomatization and uncontrolled anxiety, the REM nightmare is associated with desomatization and controlled anxiety.

STAGE 2 NIGHTMARES

We have observed a relatively small number of arousals with varying degrees of anxiety during stage 2. These mostly occur in subjects who also have stage 4 nightmares. The degree of anxiety is moderate in intensity and the cardiorespiratory response is somewhat greater than that observed in the REM anxiety dream. The content of the stage 2 nightmare also is intermediate between the types of content that occur in the REM anxiety and the stage 4 nightmare. The latter almost always is associated with a single frightening scene (falling, being crushed, choking) that develops simultaneously with the scream or other vocalization.

Additionally, a secondary content may be elaborated during the hallucinatory phase centering around the physiological response, such as increased heart rate or the subject's finding himself alone and in the dark. In the majority of stage 4 nightmares, murderous aggression is turned on the subject but sometimes aggression is turned outward toward the object. The terror experienced is related to persecutory threats involving death. The REM anxiety dream on the average occurs after a REM period has been ongoing for 20 minutes and develops out of a prolonged and elaborate dream.

Primary process mechanisms are utilized in all three types of nightmare. The manifest content of many REM nightmares appears as threatening as some of the stage 4 nightmares, but the degree of fright and the concomitant physiological response is very much less.

REFERENCES

1. Broughton, R. J. Sleep disorders: Disorders of arousal? *Science* 159:1070, 1968.
2. Gastaut, H., and Broughton, R. J. A Clinical and Polygraphic Study of Episodic Phenomena During Sleep. In J. Wortis (Ed.), *Recent Advances in Biological Psychiatry,* Vol. VII. New York: Plenum Press, 1965.
3. Shapiro, A., Goodenough, D. R., Biederman, I., and Slesar, I. Dream recall and the physiology of sleep. *J. Appl. Physiol.* 19: 778, 1964.
4. Snyder, F., Hobson, J. A., Morrison, D. F., and Goldfrank, F. Changes in respiration, heart rate, and systolic blood pressure in human sleep. *J. Appl. Physiol.* 19:417, 1964.

The Incubus Attack

ROGER J. BROUGHTON

Contrary to expectations, it was found [1, 4] that the classic incubus attack of adults, like pavor nocturnus of children, enuresis nocturna, and sleep-walking, begins in slow wave sleep, not in REM sleep. This finding has recently been confirmed by Fisher et al. [2, 3]. Discussion now reigns as to whether causal psychological activity recurs preceding each attack and generates it, or whether previous psychological factors produce physiological changes which predispose to the attack during arousals which can be provoked by other factors.

The studies agree essentially upon all of the subjective, behavioral, and polygraphically recorded features of the incubus episode.

Subjective features. Subjective features of the incubus attack are intense anxiety, palpitations, respiratory oppression or choking, feelings of paralysis (perhaps only difficulty in breathing), sensation of impending doom, and hallucinations limited to a single scene. These sudden terrifying events are quite different from the true terrifying dream or dream anxiety attack, also referred to as a nightmare by both lay and medical persons. The latter culminates a prolonged, organized, and developing dream sequence and occurs in REM sleep. The clinical differences between the two were recognized by Jones [5].

Objective features. A scream, often harrowing, signals an incubus episode. Other indications are motor activity, sometimes very intense and occasionally leading to sleep-walking; initial confusion, incoherency, and unreactivity, the episode seemingly having to "run itself out" before full contact can be made.

Polygraphic features. Onset in slow wave sleep, usually of the first cycle, with immediate desynchronization of the EEG occurs during the episode, as do marked tachycardia (the heart rate often doubling and the EKG sometimes showing extrasystoles); abrupt respiratory changes with initial expiration and the explosive cry, then tachypnea or apnea; decrease in skin resistance; eye movements; and a marked increase in muscle tone.

A number of other features have also been noted, such as a decrease in incidence in the laboratory compared to the home. But none of these are crucial in deciding upon the precipitating mechanism at the time of the attack. Moreover, many problems of analysis are present in such studies. The mental content of the attack might be determined in toto by the concurrent physiological alterations (somatization); some reported features might have a postsleep genesis; amnesic effects of arousal might make relevant mental activity difficult or impossible to retrieve; the single fragmentary scene might be produced by activation of sensory or memory systems during the arousal or even represent a return to a waking conflict or obsession now perceived through a clouded sensorium. Most of these possibilities have been considered in a recent review [1], as have the two main psychogenic mechanisms which could precipitate the attacks at the time of their occurrence, i.e., causal ongoing NREM mentation becoming intensely anxiogenic, or the sudden release of emotional conflicts which otherwise are suppressed, due to a lowering of protective mechanisms in the deepest stages of slow wave sleep.

Because the attacks generally occur during arousals from slow wave sleep in the first or second cycle, are associated with a marked increase in axial muscle tone from their very onset, and do not appear to alter the distribution of REM sleep throughout the night, the possibility that psychological or physiological components of REM sleep are the basis of the attacks can safely be rejected.

DISORDER OF AROUSAL

I have suggested elsewhere that the transient incubus attack, like the other slow wave sleep episodes, might be considered as a *disorder of arousal* and be due to unresolved conflicts producing physiological changes of a type which predispose to the attack pattern during arousal, particularly slow wave sleep arousal. The main reasons for preferring such a precipitating mechanism to a recurrent anxious dream, or other hypotheses implying an immediately preceding psychogenic origin, are the following:

1. Physiological changes are in fact present at the time of the attack which can explain most, if not all, of its symptoms (somatization): i.e., marked tachycardia and sometimes extrasystoles giving intense anxiety; increased muscle tone maximum in the body axis—perhaps the main cause of the sudden expiration and explosive cry; along with respiratory changes, leading as well to feelings of suffocation, choking, and possibly paralysis.

2. The attacks occur mainly during the normal cyclic slow wave arousal and appear to be a marked intensification of it, particularly of the cardiorespiratory aspects. On the other hand, ongoing mental activity might be expected to develop to a crescendo at any time in NREM sleep and not during a particular, relatively brief and recurrent component of it.

3. The onset in slow wave sleep allows a maximum increase in vigilance and in level of cardiorespiratory functions, as these are lowest at this time. The latitude allowed arousal is therefore the greatest possible. Interestingly, the incidence of the attacks decreases with age in parallel to a diminution of the amount of slow wave sleep.

4. The very striking abruptness of onset of the attack with massive alterations in cerebral, autonomic, and motor status does not particularly suggest culmination of ongoing NREM mental activity, which might be expected to produce a more progressive activation.

5. There are physiological changes independent of the attack of a type which would predispose to it during any arousal. In particular, incomplete arousal, whether spontaneous or provoked by mild stimuli, which does not lead to awakening or to an attack, is associated with a greater than usual rise in heart rate, the cardiac status having been described as "hyperreactive." It may well be

that muscle tone also augments disproportionately, although this has not yet been determined.

6. Perhaps most importantly, exteroceptive stimuli delivered in slow wave sleep may precipitate awakening and the attacks. It seems improbable that such stimuli would be repeatedly delivered at just the precise moment when independent ongoing mental activity was about to lead to an attack. It therefore strongly suggests that it is the altered arousal per se which triggers them.

Alteration in Arousal Mechanism as Cause of Attacks

Rather than hypothesizing recurrent traumatic mentation in slow wave sleep, it appears more parsimonious and more in keeping with the evidence to opt for an alteration in the arousal mechanism which, however, is manifestly of psychogenic origin. Such a combination is certainly not without parallel in wakefulness. Perhaps a useful comparison might be the enhanced startle response seen in some anxious individuals and which varies in incidence and intensity with their anxiety. In this instance, the psychogenic basis of the disorder would not be questioned (even although a genetic or acquired physiological predisposition might also be of importance), nor would the role of exteroceptive stimuli in precipitating the startle episode. The rather longlasting confusion of awakening from slow wave sleep seen in subjects with nightmares, of course, makes the situation more complex. But the comparison may still be valid.

A basic psychogenic etiology combined with physiological precipitation does not, of course, negate the possibility that some of the mental activity described during awakening after the attack may be related to the individual's underlying conflicts, either directly or symbolically. Nor might one be surprised to retrieve related mental activity in wakefulness, REM dream reports, or reports following NREM sleep awakenings.

The basic issue is not whether individuals suffering from the classic nightmare attack have had intensely traumatic experiences in their past or have unresolved emotional conflicts with intense anxiety retrievable in various states of consciousness, but rather whether these very striking incubus episodes represent recurrent anxious mentation or a psychosomatic arousal disorder. The evidence at hand appears to favor the latter.

REFERENCES

1. Broughton, R. J. Sleep disorders: Disorders of arousal? *Science* 159:1070, 1968.
2. Fisher, C., Byrne, J. V., and Edwards, A. NREM and REM nightmares. *Psychophysiology* 5:221, 1968.
3. Fisher, C., Byrne, J. V., and Edwards, A. NREM and REM Nightmares. Paper read at the Association for the Psychophysiological Study of Sleep, Boston, 1969.
4. Gastaut, H., and Broughton, R. A clinical and polygraphic study of episodic phenomena during sleep. *Recent Advances Biol. Psychiat.* 8:197, 1965.
5. Jones, E. *On the Nightmare*. London: Hogarth, 1949. Pp. 1–349.

A Note on the Nightmare

ERNEST HARTMANN

Nightmares, according to recent evidence, are horses of at least two very different colors: a heavy, shapeless black beast crushing the sleeper's chest as he awakens in terror, and a more ordinary reddish mare galloping off with the sleeper on a frightening and yet relatively familiar dream journey. The first is the classic incubus attack occurring early in the night during arousal from slow-wave sleep, described by Broughton and his group [2, 5]. The second is the frightening dream, the D-state nightmare or REM nightmare usually occurring later during the night, described by Fisher's group [3].

This note merely documents the frequency, or rather infrequency, of these nightmares in several thousand nights of laboratory sleep study and presents a hypothesis on the conditions giving rise to the D-state nightmare.

Our laboratory has studied a total of about 2000 nights of sleep in human subjects. Some of these involved artificial awakenings, or unusual pharmacological or medical conditions, to be discussed later; but in over 500 nights of sleep in normal adult subjects, sleeping without medication for uninterrupted nights in the laboratory, only once did a subject report a spontaneous awakening due to a nightmare. This was a "long frightening dream" type of nightmare from a D-period awakening and occurred in a young woman just before the onset of menses. No incubus attacks were reported in this group. The subjects were on good terms with the experimenters and were very willing to report any unusual event during the night, so that we believe any nightmares recalled by the subjects would have been recorded. This is borne out by the fact that a number of nightmares were recalled under other laboratory conditions, to be discussed.

In several studies normal subjects in our laboratory were awakened 5 or 10 minutes after the onset of a D-period at various times during the night. Such awakenings tended to result in relatively banal dream reports, and in over 400 such awakenings there has not been a single report which could be called a nightmare. I have consulted four additional laboratories which frequently study subjects after awakenings of this kind, and there is universal agreement that a nightmare or frightening dream after such laboratory awakenings is almost never found: from approximately 5000 awakenings in these laboratories, not over 10 minutes after the beginning of a D-period, I have had reports of at the very most two frightening dreams which might possibly qualify as nightmares.

Thus in relatively normal adults, in the sleep laboratory at least, it appears that nightmares are extremely rare, either as spontaneous interruptors of sleep, or as reports from the usual experimenter-induced awakenings 5 or 10 minutes after the onset of a D-period.*

* It should be kept in mind that the subjects studied in sleep laboratories do not represent a cross-section of the population at large. First of all, young

In our studies involving uninterrupted nights in pathological conditions or with pharmacological agents, the situation is different: There were 11 identifiable nightmares producing spontaneous awakenings in about 500 nights. All, with one questionable exception, were of the D-state nightmare type. Three of these occurred in manic-depressive patients. One occurred 20 minutes after the onset of a D-period marked by a very high eye movement density and few body movements. One was from a night containing only 2½ hours sleep of which one-third was taken up by a long D-period ending in an awakening. A sleeping medication—Doriden—had been discontinued two days before. One episode was in a night with a great deal of awakening and interruption during which the subject changed from depression to mania; the exact onset of the nightmare was not clear. One definite nightmare occurred in a cardiac patient being studied for possible arrhythmia during the night. She had a D-state nightmare at 6:00 A.M., 50 minutes after the onset of an active D-period associated with many eye movements and with some ventricular extrasystoles. In drug studies, several nightmares were reported by our subjects both in and out of the laboratory one or two nights after the discontinuation of sleeping medication and antidepressant medication; this is consistent with reports by Kales et al. [11, 12].

Thus in our sleep laboratory the incubus attack is a rare or almost nonexistent phenomenon, even under unusual conditions, but the D-nightmare or REM nightmare is not quite so rare, and when it occurs my impression is that it awakens the subject out of a long active D-period, often at a time when D-pressure could be expected to be high. The only nightmare, mentioned above, reported by an apparently normal subject sleeping an uninterrupted night in the laboratory, awakened a young woman from a 25-minute D-period just one day before the onset of her menstrual period, at a time when

adults, especially male college students, are overrepresented in the sleep laboratory. More importantly, "normal" subjects were studied, which usually meant some psychiatric or psychological test screening, varying with the laboratory and the study. In some studies a person reporting a history of nightmares might have been excluded for that reason, although I recall no such exclusions in my own studies.

our studies [9] indicate that D-pressure may be high, and when D-pressure was certainly high in this specific case, as evidenced by her showing a 32 percent D-time—the highest in her 27 laboratory nights—and an extremely high mean eye movement density of 10 eye movements per page.

The fact that children, who appear to have an unusually great need for D-time, typically report far more nightmares than adults also supports the notion that nightmares occur in situations characterized by high D-pressure.

Interestingly, a number of adults who had never recalled nightmares under ordinary conditions reported to me that they had nightmares as they were recovering from a recent attack of Asian flu. I have heard many similar anecdotal reports of nightmares after a few days of febrile illness. Since fever and febrile illness appear to reduce D-time and to produce D-deprivation [13], it is likely that the nights when nightmares are reported are periods of recovery from deprivation, which would be associated with high D-pressure and long D-periods.

Nightmares are frequently reported in the period of withdrawal from addiction to barbiturates, amphetamines, or alcohol [6, 8, 15, 16], a time when high D-pressure and long D-periods are found; nightmares are seldom reported when the subject begins taking these substances. On the other hand, reserpine has often been reported to produce nightmares soon after the initiation of medication [1, 19, 20]. We have shown [10] that reserpine is unique among clinically used agents in that it actually increases D-time in man. Therefore nightmares again are associated with periods when D-time and D-pressure are high—during medication with reserpine and after discontinuation of medication with many other drugs. Poisoning by long-lasting anticholinesterase compounds has recently been shown to produce an increased D-time in man [17], this condition has previously been associated with frequent nightmare reports [7].

I am suggesting then that long D-periods and increased D-pressure are often associated with nightmares. However, there may be additional relevant factors involved in pathological or pharmacological conditions, since recovery from simple mechanically produced D-deprivation seems to result in nightmare reports less frequently than the various pathological deprivation conditions. The difference could be merely that in the latter conditions there is a greater tendency to awaken than in the situation of a healthy normal subject generally sleeping very soundly during recovery from mechanical D-deprivation.

Studies by Foulkes and others [4, 18] indicate that within a D-period there is a certain development of content so that awakenings further into the D-period produce more vivid, bizarre, and emotional content. In my experience reports from very long (> 30 min.) D-periods frequently contain at least some anxiety. I should like to suggest that every D-period as it lengthens (toward 20, 30, 40, or more minutes) develops an increasing possibility of producing a nightmare report upon awakening. This possibility will be strengthened when D-pressure is especially high, probably producing intensive vivid content and physiological activation, and when physical or psychological factors are present which may both stimulate stressful material in the dream and increase the possibility of awakening.

REFERENCES

1. Azima, H. The possible dream inducing capacity of the whole root of rauwolfia serpentina. *Canad. Psychiat. Ass. J.* 3:47, 1958.
2. Broughton, R. J. Sleep disorders: Disorders of arousal? *Science* 159:1070, 1968.
3. Fisher, C., Byrne, J. V., and Edwards, A. NREM and REM nightmares. Paper read at the Association for the Psychophysiological Study of Sleep (APSS), Boston, 1969. Abstract in *Psychophysiology* 6:252, 1969.
4. Foulkes, D. *The Psychology of Sleep*. New York: Scribner's, 1966.
5. Gastaut, H., and Broughton, R. A clinical and polygraphic study of episodic phenomena during sleep. *Recent Advances Biol. Psychiat.* 8:197, 1965.
6. Greenberg, R., and Pearlman, C. Delirium tremens and dreaming. *Amer. J. Psychiat.* 124:37, 1967.

7. Grob, D., Harvey, A., Langworthy, O., and Lilienthal, J. The administration of di-isopropyl fluorophosphate (DFP) to man. *Bull. Hopkins Hosp.* 81:257, 1947.
8. Gross, M. M., and Goodenough, D. R. Sleep Disturbances in the Acute Alcoholic Psychoses. In *Psychiatric Research Report 24*, American Psychiatric Association, 1968. Pp. 132–147.
9. Hartmann, E. The D-state (dreaming sleep) and the menstrual cycle. *J. Nerv. Ment. Dis.* 143:406, 1966.
10. Hartmann, E. Reserpine: Its effect on the sleep-dream cycle in man. *Psychopharmacologia* (Berlin) 9:242, 1966.
11. Kales, A., Ling Tan, T., Scharf, M., Kales, J., Malmstrom, E., Allen, C. and Jacobson, A. Sleep Patterns with Sedative Drugs. Paper read at APSS, Denver, 1968.
12. Kales, A., Scharf, M., Ling Tan, T., Jacobson, A., Allen, C., and Malmstrom, E. Summary of Short-term Effects of Hypnotics on Sleep Patterns. Paper read at APSS, Boston, 1969.
13. Karacan, I., Wolff, S. M., Williams, R. L., Hursch, C. J., and Webb, W. B. The effects of fever on sleep and dream patterns. *Psychosomatics* 9:331, 1968.
14. Lewis, S. A., Oswald, I., Evans, J. I., and Akindele, M. O. Heroin and Human Sleep. Paper read at APSS, Boston, 1969. Abstract in *Psychophysiology* 6:259, 1969.
15. Oswald, I. Drugs and sleep. *Pharmacol. Rev.* 20:273, 1968.
16. Oswald, I., and Priest, R. G. Five weeks to escape the sleeping-pill habit. *Brit. Med. J.* 4:317, 1965.
17. Stoyva, J., and Metcalf, D. Sleep Patterns Following Chronic Exposure to Cholinesterase-inhibiting Organophosphate Compounds. Paper read at APSS, Denver, 1968. Abstract in *Psychophysiology* 5:206, 1968.
18. Verdone, P. Variables Related to the Temporal Reference of Manifest Dream Content. University of Chicago Ph.D. Dissertation, 1963.
19. Wilkins, R. Clinical usage of rauwolfia alkaloids including reserpine. *Ann. N.Y. Acad. Sci.* 59:36, 1954.
20. Winsor, T. Human pharmacology of reserpine. *Ann. N.Y. Acad. Sci.* 59:61, 1954.

Effects of Sleep and Dream Research on the Handling of Dreams in Psychoanalytic Practice

---

*Has the dream in practice turned out to be the royal road to the unconscious? Has the psychophysiological research on sleep and dreaming had any effect on the way dreams are handled in psychoanalytic practice? On dream interpretation?**

The Royal Road to the Unconscious: Changing Conceptualizations of the Dream

HELEN B. LEWIS

The *unconscious* is a shorthand term for a complicated set of repression-connected events which Freud [13] hypothesized to be powerful enough to instigate dreaming during normal sleep and neurotic symptoms under less clearly understood awake conditions. The unconscious described the activation of a repression-connected psychical system dominated by a requirement for affect (instinct)

* The reader interested in this question may wish to refer also to papers by Jones (p. 221) and Cartwright (p. 227).

discharge. When this psychical system was stirred before sleep by some daytime events connected to it (by feeling congruence or verbal bridge), dreaming resulted, as a compromise-formation of consciousness. This compromise-formation served to express and disguise repressed childhood experience, while allowing the person to continue sleep. During waking conditions, the repression-connected psychical system was particularly likely to gain the field when the person was coping with "strangulated affect." On these occasions neurotic symptoms resulted, following the same model of compromise-formation or "primary-process" transformations of repressed experience which could be discerned in dreams.

Freud [13] thus used the same set of repression-connected events as a model for the explication of dreaming and of neurotic symptoms. Specifically, he assumed that the "psychical mechanism employed by neuroses . . . is present already in the normal structure of the mental apparatus" (p. 607). One difference between dreams and neurotic symptoms was that the circumstances resulting in the arousal of the psychical system were clearer in dreams than in neurotic symptom formation. But since dreaming was an everyday, non-pathological model of the functioning of the unconscious, it was the royal road to the unravelling of "what is suppressed (which) continues to exist in normal people as well as abnormal" (ibid., p. 608).

CONSEQUENCES OF DISCOVERY OF REM PERIODS

The discovery of cyclically recurring stage 1-EEG-REM periods (D-periods) accompanied by reports of dreaming throws doubt upon Freud's notion of the unconscious as the cause or instigator of dream episodes. It does not seem reasonable to suppose that REM periods are instigated by the day's residue connected to the evoked unconscious. If this were the case, for example, the number of REM periods per night or the time spent in REM sleep should be positively related to the degree of the preceding day's emotional upset. Instead, the time spent in REM sleep is, if anything, negatively related to the amount of preceding daytime stress [1]. REM periods, during which dreams occur, seem to be a function of some unknown biological factor rather than a signal of the evoked unconscious.

The unconscious had explained three sets of phenomena—dream instigation, dream content, and dream forgetting—in a single, elegant construct. One consequence of the divorce between the unconscious and dream instigation is that the unconscious is also no longer the single explanation for dream content and dream forgetting. One way of recasting the role of the unconscious is to assume that, although it is not powerful enough to instigate REM episodes, it is a prepotent force which is likely to invade ready-waiting REM dream time, just as its activation can intrude symptoms in waking life. There is evidence [1], for example, that REM periods following the showing of a stress film before sleep show greater REM density than REM periods following neutral films. There is also evidence from several studies that REM period density is positively associated with such dream content features as bizarreness, visual imagery [20], emotionality [28], aggression [17], and dream intensity [22]. REM periods which show greater REM density and more charged dream content may be those which have been invaded by the unconscious.

In this formulation, however, it is apparent that some but not all REM dreams may be invaded by the unconscious, unless one postulates a special affinity between REM dreams and the unconscious such that REM dreaming time *always* picks up an *always* activated unconscious. If one adopts the postulate that some but not all dream episodes are invaded by the unconscious, then it follows that the content of these dreams should be different from the content of dream episodes not so invaded. We may postulate, further, that only some dreams, i.e., those invaded by the unconscious, should be particularly vulnerable to loss for that reason. In this formulation, the dream road to the unconscious has lost one of its "royal" characteristics, i.e., exclusive connection.

The formulation that the activated unconscious is a prepotent stimulus fits the common clinical observation that the unconscious can disturb sleep. One mode of disturbed sleep which has been studied in the laboratory is "light sleep." Light sleepers, as Zimmerman [34] has shown, report dreams on 71 percent of their NREM awakenings, as compared to 21 percent of NREM awakening dream reports from "deep sleepers." Light sleepers (chosen for a relatively low threshold of arousal) had higher pulse rates, respiration rates, and body temperature than deep sleepers, and they seemed to be dreaming almost all night. This finding suggests that the unconscious may instigate some NREM dreaming, via its instigation of some light sleep.

Studies using the EEG monitoring techniques have shown that dreams occur at sleep onset [10, 29]. These findings, together with Zimmerman's findings on light sleepers, remind us that some dreams may be the products of the sleep-waking borderline state, perhaps of the "labile balance" which Silberer [25] postulated was the time of hallucinations. Some of these dreams might be instigated by the unconscious, as well; and the unconscious may be the instigator of some borderline states.

In compensation for the loss of a single system of explanation for dreams, the discovery of REM periods makes it more feasible to collect dreams as they happen and to perform experimental manipulations of the emotional circumstances influencing them. It has already been possible, for example, to retrieve REM period dreams following presleep stress and neutral film showings [11, 33]. The results of a systematic study of the effects of stress and neutral films on dreaming are now being analyzed [31].

Another kind of study has made use of life circumstances which produce stress, such as needing surgery [18] or participating in a group therapy session [16], to study the effects of these stress conditions on dream content. Still another kind of study has shown that the hallucinatory content of dreams is increased when the patient is in an acute phase of psychosis, while the communicative content of dreams increases with patient's clinical improvement [12]. In still another kind of study [2] the influence of stress and neutral films on an experimentally induced hypnagogic state was studied, and the content of ensuing dreams could be traced from the presleep events through the reverie state and into the dream.

Another consequence of the discovery of REM period dreaming is that it fosters the study of psychophysical correspondences. One example of the kind of issue which is being pursued in our study [31] using stress and neutral films is the correspondence between such affective characteristics of dream content as anxiety, depression, and aggression, and such physiological characteristics as REM period respiration, eye movement density, and arousal threshold.

EFFECTS OF CHANGED CONCEPTUALIZATIONS ON PSYCHOANALYTIC PRACTICE

A change in conceptualizing the cause of dreaming is likely to affect psychoanalytic practice with respect to dreams in at least four different ways: (1) in the concept of a "need to dream"; (2) in the concept of manifest and latent dream content; (3) in the interpretation of dream forgetting; and (4) in a concept of dreaming as an ego function.

Need to Dream: The Function of Dreaming

A corollary of the hypothesis that dreaming was instigated by the reactivation of the unconscious was that the need to dream was a sporadic affair, occurring only when the unconscious threatened to interrupt sleep. We now know that dreaming during the REM period is part of a "third state," a complex of organismic functioning not limited to the discharge of occasional psychic wounds.

Since the discovery of the cyclically recurring third state, there have been a number of attempts to formulate a theory of the function of dreaming. Some of these have focused on the explanation of the occurrence of REM episodes; others on the function of dream content. Snyder [26], for example, suggested that REM periods are a survival of the evolutionary value of the animal's alertness to danger during sleep. Roffwarg et al. [24] have suggested that REM periods are feedback of endogenous stimulation that helps the maturation of the central nervous system. Ephron and Carrington [4] have suggested that REM episodes function to help the organism maintain some kind of cortical homeostasis during sleep's general slowdown of functioning. Lerner [19] has suggested that the content of dreams serves the function of instating kinesthetic fantasy which is diminished by motor inactivity during sleep and necessary for the maintenance of the intact body image. Breger [3] has suggested that the function of dreams is the assimilation and mastery of aroused (conflict) material into the "solutions" embodied in existing memory systems.

None of these proposed functions of REM period dreaming is mutually exclusive of other proposed functions; each has used a different starting point of observation about REM period dreaming. All the proposed functions, save Breger's, are compatible with a "fingers wandering over the keys of a piano" model of dream content, except that Lerner's theory would require that kinesthetic piano keys be struck more often than other kinds of keys. The new information suggesting a physiological need to dream thus reinstates a random model of dream content as accounting for some dreams, while conflict solution may account for the content of others, and affect discharge for still others.

Manifest and Latent Content

The logic of a theory which postulated that the unconscious instigated dreaming did not permit the existence of any dream, however banal its appearance, which did not have connections to the unconscious, since by fundamental postulate, without the activated unconscious, a dream would not have come into existence. This line of reasoning, that the manifest content of a dream *must* reflect the unconscious, was not the result of some rigidity in thinking or some holding on to an "official" position, as Erikson [5] put it, but rather an outgrowth of basic postulate. The knowledge that the unconscious does not instigate all dreaming releases the manifest content from the straightjacket of necessary connection to latent content.

The notion that the unconscious is a prepotent stimulus which is likely to invade ready-waiting dream time assumes that the unconscious takes precedence over other states as a determiner of dream content. In this model, however, there is no intrinsic reason why in the absence of conflict relatively indifferent events may not get into waiting dream time. A contented person might have contented dreams, continuing his daytime psychic state. A recent survey [27] of the content of 635 REM period reports, obtained from 58 young adults over 250 laboratory nights, concludes that REM dream reports are generally "clear, coherent, believable accounts of realistic situations in which the dreamer and other persons are involved and usually talking about them." Snyder et al. thus find themselves in agreement with the characterizations made of dreaming by interspectionist psychologists who studied dreams at the turn of the century. That the unconscious is represented even in realistic, coherent dreams is quite possible; but it is not axiomatic. An important issue for the clinician may thus be the distinction between dreams which express benign or trivial events and those which express the unconscious. Information about this question may be useful in separating the clinical wheat from the chaff. It may also focus the clinician's attention more on the incidence and subsidence of emotional disturbance.

An observation which Freud made about manifest dream content was that it seemed to be made up of composite ideas, like a composite of superimposed photographic plates. This quality of manifest dream content Freud attributed both to the lower level of consciousness which obtains during sleep, and to the special nature of ideation when it is governed by repression-connected forces, i.e., by "primary process." Ideation which expresses strangulated affect, and in a state of sleep, is regressed on two counts. For both sets of reasons, i.e., reduced intellectual level and repression-connected source, the manifest content of dreams must be taken apart, element by element.

The instigation of dreaming aside from the unconscious also releases the manifest content of dreams for translation by means other than the breakup of elements, especially in instances when the dream is about the activated unconscious. In the latter instance, the connection of these separate elements to some repression-source may be a mistranslation of the dream which should be understood more directly, or more as an ordinary, holistic experience.

Still another meaning which has accrued to the concept of latent content is the notion of the uniqueness of the individual's stream of consciousness which is sampled in his dreams. The manifest dream contains personal allusions to feelings and to biographical events which cannot be identified without their unique connection to the dreamer's personal life. Theoretically, the individual's unique web of associations could be connected in a dream to a trivial event, as well as to the unconscious. But whether a dream is about conflict or about a trivial event, what it is about may not be identifiable if we cannot correctly identify the references in the dreamer's thought to his personal life. This concept of the latent meaning of a dream remains unchanged.

In describing the varieties of dream work, Freud distinguished between universal symbols and condensations, distortions, displacements occurring in the individual's associative connections. This distinction is reminiscent of the distinction between the gestalt representation of ideas, for example phallic symbols which rest upon a congruence in shape between object and symbol, and connections reflecting "random" emotional links between objects and their representations. Freud observed that the majority of symbols in dreams are sexual in nature, that they yield no associative connections, and that they can be translated "at sight" with knowledge of the day's residue.

The possibility that some dreams may not be connected to the unconscious, while some are, opens up the question of when symbolic translation should be made of the manifest dream content, and when the manifest content, more directly interpreted although with knowledge of the individual's associative web, is sufficient to understand the dream's meaning. Presumably, under conditions when the unconscious has been stirred and has invaded a dream, and specifically where sexual impulses have been stirred, symbolic translation may be the appropriate mode of rendering dream thought. Under conditions when the unconscious is not activated, symbolic translations of manifest dreams may be mistranslations.

In the study of stress and neutral film showings before sleep [31] some of these questions are being approached experimentally. In pursuit of the difference between dream content after charged and neutral films, a "blind" judge, who does not even know that the dreams he is reading were preceded by film showings, has been given a prepared inventory of themes commonly accepted as expressing castration, homosexuality, masturbation, and so on. Our expectation is that more themes of dreams after charged films will be inventoried as charged than after neutral films.

An "open" study of the dreams which occurred after the subincision and birth films, i.e., with knowledge of the film stimulus and the dreamer's association, shows the dreams after the charged films to be full of symbolic representations. For example, after the subincision film, there were dreams containing such generally recognized castration and homosexual symbols as an airplane crash, blindness, having a flat tire, broken glasses, holding a floppy rubber scoop, being a captive, going over Niagara Falls, two guys biting each other's backs. Each example cited comes from a different dream text after the subincision film, and all but the first two examples come from different subjects.

Another analysis we are pursuing rests upon our observation that the dreams after charged films were more likely than after neutral films to contain references to the subjects' early childhood memories. As a check on our hypothesis, a blind judge is being offered biographical interviews containing childhood memories reported by each subject and asked to specify references to early memories in his dream texts.

The Interpretation of Dream Forgetting

Considering the fact that each of us has on the average about four REM periods in an ordinary 8 hours of sleep and that even the most gifted dream recallers among us remember one or at the most two of their dreams in the morning, it is fair to say that we routinely forget at least half, if not the bulk of our dream experiences every night. The forgetting of dreams is thus a normal occurrence for which repression cannot be a general explanation.

As a result of laboratory studies of on-the-spot recall and forgetting of dreams at REM period awakenings, dream recall has been shown to be subject to ordinary conditions governing memory: degree of alertness or arousal during registration of the dream experience, and during its recall; recency of dream episode; organization of the dream experience, and the like. Of particular interest to the clinician is the evidence from laboratory studies [14] which indicates that both people who regularly recall their dreams at home and those who do not, have the same number of REM periods per night and are not different in any EEG characteristics. The difference between dream recallers and nonrecallers is thus a difference mainly in their habit or capacity to recall their REM period experiences. The only dream content characteristic which differentiated the dreams in the laboratory of good recallers from those of poor recallers was a difference in the frequency of representation of the self in the dream [20]. Those subjects who were accustomed to recall their dreams at home had more dreams in the laboratory in which the self was the protagonist of the action. The memory function thus involved seems to fit a familiar pattern in which better organized material (in this case organized around the self as protagonist) is easier to remember. This kind of result suggests that the recall of dreams is a function of personal characteristics of the dreamer, and would likely reflect his capacity to recall other kinds of material as well as his recall of dreams.

At the same time there is evidence from laboratory studies that anxiety is also a potent factor in reducing dream recall. Instances in which anxiety determines dream forgetting seem to have a distinguishing quality. In contrast to REM period awakenings early in the night from deep sleep which yield reports from the subject that "nothing" was going through his mind, there are REM period awakenings in which the subject says that he was surely dreaming but has just "lost" the dream, so-called ND reports. Although these instances are relatively rare in the laboratory, the REM period from which they issue have been shown to be characterized by unusual respiratory irregularity [14], suggesting the presence of anxiety as the dream repressor. After stress films, more dream reports which had been given at on-the-spot awakenings were totally lost to spontaneous re-recall in the postsleep inquiry after neutral films, again suggesting a connection between anxiety and dream loss [31].

Anxiety not only destroys dream recall in some instances but has also been shown [9, 17] to occur in association with those (relatively infrequent) REM periods late at night which are not accompanied by penile erection. The dream reports which came from REM periods in which there was no or irregular erection were characterized by significantly more anxiety than REM dream reports accompanied by full erection.

Dreaming as an Ego Function

Like the biologically given functions of language and perception, the REM period is characteristic of all human beings and occurs regardless of their conflict state. Total REM time runs a developmental course in human beings, decreasing and stabilizing from approximately 50 percent of sleep time at birth to 20 percent at age 3 or 4 [23] and decreasing again at age 50 and later [8]. Findings on patients with chronic brain syndrome show that altered REM mechanisms play a role in the behavioral disturbances associated with this organic condition. In contrast, the association between functional psychosis and altered REM behavior is much more indirect [7]. Using the degree of eye movement as an index of REM sleep, Feinberg [6] found that feebleminded persons have less REM sleep. These findings on chronic brain syndrome and on the feebleminded have led Feinberg to suggest that sleep (including REM sleep) involves brain functions vital for intelligence and cognition. Ironically, the REM period is thus a candidate for the list of conflict-free autonomous ego functions.

Perhaps the most salient characteristic of the unconscious is that it is a psychical system dominated by strangulated affect. Although strangulated affect cannot instigate REM periods, it may infiltrate them and fashion dream content so as to obtain discharge. This kind of hypothesis has a psychophysical parallel in the evidence that the REM period involves some kind of physiological discharge process. Moreover, the biochemistry of REM period discharge implicates some substances which are linked to the physiology of emotional states. Buried in the hypothetical ego function of REM period dreaming, then, there may be much information about the mechanisms of affect discharge.

Another consequence of the view of dreaming as an ego function is that it encourages the study of individual differences in dreaming. Although individual differences in dreaming were studied before the discovery of REM periods, as, for instance, Hall and Van de Castle's [15] normative studies, the theory that dreams were instigated by the unconscious led to the view that the study of individual differences in dreaming, without reference to the unconscious, was unproductive. In this connection the construct *psychological differentiation* [30, 32] may be a particularly useful tool with which to pursue individual differences in dream behavior. Connections have been observed between field-dependence (which reflects differentiation) and such dream phenomena as the frequency of eye movements, susceptibility to the effects of dream deprivation, dream recall, and dream content. I have elsewhere reviewed some of these studies [21] and Witkin reviews some of the evidence in his contribution to this issue.

These studies lend support to the view that the functioning of the unconscious in dreams is mediated, as it is in other behavior, by differences in ego organization. This kind of approach to dreaming must supplement, but need not supplant, the notion that dream content expresses the unconscious. Strangulated affect still represents a code by which many dreams can be translated; the organization of the ego provides another set of clues.

REFERENCES

1. Baekeland, F., Koulack, D., and Lasky, R. Effects of a stressful presleep experience on electroencephalograph-recorded sleep. *Psychophysiology* 4:436, 1968.
2. Bertini, M., Lewis, H. B., and Witkin, H. A. Some preliminary observations with an experimental procedure for the

study of hypnogogic and related phenomena. *Arch. Psicol. Neurol.* 6:493, 1964.

3. Breger, L. The function of dreams. *J. Abnorm. Psychol.* (Monograph) 72:1, 1967.
4. Ephron, H. S., and Carrington, P. Rapid eye movement sleep and cortical homeostasis. *Psychol. Rev.* 73:500, 1966.
5. Erikson, E. H. The dream specimen of psychoanalysis. *J. Amer. Psychoanal. Ass.* 1:5, 1954.
6. Feinberg, I. Eye movement activity during sleep and intellectual function in mental retardation. *Science* 159:1256, 1968.
7. Feinberg, I. The ontogenesis of human sleep and the relationship of sleep variables to intellectual function of the aged. *Compr. Psychiat.* 9:138, 1968.
8. Feinberg, I., Koresko, R., and Heller, N. EEG sleep patterns as a function of normal and pathological aging in man. *J. Psychiat. Res.* 5:107, 1967.
9. Fisher, C. Dreaming and Sexuality. In M. Schur, A. Solnit, R. M. Lowenstein, and L. Newman (Eds.), *Essays in Honor of Heinz Hartmann's Seventieth Birthday.* New York: International Universities Press, 1966.
10. Foulkes, D. Dream reports for different states of sleep. *J. Abnorm. Psychol.* 65:14, 1962.
11. Foulkes, D., and Rechtschaffen, A. Presleep determinants of dream content: Effect of two films. *Percept. Motor Skills* 19: 983, 1964.
12. Freedman, N., Grand, S., and Karacan, I. An approach to the study of dreaming and changes in psychopathological states. *J. Nerv. Ment. Dis.* 5:399, 1966.
13. Freud, S. The Interpretation of Dreams. In *The Standard Edition of the Complete Psychological Works of Sigmund Freud,* tr. and ed. by J. Strachey with others. London: Hogarth and the Institute of Psycho-Analysis, 1953. Vol. V.
14. Goodenough, D. R. Some Recent Studies of Dream Recall. In H. A. Witkin and H. B. Lewis (Eds.), *Experimental Studies of Dreaming.* New York: Random House, 1967. Pp. 128–147.
15. Hall, C. S., and Van de Castle, R. *The Content Analysis of Dreams.* New York: Appleton-Century-Crofts, 1966.
16. Hunter, I., and Breger, L. The Effect of Presleep Group Therapy upon Subsequent Dream Content. Paper read at Association for the Psychophysiological Study of Sleep (APSS), Santa Monica, Cal., 1967.
17. Karacan, I., Goodenough, D. R., Shapiro, A., and Starker, S.

Erection cycle during sleep in relation to dream anxiety. *Arch. Gen. Psychiat.* (Chicago) 15:183, 1966.

18. Lane, R. W., and Breger, L. The Effect of Preoperative Stress on Dreams. Paper read at APSS, Santa Monica, Cal., 1967.
19. Lerner, B. Dream function reconsidered. *J. Abnorm. Psychol.* 72:85, 1967.
20. Lewis, H. B., Goodenough, D. R., Shapiro, A., and Sleser, I. Individual differences in dream recall. *J. Abnorm. Psychol.* 71:52, 1966.
21. Lewis, H. B. Some Clinical Implications of Recent Dream Research. In L. Abt and B. Riess (Eds.), *Progress in Clinical Psychology*. New York: Grune & Stratton, 1969.
22. Pivik, T., and Foulkes, D. Dream deprivation: Effects on dream content. *Science* 153:1282, 1966.
23. Roffwarg, H., Dement, W. C., and Fisher, C. Preliminary Observations of the Sleep-Dream Pattern in Neonates, Infants, Children and Adults. In E. Harms (Ed.), *Monographs on Child Psychiatry*. New York: Pergamon Press, 1964.
24. Roffwarg, H., Muzio, J., and Dement, W. C. Ontogenetic development of the human sleep-dream. *Science* 152:604, 1966.
25. Silberer, H. Report on a Method of Eliciting and Observing Certain Symbolic Hallucinations-Phenomena. In D. Rapaport (Ed.), *Organization and Pathology of Thought*. New York: Columbia University Press, 1951.
26. Snyder, F. Toward an evolutionary theory of dreaming. *Amer. J. Psychiat.* 2:121, 1966.
27. Snyder, F., Karacan, I., Tharp, V., Jr., and Scott, J. Phenomenology of REM Dreaming. Paper read at APSS, Santa Monica, Cal., 1967.
28. Verdone, P. Temporal reference of manifest dream content. *Percept. Motor Skills* 20:1253, 1965.
29. Vogel, G., Foulkes, D., and Trosman, H. Ego functions and dreaming during sleep onset. *Arch. Gen. Psychiat.* (Chicago) 14:238, 1966.
30. Witkin, H. A., Dyk, R., Faterson, H., Goodenough, D. R., and Karp, S. A. *Psychological Differentiation*. New York: Wiley, 1962.
31. Witkin, H. A., Goodenough, D. R., Lewis, H. B., Shapiro, A., and Koulack, D. Unpublished studies.
32. Witkin, H. A., Lewis, H. B., Hertzman, M., Machover, K., Meissner, P., and Wapner, S. *Personality Through Perception*. New York: Harper, 1954.

33. Witkin, H. A., and Lewis, H. B. The relation of experimentally induced presleep experiences to dreams. *J. Amer. Psychoanal. Ass.* 13:819, 1965.
34. Zimmerman, W. Psychological and Physiological Differences Between "Light" and "Deep" Sleepers. Paper read at APSS, Santa Monica, Cal., 1967.

The Dream in Psychoanalytic Practice

JAMES C. SKINNER

I have been asked to discuss whether the enormous amount of recent information from the laboratories of sleep and dreaming has affected the psychoanalytic interpretation of the dream or the psychoanalytic use of the dream. A precise answer to this question would require an elaborate investigation of the attitudes and techniques of psychoanalysis throughout the country. My answer is based on my own experience, that of my students in psychoanalysis, and also on an examination of the nature of the research itself.

On this basis my response is that there has been very little change in the psychoanalytic interpretation of the dream in the clinical practice of psychoanalysis. The technique of interpretation is familiar to us from Freud's description of the process and from our daily experience in psychological interpretation of behavior and symptom. We profess belief in the existence of that kernel which Freud said existed within the dream—the infantile wish. In actual practice, we often are content to utilize the manifest dream as confirmation to ourselves and our patients of current conflicts and preoccupations. Sometimes we, in fact, tease out the "latent dream" but one usually far removed from any truly infantile wish. Erikson [1] has comforted and supported us in our often guilt-laden preoccupation with the manifest dream; and Richard Jones [6] has assured us that Freud himself paid only lip service to the wellspring of the dream in his delineation of the technique of interpretation. Current research in sleep and dreaming has nothing to say concerning the technical use of the dream in psychoanalysis.

NEW PERSPECTIVES ON THE DREAM

If, however, the attitude the analyst adopts toward the dream as a psychological phenomena is examined, there are, I believe, certain changes.

Some years ago, when the sleep-dream cycle (REM cycle) was first described, it appeared quite possible that the psychological experience of dreaming which accompanies this cycle would be reduced to an interesting artifact of a crucial neurophysiological process. As research proceeded, it appeared more and more likely that the REM cycle was crucial in some way for the total biological functioning of the organism, but that the dream which accompanied it might be only a kind of fringe benefit to psychiatrists. The dream could still be analyzed and would still have meaning as an example of the issues current and active in the patient's mind, but it could hardly be thought of as representing the critical transaction between the unconscious and the preconscious which Freud describes in Chapter 7 in *The Interpretation of Dreams* [3]. Very recently, however, new information from the laboratories gives the dream itself more importance.

If one of the current models of the REM cycle, in its relationship to sleep, turns out to be valid, then these periods of REM represent increased drive activity, followed by periods of quiescence [7]. If this is true, then the hallucinated dream represents a true reflection of this drive activity and, as Freud suggested, may be crucial in its management. It has been suggested [4] even more recently that there are regular cycles of drive activity throughout the waking daytime life of the individual—cycles accompanied by behavior which seems calculated to reduce these drives. The result of this, once again, is to increase the importance of the dream as a crucial psychological process involved in the psychological economy of the organism. It seems quite possible that just as the REM cycle, in its neurophysiological aspects, is crucial to the health of the organism, so is the dream which accompanies it of unique importance in our emotional health.

Most of the issues I have so far discussed are reviewed admirably in Chapter 13 of Hartmann's *The Biology of Dreaming* [5]. With the exception of the relevance of the daytime drive cycle, Dr. Hartmann reviews the import of current research to psychoanalytic dream interpretation and dream psychology. He remarks upon the need and opportunities for further research into areas which are of more direct relevance to the psychoanalytic interpretation of the dream and its use in psychoanalysis. What possible modifications of interpretive technique could arise from such investigations? What inquiries could lead to a different use of the dream in analysis? I should like to suggest one promising direction: a reexamination of the familiar concept of the dream as a predominantly visual experience which must be translated back into the form of verbal thought.

As we know, Freud [3], in his section on *secondary revision* in the sixth chapter (and again in Chapter 7) of *The Interpretation of Dreams* was concerned with the regressive movement of desire. He described the movement of ideas through the various stations of the mental apparatus until they reached the memory traces, which he described as predominantly visual. He conceived of the dream thought as moving farther backward through these memory traces to the point at which the perceptual apparatus lay, and there receiving visual representation of hallucinatory intensity. In this way the wish was fulfilled in visual imagination and in its most infantile form. Freud [3] says on regression:

> Intentional recollection and other constituent processes of our normal thinking involve a retrogressive movement in the psychic apparatus from a complex ideational act back to the raw material of the memory traces underlying it. In the waking state, however, this backward movement never extends beyond mnemonic images; it does not succeed in producing a hallucinatory revival of the perceptual images [p. 543].

It is clear that he considers the memory traces, to which recollection returns, to be essentially visual images. The distinction is that in the dream there is an arousal of perceptual images.

We call it regression, when, in a dream, an idea is turned back into the sensory image from which it was originally derived (ibid.).

Later he says:

I may also recall that one of the facts arrived at in the Studies of Hysteria was that, when it was possible to bring infantile scenes (whether they were memories or fantasies) into consciousness, they were seen as hallucinations and lost that characteristic only in the process of being reported. It is, moreover, a familiar observation that even in those whose memory is not normally of a visual type, the earliest recollections of childhood retain far into life the quality of sensory vividness (ibid., p. 546).

The work of Dr. Fisher and his associates [2] in studying subliminal visual stimulation and dreams is well known. In the course of his experiments with patients who were presented an image for so brief an exposure that they had no conscious perception of its nature, aspects of the picture appeared both in free drawings, which were elicited following the exposure, and in the manifest content of their dreams. Dr. Fisher's interest was in demonstrating the existence of this phenomenon and in suggesting the importance of visual perceptions from the preceding day, which were not consciously perceived, in the construction of the dream. He has been able to demonstrate, as Freud suggested in a passing remark, that some of the day residue which goes into the construction of the dream is received at a subliminal level and that some of the dream work of condensation, displacement, and so on, goes on during the day before the night of actual dreaming. In the course of demonstrating this phenomenon, Dr. Fisher has also been able to show that the transformations which the subliminally perceived material undergoes are closely related to the primary process transformations of the latent dream thoughts themselves.

I mention Dr. Fisher's work in connection with my own thesis because he, too, was concerned with a recovery of visual imagery through the process of asking the patient to draw. He mentions that perhaps more than half of the pictorial elements of the dream are identified as coming from consciously perceived images, rather than from subliminal perceptions. My interest is in the former—those images and those pictorial qualities of the dream which are imperfectly rendered into language and which may either directly represent earlier experiences which play an important part in the meaning of the dream or may evoke further relevant associations.

In the process of interpreting a patient's dream, we ask him to tell us about the dream in words which, in part, are a description of the visual hallucination as he remembers it and, in part, a translation of visual elements into nonvisual thought. This process of translation—from the hallucinated dream to thought—has already taken place upon awakening. All of us have had the frustrating experience of attempting to encompass an elaborate and complex visual image in the narrower confines of words. In the moment of telling our dream to ourselves, we know we are compromising; we have the sharp sense of losing a great deal of the richness of the scene we perceived during the night. As Freud stated, the earliest, the infantile wish is remembered in visual form. To the extent that we ask the patient to describe in words the dream he has experienced as perception, as visual imagery—to that extent do we lose understanding of the most basic recollections and desires.

It was because of concern with this particular problem, and the recurrent frustration I and my patients have experienced in attempting to translate a rich and complex visual imagery into the narrower secondary process of waking life, that I have attempted a way of partially avoiding this second step of translation. Freud postulated the translation of the thought into the perceptual hallucination, and then described the technique of translating back from the perceptual hallucination to the thought. Ordinarily as one proceeds with the interpretation of a dream, the patient's attention is drawn to one after the other of the visual elements remembered from the dream; it is to these that he associates. However, by the time the dream is reported, many of these visual elements have already been translated into thought and, as such, are diminished in complexity. One hopes to recover the lost complexity by virtue of the chain of associations.

Recently I have been experimenting with a way of avoiding this loss. In those dreams which my patients report which contain remembered images of objects, buildings, arrangement of objects within space, machines, unusual gestures, strange animals, curious landscapes, or particular designs, I ask the patient to draw that portion of the dream on a blackboard in my office. In my still limited experience with this procedure, I have found that the drawing portrays what appear to be important clues to the latent dream which are not reached in the verbal associations and perhaps never would have been elicited. The patient frequently has a strong sense of recovering something which was clearly there in the hallucinated dream but which, in the process of secondary revision, in the need to combine and order the material, was lost. In my experience with my patients' dreams and with my own, it frequently occurs that the drawn image has clear relevance not only to immediate events and concerns but also to very early memories from childhood. Even in those dreams in which motion and action are dominant, it has proved possible for the patient to produce a number of what might be considered "still photographs," which—though lacking motion—are rich in other elements.

I mention this work in which I am currently engaged because it seems to me to be pertinent to the question I have been asked. In order to discuss the extent to which current research in dream and sleep has affected the practice of psychoanalytic dream interpretation, it is necessary to point out the areas which have been untouched by this research. There are inquiries still to be undertaken which, indeed, would have profound effects on the use of the dream in psychotherapy. For instance, if it turns out to be consistently true, as my work so far suggests, that the visual dream as reproduced by the patient contains some of the earliest memories, conflicts, and desires, then one must ask if the current method of dream interpretation, which depends so heavily on translation into verbal concepts, is the most useful form to use.

There are other questions, the answers to which might make significant differences in the psychoanalytic practice of dream interpretation. One of these questions, which has already been mentioned, has to do with the importance of the dream itself, quite apart from the REM cycle. On the basis of what has so far been discovered, it is still possible to view the REM cycle as a significant activity and the experience of dreaming as an interesting but not a psychologically or biologically significant event. One would still not be surprised to find that this hallucinatory experience has meaning, can be placed in relevance to the rest of the patient's life, and may be useful in underlining or understanding some problems or aspects of his psyche. Even as an incidental accompaniment of the neurophysiological drive-activating cycle, the dream can be useful in the treatment of a patient.

This, however, says nothing about the use of the dream *to* the patient, apart from the psychoanalytic situation. What we would like to know is whether or not the experience of dreaming is in itself helpful, integrating, or necessary to an individual. Experiments which suggest that hallucinations during waking life are related to dream deprivation may only prove the importance of the REM cycle, and not the importance of the hallucinated, psychological experience of dreaming. What about the dreams of which one has no memory and yet for which we have evidence at regular intervals throughout the nighttime? Are these unremembered dreams still of significance in the patient's psychological economy? Are they useful to him in some way, whether or not they are recalled? It would be helpful if there were ways to interfere with the psychological process of dreaming and yet allow the REM cycles to continue unchanged.

My answer to the question, then, of whether or not current research in dream and sleeping has substantially affected the psychoanalytic attitude toward the dream and its use in psychoanalytic practice is no. But in answering that question I have attempted to point out that there are other directions of investigation which may result in information that *will* profoundly affect the way the dream is interpreted, and the significance attached to it in the treatment process. Some of this relevant inquiry does not need the complicated apparatus of the sleep laboratory but can be done with simplicity and validity in the clinical practice of psychoanalysis.

REFERENCES

1. Erikson, E. The dream specimen of psychoanalysis. *J. Amer. Psychoanal. Ass.* 25:56, 1954.
2. Fisher, C., and Paul, J. H. Subliminal visual stimulation and dreams. *J. Amer. Psychoanal. Ass.* 7:1, 1959.
3. Freud, S. *The Interpretation of Dreams.* New York: Basic Books, 1955.
4. Friedman, S. Oral activity in mild chronic schizophrenia. *Amer. J. Psychiat.* 125:6, 1968.
5. Hartmann, E. *The Biology of Dreaming.* Chicago: Thomas, 1967.
6. Jones, R. Dream interpretation and the psychology of dreaming. *J. Amer. Psychoanal. Ass.* 13:2, 1965.
7. Snyder, F. Toward an evolutionary theory of dreaming. *Amer. J. Psychiat.* 123:2, 1966.

The Manifest Dream, the Latent Dream, and the Dream Work

*Do we know anything more about the dream itself (manifest dream) than we did 15 years ago? Anything more about the formation of the dream, the dream work, the latent dream?**

The Transformation of the Stuff Dreams Are Made Of

RICHARD M. JONES

We know substantially more than we did fifteen years ago about the manifest dream, the latent content, and the dream work. Most of this new knowledge has been produced by studies of the relation of experimentally induced presleep experiences to dreams as exemplified by the investigations of Pöetzl [9, 10], Fisher [3], Shevrin and Luborsky [11], and most recently by the elaborate sleep-

* The reader interested in this question may wish to refer also to papers by Baekeland (p. 49), Foulkes (p. 147 and p. 165), Witkin (p. 154), Van de Castle (p. 171), Fisher (p. 183), Broughton (p. 188), Hartmann (p. 192), Lewis (p. 199), Ephron and Carrington (p. 344), and Stoyva (p. 355).

monitored investigations of Witkin and Lewis [13]. Space does not permit a detailed review of these findings here; suffice it for illustrative purposes to note some of the more suggestive tentative findings reported by Witkin and Lewis: (1) Dreams following emotionally charged presleep stimuli tend to highlight the more prominent elements of such stimuli, while dreams following neutral presleep stimuli tend to highlight the more peripheral elements of such stimuli. (2) Subjects' attitudes and conflicts in respect to the experimenter and the laboratory situation tend to be worked over in dreams much as are the more charged elements of the experimental stimuli. (3) Although the specific contents of an individual's symbolic handling of conflict material in his dreams varies almost limitlessly, consistencies of pattern or style are sometimes discernible. For example, one person may consistently represent upsetting presleep stimuli by way of reversing them in his dreams, while another person may consistently represent upsetting presleep stimuli by way of placing the most noxious items in stories or dreams within dreams, while still another may favor the strategem of being in the dream in spirit but not in person—and so on. (4) Dreams which tend to be forgotten are more likely to follow threatening presleep stimuli, as measured by simultaneous autonomic reactions, than to follow nonthreatening stimuli. (5) Symbolic equations which are among the most transparent to the observer are frequently those which the dreamer himself denies. (6) Dreams following neutral stimuli are more likely to reflect the person's present life experiences, while dreams following emotionally charged stimuli are more likely to tap memories of early childhood experiences.

These and other investigations have sought to bring the refinements of electronic sleep monitoring methods to bear on the study of the relationship between recently problematic perceptual and cognitive events (day residue) and enduringly problematic memories (latent content) by the symbolizing processes characteristic of sleep (dream work). The most significant effect of such work has been to restore the perspective which several generations of psychologists lost sight of despite this early warning by Freud [4]:

> . . . now that analysts at least have become reconciled to replacing the manifest dream by the meaning revealed by its interpretation, many of them have become guilty of falling into another confusion which they cling to with equal obstinacy. They seek to find the essence of dreams in their latent content, and in so doing they overlook the distinction between the latent dream thoughts and the dream work. At bottom, dreams are nothing other than a particular *form* of thinking, made possible by the conditions of the state of sleep.

Erikson [2] sought to remind a later generation of psychologists of this warning in these words:

> The psychoanalyst, in looking at the surface of mental phenomena, often has to overcome a certain shyness. So many in his field mistake attention to surface for superficiality, and a concern with form for lack of depth. But the fact that we have followed Freud into depths which our eyes had to become accustomed to does not permit us, today, to blink when we look at things in broad daylight. Like good surveyors we must be at home on the geological surface as well as in the descending shafts. . . . Unofficially, we often interpret dreams entirely or in parts on the basis of their manifest appearance. Occasionally, we hurry at every confrontation with a dream to crack its manifest appearance as if it were a useless shell and to hasten to discard this shell in favor of what seems to be the more worthwhile core. When such a method corresponded to a new orientation, it was essential for research as well as for therapy; but as a compulsive habituation, it has since hindered a full meeting of ego psychology and the problems of dream life.

THE TRANSFORMATION PERSPECTIVE

I think, however, that these fundamental distinctions had to continue to wear thin as long as the study of dreaming had to be pursued exclusively by clinicians whose perception of their data is, of professional necessity, persistently colored by preconceptions about "latent contents." Not until the means were at hand to support the study of dreaming by investigators working with subjects, as well as by clinicians working with patients, did the question have to be faced whether manifest dream reports, i.e., the laboratory worker's most uncontaminated observations, would be looked upon as valid reflections of nature, or whether these were to be perceived as merely artifactual reflections of nature that had to have their inherent "distortions" corrected by reference to their "disguised" latent contents before they could be trusted to serve as sources of scientific evidence and inference. The answer to this question has by now become clear: Tracing the components of a manifest dream to their "disguised" associations with repressed infantile memories and the derivatives of these repressed infantile memories is *one* valid approach to dream analysis and, as such, will continue to add to our knowledge of the processes of dreaming—particularly in their connections with the processes of neurosis. However, this is but one of many conceivable approaches to equally valid and valuable forms of dream analysis. Surely it can no longer be assumed that dreaming serves neurotic defense purposes only. Indeed, we may now legitimately resolve to substitute the term *transformation* whenever we encounter the terms *disguise, distortion,* or *censorship* in dream literature.

Speaking from within the theory of dreaming, i.e., leaving the interests of dream interpretation aside, this is hardly a revision, since it was the meaning Freud preferred when his concern with questions of dream *formation* was unambiguous:

> Two separate functions may be distinguished in mental activity during the construction of the dream: production of the dream-thoughts, and their *transformation* into the content of the dream.

However, as documented elsewhere [6], Freud's formulations of the dream work were sometimes lax in that they confused the theory of dreaming with the theory of dreams, with the result that he sometimes referred to "distortion" or "censorship" when "transformation" would have carried his meaning better.

To illustrate: A young woman reported a dream in which, in a state of high excitement and suspense, she was attempting to put a wild horse into a corral. While thus engaged she kept thinking how nice it would be if the horse was not a hired one but was her very own. She was also impressed in the dream with the horse's penis.

Surely, we would not stir much controversy among a group of clinicians were we to suggest that the repressed infantile wish expressed in the process of this dream's formation was a wish for a penis of the dreamer's own. A really intuitive dream interpreter, say a Wilhelm Steckel, might surmise in addition that the day residue was a recent memory of having had sexual intercourse, and perhaps also that her lover was somehow less than "eligible."

There was no way to test the hypothesis as regards the repressed infantile wish. There almost never is. But there was a way to confirm the view that transformation, rather than disguise, is the more useful view of this dream's "work." This was accomplished by the simple means of listening to the dreamer's own interpretation of her manifest dream: It was a "wonderful dream," and wasn't it clever the way it gave another picture of having had intercourse with her lover the night before. There had been moments when she was not sure she could keep him in the "corral," and it was now difficult to determine whether the dream more accurately depicted her sexual impatience or her more general impatience concerning the lover's impending divorce.

Another person may have had the identical dream, awakened in fright, and not have had the slightest idea what waking experiences the dream referred to. We might well, then, have spoken of the manifest dream as having a disguised latent meaning. But let us be very clear where the element of disguise enters into the sequence. It is in the dreamer's waking reaction to the dream, whether this involves clinical interpretation or not. It does not necessarily enter into the process of dreaming as such. In other words, the process of dreaming does involve the transformation of mental contents, whether recent or infantile, into new forms; but the onus of distortion, whether it be slight or massive, falls upon the waking state, a state in which dreams may be interpreted but not formed. In speaking of dream formation, therefore, we are on more solid ground if we accustom ourselves to thinking of the dream work as transformative rather than distortive. The resulting transformations may subsequently be understood by the waking psyche in such ways as make them classifiable as disguises. But they may also be understood by the waking psyche in such ways as make them classifiable as revelations or expressions or inspirations or compensations or creative insights or what have you.

Reenter, now, with renewed credentials of respectability such methods of dream analysis as have been described by Jung [8], Angyal [1], Ullman [12], Jones [5, 7], and others who have been concerned to relate an understanding of dreams to an understanding of normal growth and development as well as to an understanding of neurosis.

REFERENCES

1. Angyal, A. *Neurosis and Treatment.* New York: Wiley, 1965.
2. Erikson, E. The dream specimen of psychoanalysis. *J. Amer. Psychoanal. Ass.* 2:139, 1954.
3. Fisher, C. Dreams, images, and perception: A study of unconscious–preconscious relationships. *J. Amer. Psychoanal. Ass.* 4:5, 1956.
4. Freud, S. The Interpretation of Dreams (1900). In *The Standard Edition of the Complete Psychological Works of Sigmund Freud,* tr. and ed. by J. Strachey with others. London: Hogarth and the Institute of Psycho-Analysis, 1953. Vol. IV–V, p. 506.
5. Jones, R. M. *Ego Synthesis in Dreams.* Cambridge, Mass.: Schenkman, 1962. P. 43.
6. Jones, R. M. Dream interpretation and the psychology of dreaming. *J. Amer. Psychoanal. Ass.* 13:304, 1965.
7. Jones, R. M. The psychoanalytic theory of dreaming—1968. *J. Nerv. Ment. Dis.* 147:587, 1968.
8. Jung, C. J. *Modern Man in Search of a Soul.* New York: Harcourt, Brace & World, 1933.
9. Pöetzl, O. Tachystoskopish provozierte optische Halluzinationen bei einem Fall von Alkoholhalluzinose mit ruckgebildeter zerebraler Hemianopsie. *Jb. Psychiat. Neurol.* 1915. Pp. 141–146.
10. Pöetzl, O. Experimental erregte Traumbilder in Ihren Beziehunger zum indirekten Shenen. *Z. Neurol. Psychiat.* 37:278, 1947.
11. Shevrin, H., and Luborsky, L. The measurement of preconscious perception in dreams and images: An investigation of the Poetzl phenomenon. *J. Abnorm. Soc. Psychol.* 56:285, 1958.

12. Ullman, M. Dreaming, altered states of consciousness and the problem of vigilance. *J. Nerv. Ment. Dis.* 133:529, 1961.
13. Witkin, H., and Lewis, H. The relation of experimentally induced pre-sleep experiences to dreams: A report on method and preliminary findings. *J. Amer. Psychoanal. Ass.* 13:819, 1965.

The Relation of Daytime Events to the Dreams That Follow

ROSALIND DYMOND CARTWRIGHT

The new sleep research offers psychologists the possibility of understanding man's behavior in ways never before possible. There is now the opportunity of obtaining more direct access to unconscious processes as they operate, not in the person with disturbances, but in the normal individual where they are presumably functioning in proper relation to the rest of mental life. The new technology gives us both the method for obtaining large samples of unconscious mental activity to better understand its nature and the chance to study the interplay between conscious and unconscious thought. It has now become possible to do this by tracing the sequential course of mentation from daytime into the dreams of the nighttime and then on into the subsequent day.

Ever since we accepted the position that human responses are shaped to some degree by factors outside of those the person can or will report directly, psychologists have been at work devising methods for getting around the limitations of the conscious self-report. Many experimental methods have been developed to reduce the contribution of stimulus pull from the outer world of reality in order to increase the contribution of stimuli from the inner world. All these have in common the aim of lowering the degree of conscious control the individual exerts in shaping his response toward a socially determined one. In this way it is hoped that the behavior will more clearly show some of the underlying feelings and motives, the cognitive maps and perceptual habits which influence responses but are outside of awareness. Projective tests, free association techniques, hallucinogenic drugs, sensory restriction have all become part of our bag of experimental tricks to reduce the input of external cues so that the behavior sampled will be determined more by internal factors. How much better it would be if we could watch the mind at work when this state of affairs is the natural one.

The EEG-EOG technology for monitoring sleep has given us neurophysiological marker variables which indicate, with high reliability, when samples of mental activity can be drawn which differ markedly from those available during wakefulness. During the day our perceptions are more or less accurate representations of outer reality with some distortion from inner factors. During the night the reverse is true: our dream perceptions are reflections of our inner world, with outer reality recognizable very little. During the day our mental activity is directed outward toward integrating our behavior with reality. To do this we must represent what is "out there" accurately in perception and relate it to how it can best serve both our immediate and long-term needs. During the night when constant active responses are no longer required of us, the spotlight of attention can move from the outer world to the inner. The perceptions need no longer be factually accurate and clearly they are far from that. What function is served by the regularly recurring episodes of dreaming where the style of thought is so unrealistic that we find it alien has puzzled man throughout his history. It now seems possible to approach this question by more systematic analysis with greater hope that headway can be made.

The psychologist has two clear tasks: (1) to describe, organize, and analyze the material from the unconscious now that large quantities of this primitive stuff can be trapped in its natural habitat, and (2) to relate it to the rest of mental life as we know it. The possible relations between conscious and unconscious mental life are many. In dreaming we may continue the mental life of the preceding day—or not. If we do, if may be done rather poorly since the method available is the primitive, alogical, picture language of early childhood. In this case the contribution of dreaming to daytime behavior would be expected to be small and of low quality. In contrast, dreaming may represent a time and method uniquely suited to the task of bringing daily experience to terms with emotional factors and memories which are bypassed in the press of the action-oriented day. In this case the effect of dream experience might be expected to be larger and more positive.

It may be, however, that dreaming mentation is strictly fortuitous and random, more like a series of Rorschach ink blots to which we later add meaning of a sort, depending on our current concerns, but which is random sensation unrelated inherently to any continuing mentation line from the day. If this turns out to be the case, the study of the content of dreams will not unlock any great insights into the human mind, and psychologists can go back to sleeping nights and working with daytime data.

Our experience to date is too limited to provide a basis of choice between these positions or to support some other conceptual formulation. Experimental work set up to discriminate between these possibilities is, at present, zero. Our evidence is fragmentary and at best deals more with the influence of daytime experimental stimuli on nighttime dreaming mentation than with the effect of the dreams on later behavior.

In a recent study in our own laboratory 10 young male adult graduate students were exposed to a stag movie during the day. The REM content reports were collected for 1 night before and for the 4 nights subsequent to this to trace the effect on dreaming of a strongly affect-arousing visual stimulus. The dreams of the night before seeing the movie were used as a control sample against which to measure the effect of the film on dream content. The subject's own sexual history and personality were assessed as relevant background factors and the immediate physiological response to the film was recorded by measuring the heart rate and 17-hydroxycorticosteroid changes in the blood. Thus the effect of a particular known event during the day could be traced into the dreams of the night and related to the subject's potential set to respond, his immediate physical reaction, and his dream fantasy response. Data relevant to daytime behavioral effects following the dreams were limited to a collection each day of the subject's associations to the dreams of the night before during a one-hour interview with a psychiatrist. Thus this study, too, is not adequate to speak to the whole of the paradigm but only to add to our small pool of knowledge of the effects from day into night. The effects were many and varied, some of which have already appeared in the literature [1, 3] and will only be summarized here briefly:

1. In comparison with the night of dream content collection before seeing the film, the first night after the film showed a significant increase in failure to recall content from REM awakenings. The film clearly had a great impact but it is impossible to assess it from the content of the first postfilm night because of the massive "repression."

2. Direct incorporation of the film characters, settings, and activities into the REM reports was highest on the second postfilm night showing that it took some time for the data to be assimilated and utilized in fantasy.

3. Direct incorporation into the dream of the daytime experience of the subjects in the experimental situation—the laboratory setting, personnel, and activities—was greater than the direct incorporation of the stag film.

4. Based on the Hall and Van de Castle [2] norms, there was a significantly higher proportion of use of common sexual symbols in the dreams of these subjects than in the dreams of a similar sample of young men who had not seen the film. Findings 3 and 4 taken together seem best summed up this way: The influence of the daytime events on the nighttime fantasy was direct for the more neutral events and more indirect (symbolic) for the affective material.

5. Subjects who had an immediate anxiety response to the film, in terms of an increase in the 17-hydroxycorticosteroids or heart rate increase, or both, showed the greatest increase in failure to recall dream content that night. This failure of recall was also strongly related to direct incorporation from the film into the dreams. This

seemed to show that those for whom the film was anxiety arousing had an all-or-none response in dreams.

6. Subjects who brought to the experience a background of interest in sex and sexual experience, as judged from their personal histories, had a more modulated response. Incorporation for them was symbolic rather than direct, and they had many direct associations to the film from their waking interview on the previous night's dream reports.

Clearly the effect of the daytime experience on the nighttime fantasy and the subsequent daytime associations to it was influenced by the saliency of the stimulus in the life of the person and by his immediate physiological responsiveness. Those for whom sex held interest and who had some heterosexual experience seemed most able to code the material into common cultural symbols and relate it in dreams to other experiences and memories, then to decode it relatively easily during wakefulness. Those who had little acquaintance with sex or for whom sex was of low saliency seemed to have no readily available fantasy nexus to handle this input. For these subjects the film material was blocked or came through directly at night and was not productive of morning associations.

This study has taught us something of the complexity of relating the nighttime fantasy data to what precedes and follows from it in wakefulness. It has also given us cause to believe that this subject can be approached experimentally with high hopes of a productive yield.

REFERENCES

1. Cartwright, R., with Bernick, N., Borowitz, G., and Kling, A. The effect of an erotic movie on the sleep and dreams of young men. *Arch. Gen. Psychiat.* (Chicago) 20:262, 1969.
2. Hall, C., and Van de Castle, R. *The Content Analysis of Dreams.* New York: Appleton-Century-Crofts, 1966.
3. Kling, A., Cartwright, R., Bernick, N., and Borowitz, G. Physiological, Psychological, and Symbolic Correlates of Sexual Arousal in Man. In H. Giese (Ed.), *Sex and Fantasy.* Hamburg, Germany: Rowholt, 1969.

Dream Research and Psychoanalytic Theory

*Does all the recent psychophysiological research on sleep and dreaming have any effect on psychoanalytic theory? On other psychological theory?**

Psychoanalytic Dream Theory Reexamined

DAVID R. HAWKINS

An enormous recrudescence of interest in dreaming was stimulated by the findings of Dement and Kleitman [4] that dreaming occurred regularly during the night in connection with rapid eye movements and a particular type of EEG pattern subsequently known as stage 1. Not only were there many neurophysiological findings related to the dreaming or D-state of sleep, but the method for waking subjects whenever dreaming occurred promised much easier access in both breadth and depth to the study of dreams. It looked for a while as if the "royal road to the unconscious" was about to become a multilane super-interstate throughway. Un-

* The reader interested in this question may wish to refer also to papers by Baekeland (p. 49), Karacan and Williams (p. 93), Foulkes (p. 147), Lewis (p. 199), Jones (p. 221 and p. 335), Pearlman (p. 329), and Ephron and Carrington (p. 344).

fortunately, not much useful traffic has developed. I will discuss why this is so.

It was inevitable that the new insights and methodology would lead to a reexamination of psychoanalytic dream theory. Indeed, one of the earliest experiments performed by Dement [3] was addressed to the concept that the function of dreams is to discharge the unconscious. A selective deprivation of the D-state and therefore of dreaming should lead to psychological distress with perhaps the buildup of instinctual drives and anxiety. The initial study strongly indicated a buildup of neurophysiological or neurochemical need for D-state sleep, and there was a suggestion of increased tension and irritation in the subjects. Subsequent studies both in human beings and other mammals have confirmed that there is a mechanism to insure the D-state or REM stage of sleep and that it responds to deprivation with increased urgency for this stage of sleep. These studies have not clearly demonstrated psychological difficulties.

Most of the studies in this area have taken the approach of studying the mean function of a group rather than remembering the importance in human behavioral research of paying attention to individual differences. Cartwright and her colleagues [2] alone in this area of study have paid attention to the individual and have clarified that there are differing responses both neurophysiologically and psychologically to D-state deprivation. It is Cartwright's hypothesis that "dreaming mentation is continuous but can only occupy awareness under certain conditions, i.e., a heightened level of arousal and a reduction of the usual sensory input."

Trosman [16] first formally discussed the implications of new dream research for psychoanalytic theory. I agree essentially with his points of view but have tried to develop the relationship further in three papers [9–11], the contents of which will be summarized briefly here. Freud stressed that the dream is a fully valid physical act which plays a meaningful role in the individual's psychic life. We know from the new research that there is a special stage of sleep, the D-state, which occurs in every human being and which is accompanied by dreaming. To date we have not unequivocally established a meaningful role for the dream. Psychophysiological studies cannot do this; however, the capacity to awaken human beings during the D-state and obtain detailed reports may help us with this problem. The investigations of Witkin [17] and his associates seem the most useful and comprehensive in this regard. Briefly, they present highly emotionally charged moving pictures to subjects just before sleep. The subjects are then awakened and sequential dream reports are obtained. They are in effect presenting tagged stimuli whose development and impact on the psychic life of the dreamer can be studied.

The meaningfulness of dreams and their role in the psychic economy of the individual seem to the experienced analyst clearly established. However, research which will allow this to be put on a firm objective basis still needs to be pursued.

An important aspect of Freud's dream theory was that the dream represented the disguised fulfillment of a suppressed or repressed wish. Obviously, direct psychophysiological studies cannot give us the answer to this postulate, but again the methodology of access to dream reports may be of some use. It may be, however, that as we better understand neurophysiology, particularly of the limbic system, we will come to a clearer notion of motivation. Animal preparations, such as the cats studied by Jouvet [12] in which the nucleus coeruleus has been extirpated and hence the motor paralysis of the D-state interfered with, might possibly lead to some answers in this regard. If these animals could also be influenced in some way which can arouse inter alia motivations of hunger, thirst, sexual excitement, it might be possible to get at some of these questions by studying their behavior.

My own point of view on this matter is that we now are quite clear that behavior and hence thinking are motivated and that any careful study of human verbal productions or fantasy will reveal motivations or wishes. A dream would seem to be an unusually rich source for assessing underlying wishes or motivation.

A cornerstone of psychoanalytic dream theory is that the dream serves the function of being a guardian of sleep. Freud assumed that during sleep there was a lowering of repression, and consciously unacceptable drives might begin to make their presence felt. It was his concept that this usually occurred when there was beginning to be arousal, that is, during light sleep. According to Freud's concept, the unconscious drives or wishes, instead of leading to action or arousing the sleeper, were able to move in a direction opposite to that in waking thought and activate the system perception from within, thus allowing the hallucinatory experience of the dream to occur.

Our new knowledge derived from psychophysiological sleep studies, which includes information unavailable to Freud, indicates a need for revision of Freud's original hypothesis. We now know that the D-state (and presumably also dreaming) is a repetitive, virtually automatic phenomenon which, except under unusual circumstances, occupies the same amount of time each night. Hence we might think of things really the other way around and say that sleep insures dreaming. However, there may be more than a grain of truth in Freud's notion, for if we conceive of the dream now as a psychological event it would seem that the way in which the material is handled in the dream does, indeed, determine whether or not there is waking from the D-state. We know that under certain circumstances dreams which become too anxiety-filled do lead to awakening.

The other major function of dreaming, according to Freud, was to discharge the unconscious to bring it back under control of the preconscious. Freud related his discharge of "unconscious excitations" concept to the "excretion theory" of Robert [15]. Robert indicated that dreams deal with trivial daily impressions and rarely with important daily interests. His notion was that dreams serve the purpose of dealing with thoughts which have not been properly incorporated into memory during the previous day. Robert seems to have anticipated the information processing and storing aspects of dreams which I [9] and other investigators [5, 8] have recently postulated as being the function of dreaming.

Again, at present, we can't conclusively confirm or refute this notion of Freud's. It is useful to conceptualize in psychoanalytic structural terms in thinking of the activation of the D-state as permitting the ego to integrate id or instinctual drives along with problems raised during the previous day. According to this concept, the D-state would allow a playing out of the drive and rearrangement of motives in model form. That is, no action is involved, but there is an opportunity for rehearsal or trying out different ways of permitting eventual gratification of a variety of drives or needs.

Two neurophysiological findings in recent years with regard to sleep do tend to confirm early ideas of Freud. These are the demonstration by Pompeiano [14] of motor paralysis during the D-state and the finding that during the D-state there are spiking waves originating in the pons which lead to similar activity in the lateral geniculate and in the occipital cortex (optical radiation area) [1].

In his first statement about dreams in the *Project for Scientific Psychology* Freud [7] said, "Dreams are devoid of motor discharge. . . . we are paralyzed in dreams." He postulated some mechanism which left the spinal neurons in a state he called uncathected, meaning incapable of excitation and discharge. In his final statement on dream interpretation in *An Outline of Psychoanalysis* Freud [6] emphasized that it is the fact of motor paralysis which allows safe expression of generally unacceptable primitive id impulses during dreaming.

A major conceptual contribution in Chapter 7 of *The Interpretation of Dreams* was that of the role of regression in dream formation. Freud postulated that the latent dream thoughts moved in a reverse fashion through the mental apparatus to activate the system perception from within, thus accounting for the hallucinatory aspect of dreams. Spiking waves which originate in the pons travel from the lateral geniculate body to the occipital cortex in such a fashion as to signal stimuli as if arising from the retina. It is tempting to assume that this is the neurophysiological basis for Freud's postulated regressive direction of internal stimuli to the system perception. The interpretation of these apparent signals would be dependent on the psychological state of the individual. According to this notion this process would be analogous to the case in which one interprets ink blots of the Rorschach test as meaningful percepts.

There are other ways in which it would be possible to attempt to reconcile or perhaps find differences between the new psychophysiological studies and psychoanalytic dream theory. I think it fair to state that to date there is nothing in the new findings which requires a major revision of psychoanalytic dream theory, though certain changes in emphasis are indicated. There are some findings which tend to be confirmatory; however, nothing has clearly established in unqualified terms that psychoanalytic dream theory is correct.

What about dream theory as adumbrated by other schools of psychology? It seems that much the same thing may be said about these theories in relationship to the new sleep studies as about psychoanalytic theory. There are certain things which confirm and others that suggest need for modification, but to date none of the studies are crucial for various dream theories. Kirsch [13] has published a brief paper relating recent studies to Jung's theory of dreams. In his summary he states, "A very brief resume of Jung's approach to dreams has been presented emphasizing those aspects which appear analogous to the REM state. There seems to be a parallelism covering the basic hypothesis, and there is the need for a reassessment of our psychological understanding of dreams based on the recent research." At a symposium on "Dream Psychology and the New Biology of Dreaming" [13a] held at the University of Cincinnati, 1967, dream theory in the light of new research was examined. A Focal Conflict View, A Culturalist View, A Jungian View, An Adlerian View, An Existentialist View as well as a Freudian View were discussed. In general, the same conclusions were reached as I have indicated above for Freudian theory.

I believe this indicates that those who are interested primarily in the psychological aspects of dreaming and its role in the psychic economy in the individual should be conversant with the new findings. Hopefully some will utilize them and the new methodology to attempt more extended individual studies of the dream process.

REFERENCES

1. Bizzi, E., and Brooks, D. C. Relationship between pontine and lateral geniculate nuclei during episodes of deep sleep. *Arch. Ital. Biol.* 101:666, 1963.

2. Cartwright, R. D., Monroe, L. J., and Palmer, C. Individual differences in response to REM deprivation. *Arch. Gen. Psychiat.* (Chicago) 16:297, 1967.
3. Dement, W. C. The effect of dream deprivation. *Science* 131: 1705; 132:1420, 1960.
4. Dement, W. C., and Kleitman, N. Relation of eye movements during sleep to dream activity: An objective method for the study of dreaming. *J. Exp. Psychol.* 53:339, 1957.
5. Dewan, E. M. Sleep as a Programming Process and Dreaming ("D-State") as an Addressing Procedure. Paper read at Association for the Psychophysiological Study of Sleep, Santa Monica, Cal., 1967.
6. Freud, S. An Outline of Psychoanalysis. In *The Standard Edition of the Complete Psychological Works of Sigmund Freud,* tr. and ed. by J. Strachey with others. London: Hogarth Press and the Institute of Psycho-Analysis, 1964. Vol. XXIII, p. 141.
7. Freud, S. The Origins of Psychoanalysis (partly including: A project for scientific psychology) (1895). *Standard Edition.* London: Hogarth, 1966. Vol. I.
8. Greenberg, R., and Leiderman, P. H. Perceptions, the dream process and memory: An up-to-date version of notes on a mystic writing pad. *Compr. Psychiat.* 7:517, 1966.
9. Hawkins, D. R. A review of psychoanalytic dream theory in the light of recent psycho-physiological studies of sleep and dreaming. *Brit. J. Med. Psychol.* 39:85, 1966.
10. Hawkins, D. R. Implications for psychoanalytic theory of psychophysiologic sleep research. *Med. Psicosom.* 12:290, 1967.
11. Hawkins, D. R. The Challenge Posed to Dream Theories by the New Biology of Dreaming: A Freudian View. In M. Kramer (Ed.), *Dream Psychology and the New Biology of Dreaming.* Springfield, Ill.: Thomas, 1969.
12. Jouvet, M., and Delorme, F. Locus coeruleus, et sommeil paradoxal. *C. R. Soc. Biol.* (Paris) 195:896, 1965.
13. Kirsch, T. B. The relationship of the REM state to analytical psychology. *Amer. J. Psychiat.* 124:1459, 1968.

13a. Kramer, M. (Ed.) *Dream Psychology and the New Biology of Dreaming.* Springfield: Thomas, 1969.

14. Pompeiano, O. Ascending and Descending Influences of Somatic Afferent Volleys in Unrestrained Cats: Supraspinal Inhibitory Control of Spinal Reflexes During Natural and Reflexly-induced Sleep. In *Neurophysiologie des Etats de Sommeil.* Paris: Centre National de la Recherche Scientifique, 1965.

15. Robert, W. Der traum als natürnotwendigkeit erklärt (Hamburg, 1886.) As quoted in S. Freud, The Interpretation of Dreams (1900). *Standard Edition*. London: Hogarth, 1953. Vol. IV–V. 1886.
16. Trosman, H. Dream research and the psychoanalytic theory of dreams. *Arch. Gen. Psychiat.* (Chicago) 9:9, 1963.
17. Witkin, H. A. The relation of experimentally induced presleep experiences to dreams. *J. Amer. Psychoanal. Ass.* 13:819, 1966.

Is the Domain of the Psychological Still Floating?

ELIZABETH R. ZETZEL

In one of his early letters to Fliess, Freud [3] made the following statement:

> I have no inclination at all to leave the domain of the psychological, floating as it were in the air without any organic foundation, but I have no knowledge, neither therapeutically nor theoretically, beyond that conviction. So I have to conduct myself as if I had only the psychological before me.

This "as if" was an extremely crucial and important step in the initiation of psychoanalysis as an independent body of knowledge. In effect Freud was noting that he could not explain the conclusions he was reaching at that time in respect to the structure and function of the mind. This, however, did not mean that he renounced the idea that psychological events would ultimately be explained in terms of their organic basis. It suggested rather that until the time came that a correlation could be made, the development of psychological understanding would have to be viewed in terms of a psychological theoretical framework, since it could not be explained in terms of physiological structure and function.

The recent advances in many areas of neuroanatomy, neurophysiology, and biochemistry clearly suggest that the time is approaching when this correlation may be anticipated as an attainable goal. The contemporary psychoanalyst must therefore try as far as possible to be both flexible and dispassionate in an attempt to review and amend, wherever necessary, Freud's original theory in the light of new objective knowledge. The theory of dreams was the source of Freud's original model of the psychic apparatus. Chapter 7 of *The Interpretation of Dreams* (1900) [4] remains a basic contribution to psychoanalytic theory. Recent scientific work, however, has added objective knowledge relevant to sleep and dreaming through the development of scientific methods undreamed of in Freud's day. A review of Freud's original theory is therefore indicated in order to discover whether or not we have yet acquired enough objective knowledge to abandon the "as if" hypothesis on which Freud constructed his original model of the psychic apparatus. In this discussion I will mainly refer to the original text of *The Interpretation of Dreams.* I will, however, include some reference to later contributions, in particular Freud's reference to traumatic dreams as an exception to his theory of wish fulfillment and his discussion of the perceptual apparatus in a later paper entitled The Mystic Writing Pad [6].

In Chapter 5 of *The Interpretation of Dreams,* Freud discussed the characteristics of memory in dreams, indicating that he had not so far been able fully to account for them. He suggested that "Their proper place must be looked for elsewhere, *either* in the psychology of the state of sleep *or* in the discussion of the structure of the mental apparatus upon which we shall later embark." He clearly implied elsewhere that sleep was not only a psychological but a biological and physiological event. He therefore suggested that a psychological approach to the meaning of dreams required conceptual differentiation between sleeping and dreaming. In neither Chapter 7, however, nor in the later *Metapsychological Supplement to the Theory of Dreams* (1917) [5] did Freud entirely succeed in maintaining this important conceptual differentiation. In Chapter 7, for example, his suggestion that the wish to sleep was a primary instigator of the dream at least implicitly attempted to present a psychological rather than a biological explanation of sleep. In the

Metapsychological Supplement his equation of sleep with a state of primary narcissism is subject to even more questions as to how far he has used a psychological model to explain not only psychic but also biological and physiological events.

I do not wish to imply that these attempts did not prove fruitful for the later development of our psychological understanding. I would, however, like to suggest that the most significant areas in which recent research findings appear at first sight to be incompatible with Freud's constructs are those in which he himself departed from his own original frame of reference, namely "to keep only the psychological" before him. Insofar as we maintain this point of view we should only be concerned with those dreams which are either spontaneously remembered or which have aroused sufficient conscious attention on the part of the dreamer to enable him to report the fact that he has forgotten a dream. We must also remember that, as Lewin [7] indicated, dreams are not only forgotten because their content leads the dreamer to repress them; they are sometimes lost for other reasons. I won't expand this point but mainly refer to his useful differentiation between forgetting as a verb, i.e., repression of content, and forgetting as a noun, i.e., losing, which may well bear some relation to the differences between sleeping and waking life.

CONTEMPORARY EVIDENCE RE DREAMING

Contemporary research has shown that dreaming, as indicated by the physiological D-state or REM state, is to be regarded as an integral and significant component of normal sleep. The proportion of sleeping time occupied by this state makes it more than probable that a remembered dream occupies only a small fraction of any night's total dreaming sleep. Dream deprivation studies have clearly suggested that dreaming is not only primarily, or perhaps even significantly the guardian of sleep in the sense that Freud suggested; it is rather a necessary part of sleep, deprivation of which interferes with the well-being and adaptation not only of human beings but of many nonhuman species. We are thus inevitably drawn to the conclusion that dreaming sleep as indicated by the REM state must serve an adaptive biological purpose. It does not occur only in response to external or internal stimuli which would otherwise lead to arousal.

There is, in addition, a good deal of evidence to suggest that the REM state specifically lends itself to formal topographical and possibly to temporal regression. We now have objective evidence that the paths to motility are indeed particularly inhibited during the dreaming state. We also have evidence that this inhibition is associated with specific activation of the perceptual apparatus. It is not hard to believe that this complex biological state should involve modifications in respect to internal economy, including here not only the reemergence of forgotten early memories but also the otherwise defended-against impulses with which they were associated. All that we know about the material of dream work in reported dreams might thus be attributed to the biological need to go on dreaming. These dreams, anxiety dreams, and arousal dreams would point to relative failure to go on dreaming successfully. The remembered, the anxiety, and the clearly repressed dream (which can represent only a small fraction of total dream time) might thus be regarded as evidence that the regression integral to the dreaming state has, for whatever reason, threatened its own continuation. In other words, the dream we deal with as a psychological event may have been dreamed in order to preserve dreaming sleep as an important biological state of adaptation.

THE NEW KNOWLEDGE AND FREUD

Several recent investigators have suggested in this context that many of Freud's original propositions may be regarded as relevant to dreaming during the REM state. On the one hand there has been objective evidence, largely confirmatory of Freud's suggestion, that the manifest content of the remembered dream contains disguised but nevertheless recognizable perceptual memories from the recent past. Fisher [2], for example, has confirmed and expanded the reappearance of preconscious perceptions in the manifest dreams of experimental subjects. Freud originally placed particular emphasis on the 24 hours preceding the dream. Recent experimental work has shown that this period may be expanded to as much as 72 hours. Such an expansion modifies but does not contradict Freud's original thesis. Freud suggested in his later paper on The Mystic Writing Pad that perception and memory must be allocated to different areas of the central nervous system. The apparatus which perceives must in other words be unburdened by memory as it absorbs new perceptions. The accumulated evidence in respect to the enormous amount of preconscious perception which goes on at all times adds weight to the comparison he made between the repeated clearing of the receiving surface of the mystic writing pad and the laying down of permanent memory traces. The possibility must be envisaged that the REM state, during which preconscious perceptions from the recent past are incorporated into the manifest dream experience, may involve what might be described as the clearing of the perceptual apparatus. One explanation of the effects of dream deprivation on individual perception might then relate to the possibility that the dream-deprived individual's perceptual apparatus had not been offered adequate opportunity for this clearing process. This I believe remains an area for further objective investigation.

In a recent paper Meissner [8] reviewed the contributions of other workers in this field and added the results of his own research. He does not attempt, happily, to substitute the language of neurophysiology for the language of psychoanalysis. Instead he presents interesting material relevant to the D-period or REM period as a major biological state. This he reviews in respect to certain aspects of Freudian theory. My only criticism of Meissner's stimulating thesis is, first, that he may have accepted too literally the continued validity of Freud's instinct theory and, second, that his approach to repression and the dream censor does not take fully into account some of the later modifications of analytic theory. Among these I will select two for special attention.

First, the unconscious automatic nature of ego defenses means in effect that these defenses are just as much part of the censored as the underlying ego-alien wishes concerned. Meissner suggests in this context that individuals who use repression as a defense not only forget dreams, which is often true, but actually dream less than other people. Clinical experience leads me to believe that exactly the opposite is the case. Individuals who use repression as a major defense fall by and large into the group of hysterical characters or hysterical neurotics. Although such individuals often forget their dreams they are usually prolific dreamers. The nature of their dreams during the analytic process clearly reveals not only the nature of the defended-against wishes but also the fact that anxiety increases as this specific defense is increasingly threatened.

The second point I wish to discuss concerns still unresolved questions as to how far the repetition compulsion represents an exception to the theory of dreams as wish fulfillment which was Freud's original proposal. Meissner suggests that dreaming serves a useful adaptive purpose in the organization of the perceptual system and a gradual internalization of perceived memories. In this context I would like to refer to another of Freud's early letters [3] to Fliess.

As you know, I am working on the assumption that our psychical mechanism has come about by a process of stratification—the material present in the shape of memory traces is from time to time subjected to a reorganization in accordance with fresh circumstances; is, as it were, transcribed.

This statement may be reconsidered in terms of our understanding of the repetition compulsion. A brief consideration of what happens to the traumatic dreams of essentially healthy individuals is compatible with Meissner's basic hypothesis. At first such dreams repeat, without distortion, the traumatic experience. This does not continue indefinitely as the individual recovers. True, he continues to have anxiety dreams in which elements of the traumatic experience may readily be recognized. Gradually, however, the dreams change. The repetition is more and more distorted. Earlier memories are intertwined with the recent experience and the significance of the traumatic event becomes more and more understandable in the light of the dreamer's early experience and definitive character structure. In such cases the repetitive and gradually changing dreams have clearly served adaptive, progressive purposes. The need to repeat is neither pathological nor essentially regressive. Bibring [1] in his paper on the repetition compulsion referred to possible progressive implications. The REM state, by reviving recent perceptual memories, facilitates affective reexperience, gradual toning down of affect, and ultimate mastery. It is by no means impossible that the large dreaming time of the young infant serves a similar progressive adaptive purpose.

REDUCTION OF DREAMING TIME

Finally, I will comment on one interesting objective finding, namely the relatively sharp reduction of dreaming time around the age of 3 to 6. It almost seems redundant for a psychoanalyst to mention the interesting correlation between this apparently common finding and the time of the resolution, for better or worse, of the infantile oedipal situation. This time has been described by many as the period in which psychic structure becomes for the first time relatively stronger than primitive unmodified instinct. Anxiety as the signal for repression and related defenses is definitively established during this period. It may thus be suggested that this development is responsible not only for the maintenance of stable ego defenses but also for the well-recognized infantile amnesia. It might also be speculated as to how far this decisive change in internal economy which may well be facilitated by biological maturation is also related to the convincingly demonstrated quantitative reduction in dream time which occurs concurrently.

SUMMARY

In conclusion, I have been able to touch on only a few among the many interesting and stimulating suggestions offered by recent objective studies of sleep and the dream. In summary I would suggest, first, our continued need to maintain a conceptual differentiation between the dream as a meaningful psychological event and objective studies relevant to different stages of sleep. If Freud went wrong it was not in respect to the former, but in areas which pertained to the biological functions of sleep. I have referred to the interesting correlation between the time dreaming sleep diminishes and the passing of the oedipal situation. I have suggested finally that a consideration of the meaning of repetitive dreams during the mastery of traumatic experience is in keeping with the proposal that dreaming sleep is a state which serves progressive adaptive purposes in respect to the organization of memory and the capacity to tolerate and master painful affective experience.

REFERENCES

1. Bibring, E. The conception of the repetition compulsion. *Psychoanal. Quart.* 12:486, 1943.
2. Fisher, C. Psychoanalytic implications of recent research on sleep and dreaming. II. Implications for Psychoanalytic Theory. *J. Amer. Psychoanal. Ass.* 13:271, 1965.
3. Freud, S. *The Origins of Psychoanalysis* (1898). New York: Basic Books, 1954.
4. Freud, S. The Interpretation of Dreams (1900). In *The Standard Edition of the Complete Psychological Works of Sigmund Freud,* tr. and ed. by J. Strachey with others. London: Hogarth and the Institute of Psycho-Analysis, 1953. Vol. IV–V.
5. Freud, S. A Metapsychological Supplement to the Theory of Dreams (1917). *Standard Edition.* London: Hogarth, 1957. Vol. XIV.
6. Freud, S. The Mystic Writing Pad (1925). *Standard Edition.* London: Hogarth, 1961. Vol. XIX.
7. Lewin, B. The Forgetting of Dreams. In R. Loewenstein (Ed.), *Drives, Affects and Behavior,* Vol. 1. New York: International Universities Press, 1933.
8. Meissner, W. W. On dreaming as process. *Int. J. Psychoanal.* 49:1, 1968.

The D-State, Dreaming, and Memory

*Are there important connections between dreaming and memory? Or between the D-state and memory?**

The Relationship between REM Sleep and Learning: Animal Studies

WARREN C. STERN

The role of REM sleep (D-state) in understanding the physiological basis of animal behavior has only recently been investigated. The outcome of this research, important in itself, also provides a test of several theories of sleep function [3, 8, 14, 21, 26, 28]. Recent studies have reported that REM sleep deprivation (RD) impaired acquisition of tasks trained after the deprivation. In some experiments RD also disrupted the performance of tasks trained prior to the deprivation. A description and assessment of this research is the subject of this paper.

* The reader interested in this question may wish to refer also to papers by Dewan (p. 295), Hartmann (p. 308), Pearlman (p. 329), and Jones (p. 335).

All the RD studies to be discussed accomplished the deprivation by using the "inverted flower pot" or "water tank" technique. In this procedure the animal is placed on a small platform located at the water level in an escape-proof enclosure. The muscular relaxation which accompanies REM sleep, but not NREM sleep, results in contact with the water and termination of the REM period. The effectiveness of this procedure in inducing REM sleep loss has been demonstrated in cats [15], rats [10, 20], and mice [13]. The water tank procedure also induces a considerable physiological stress as measured by adrenal gland hypertrophy [18, 31], thymus gland atrophy, and increased ACTH synthesis [18]. Morden et al. [20] have advocated a large platform stress control (in the water tank apparatus) which would presumably enable the animal to curl up and obtain normal amounts of REM sleep. Most RD studies have employed this control. However, Duncan et al. [10] reported that rats confined to large platforms are deprived on the average of 50 percent of their REM sleep compared to 80 percent deprivation on small platforms. Fishbein [13] reported similar findings in mice. Thus failure to find learning differences following treatment between small and large platforms groups, as reported for active avoidance acquisition [1, 2] and passive avoidance retention [29], can be interpreted either as a failure of 50 percent versus 80 percent RD to produce differential behavioral effects or as a stress effect. Stern [29, 31] employed an alternative stress control in which rats were immersed in cold water for 1 hour per day such that their adrenal gland hypertrophy and body weight losses (restricted food intake) equaled or exceeded those of the RD condition. The 5-day cold water immersed stress controls did not show learning impairments on tasks which were impaired by 5 days of RD (described later [29]). Nevertheless it should be noted that this control employs a repeated acute stress, whereas the RD water tank stress is more continuous. Also the cold water controls may have experienced some REM sleep loss. The importance of conducting a stress control is demonstrated by the findings that in rats both the RD and cold water immersion procedures (compared to normal rats) induced equivalent increases in the rate of click-elicited startle response habituation [32]. (Webb [33] reported a similar increase in startle response habituation in totally sleep deprived rats. Dewson et al. [9] found that RD increased auditory cortex recovery cycles to clicks. This increase in neurophysiological excitability would not have predicted the reduced behavioral responsiveness to clicks.) RD and cold water immersion also produced equivalent decreases in bar pressing rates on a continuous (Sidman) avoidance task trained prior to RD [29]. Thus omission of a stress control condition could have resulted in the attribution of the startle response habituation and Sidman avoidance changes to a loss of REM sleep.

An additional control, which is frequently omitted, is a group deprived of an amount of NREM sleep equal to the duration of the REM sleep loss. This control is necessary in order to demonstrate that the RD treatment effects are specifically due to REM sleep loss. An NREM sleep loss control was conducted by Stern [29] in which rats were manually prevented from sleeping for 15 to 16 hours per day for 5 days. The 8- to 9-hour sleep period each night permitted a total sleep time (per diem) which at most equaled the total amount of sleep obtained (per diem) by the small platform rats (i.e., 8 hours per day [10]). The sleep loss controls performed like normal rats and also performed significantly better than the RD rats on active and passive avoidance acquisition [29].

EFFECTS ON PERFORMANCE OF PRETRAINED TASKS

Several studies have examined the effects of RD upon performance of a task trained prior to the deprivation. Pearlman and Greenberg [24] reported that retention performance of a partially trained passive avoidance response following 24 hours of RD by rats was impaired relative to large platform controls. Similarly, Stern [29] reported a performance impairment, compared to cold water stress controls, of a passive avoidance response trained for 6 days prior to 5 days of RD. Fishbein [11] conducted extensive one-trial trained passive avoidance studies with mice in which it was found that training followed by 3 days of RD and ½ to 3 hours recovery before retention testing produced complete amnesia for the task, whereas a 24-hour recovery period produced normal retention. Although the three preceding studies lacked NREM sleep loss controls, and the mice experiments also lacked adequate stress controls, the results were generally interpreted as an RD induced memory disruption. It is also possible to interpret these results as an RD induced performance decrement not necessarily related to memory disturbance, or as an RD induced "dissociation" or "state dependent" phenomenon similar to that described by Overton [22, 23] following certain drug treatments. A "non-memory impairment" performance decrement might result from sickness, activity level change, change in motivation, and so forth. The dissociation interpretation is suggested because the performance impairments of the preceding studies occurred when training was given in the normal state and retention testing was given in the RD state—no passive avoidance performance decrement occurred if recovery to the normal state was permitted [11]. Additional support for the dissociation proposal is the finding that in mice a 3-day RD-train–7-day RD-retention test treatment sequence did *not* produce passive avoidance performance impairment when retention testing was conducted immediately after RD (both training and retention testing were done in the RD state). However, a 1-day recovery period between RD and retention testing (return to the normal state) produced a marked performance impairment [12]. A test of the dissociation hypothesis would be provided by a treatment sequence of RD-train–RD-recovery-test–RD-test. A performance decrement should occur during recovery (as reported [12, 16]), but performance should improve when RD is reintroduced (as reported [16]). An additional interpretation problem of the RD induced memory disruption hypothesis is that, at present, performance on active avoidance tasks trained prior to RD has not been reported to be disrupted by the deprivation [1, 29]. This consideration restricts the behavioral generality of the memory disruption, generalized performance decrement, and dissociation hypotheses. The lack of active avoidance impairment also suggests the possibility that performance deficits may be specific to passive avoidance.

In summary, the interpretation that passive avoidance performance decrements following RD are due to memory disruption is only one of several possible explanations.

EFFECTS ON NEW LEARNING

A preliminary description of a learning impairment following RD has been given for Y-maze acquisition by cats [7]. However, this study contained few subjects and did not report control data. Albert et al. [1, 2] reported that active avoidance acquisition by RD rats was the same as large platform controls, but inferior to normal rats. The lack of differences between RD and large platform controls may be attributed either to the large amount of REM sleep loss in the control condition or to stress. A 2-day RD-train, 2-day RD-retention test treatment sequence produced normal shock avoidance retention in cats [4]. However, 2 days of RD preceding training may be insufficient to produce a learning impairment in cats. The effects of RD upon subsequent learning by rats was examined in a series of controlled experiments by Stern [29]. It was found that 5 days of RD preceding training (1) more than doubled the number of trials required until five consecutive avoidance responses were made in a 1-way shuttle box, (2) resulted in poorer retention of a one-trial trained passive avoidance step-down task,* and (3) produced slower acquisition of a sugar water motivated alternation discrimination in which responding was rewarded on every other trial. Acquisition of these tasks was significantly poorer in the RD condition when compared to normal rats, cold water stress controls, and NREM sleep loss controls—the latter control was not conducted for the alternation discrimination. These apparent RD-induced learning deficits were probably not due to (1) dissociation—both training and testing were conducted in the RD state, (2) altered activity levels —both active and passive avoidance were impaired, (3) lower shock reactivity—RD produces an increased reactivity to electric shock [1,

* Fishbein [12] reported normal 1-hour passive avoidance retention when training followed 3 days of RD in mice.

19, 30], and (4) a generalized nonspecific performance impairment —performance of active avoidance trained prior to RD was not disrupted [1, 29] and passive avoidance performance with a 5-second retention interval (train and test after RD) was not impaired [29]. Since the learning impairments occurred in three different tasks it is also unlikely that these effects were due to some unique property of the behavioral testing situation.

EFFECTS OF TOTAL SLEEP DEPRIVATION

Several studies have measured the behavioral effects of 8 to 48 hours of total sleep deprivation in animals. Bunch et al. [5, 6] and Licklider et al. [17] reported that sleep deprivation improved acquisition of escape responses from a water maze by rats. However, the increased reactivity to the aversive aspects of water immersion by the deprived rats led Licklider et al. to conclude that ". . . the superiority of the wakeful [sleep deprived] rats may be regarded mainly as one of performance and not . . . one of ability to learn" (p. 346). Rust [27] found that food-motivated bar pressing was not disrupted by 48 hours of total sleep deprivation in rats. Similarly, 176 hours of total sleep deprivation in monkeys did not markedly disrupt performance on a matching task trained prior to the deprivation [25]. Thus in contrast to the REM sleep deprivation studies, total sleep deprivation has not been reported to produce learning or performance impairments. It is likely that these total sleep deprivation studies have not employed sufficiently sensitive behavioral measures since partial sleep deprivation (RD) frequently results in acquisition impairments. The methodological difficulty of producing total sleep loss in animals has undoubtedly contributed to the paucity of research in this area.

SUMMARY

In summary, water tank–produced REM sleep deprivation has provided highly suggestive evidence that RD impairs the acquisition of learned behavior and perhaps the retention of responses trained prior to the deprivation. Replication of these results in additional behavioral tests and with other methods of inducing REM sleep loss is needed. The results obtained so far are in general agreement with the theoretical predictions of Moruzzi [21] and Dewan [8]. Moruzzi proposed that sleep permits recovery of "plastic" synapses so that subsequent learning during wakefulness is more efficient. Dewan [8] and Gaarder [14] have hypothesized that new memories are processed and encoded during REM sleep. However, the behavioral effects produced by RD would not be readily predicted by the ontogenetic [26], phylogenetic [28], and oculomotor exercise [3] hypotheses of REM sleep function. It may be that REM sleep has many functions and that at present no one hypothesis provides a complete description of why REM sleep occurs.

REFERENCES

1. Albert, I., Cicala, G. A., and Siegel, J. Further Studies on the Behavioral Effects of REM Sleep Deprivation. Paper read at Association for the Psychophysiological Study of Sleep (APSS), Boston, 1969.
2. Albert, I., Siegel, J., and Cicala, G. The Behavioral Effects of REM Sleep Deprivation in Rats. Paper read at APSS, Denver, 1968.
3. Berger, R. J. Oculomotor control: A possible function of REM sleep. *Psychol. Rev.* 76:144, 1969.
4. Brill, R. W., Jr., and Goodman, I. J. Effects of REM Sleep Deprivation on Memory in Cats. Paper read at APSS, Boston, 1969.
5. Bunch, M. E., Cole, A., and Frerichs, J. The influence of twenty-four hours of wakefulness upon the learning and retention of a maze problem in white rats. *J. Comp. Psychol.* 23: 1, 1937.
6. Bunch, M. E., Frerichs, J. B., and Licklider, J. R. An experimental study of maze learning ability after varying periods of wakefulness. *J. Comp. Psychol.* 26:499, 1938.
7. Dement, W. Recent studies on the biological role of rapid eye movement sleep. *Amer. J. Psychiat.* 122:404, 1965.
8. Dewan, E. M. Tests of the Programming (P) Hypothesis for REM Sleep. Paper read at APSS, Denver, 1968.

9. Dewson, J., Dement, W., Wagener, T., and Novel, K. Rapid eye movement sleep deprivation: A central neural change during wakefulness. *Science* 156:403, 1967.
10. Duncan, R., Henry, P., Karadzic, V., Mitchell, G., Pivik, T., Cohen, H., and Dement, W. Baseline Sleep and REM Sleep Deprivation in the Rat. Paper read at APSS, Santa Monica, Cal., 1967.
11. Fishbein, W. The Effects of Paradoxical Sleep Deprivation During the Retention Interval on Long-Term Memory. Paper read at APSS, Boston, 1969.
12. Fishbein, W. The Effects of Paradoxical Sleep Deprivation Prior to Initial Learning on Long-Term Memory. Paper read at APSS, Boston, 1969.
13. Fishbein, W. Paradoxical Sleep: A Periodic Mechanism for Securing and Maintaining Information for Long-Term Memory. University of Colorado Doctoral Dissertation, 1969.
14. Gaarder, K. A conceptual model of sleep. *Arch. Gen. Psychiat.* (Chicago) 14:253, 1966.
15. Jouvet, D., Vimont, P., Delorme, F., and Jouvet, M. Étude de la privation selective de la phase paradoxale de sommeil chez le chat. *C. R. Soc. Biol.* (Paris) 158:756, 1964.
16. Joy, R. M., and Prinz, P. N. Chronic postural restriction in the rat: Its effect upon sleep patterns and the acquisition and retention of a conditioned avoidance response (abstract). *Proc. West. Pharmacol. Soc.* 10:50, 1967.
17. Licklider, J. C. R., and Bunch, M. E. Effects of enforced wakefulness upon the growth and the maze-learning performance of white rats. *J. Comp. Psychol.* 39:339, 1946.
18. Ling, G. M., and Usher, D. R. Effect of REM and Total Sleep Deprivation on the Synthesis and Release of ACTH. Paper read at APSS, Boston, 1969.
19. Morden, B., Conner, R., Mitchell, G., Dement, W., and Levine, S. Effects of rapid eye movement (REM) sleep deprivation on shock-induced fighting. *Physiol. Behav.* 3:425, 1968.
20. Morden, B., Mitchell, G., and Dement, W. Selective REM sleep deprivation and compensation phenomena in the rat. *Brain Res.* 5:339, 1967.
21. Moruzzi, G. The Funtional Significance of Sleep with Particular Regard to the Brain Mechanisms Underlying Consciousness. In J. C. Eccles (Ed.), *Brain Mechanisms and Conscious Experience*. New York: Springer-Verlag, 1966.
22. Overton, D. A. State-dependent learning produced by depres-

sant and atropine-like drugs. *Psychopharmacologia* (Berlin) 10: 6, 1966.

23. Overton, D. A. Dissociated Learning in Drug States (State Dependent Learning). In D. H. Efron (Ed.), *Psychopharmacology: A Review of Progress 1957–1967*. Washington, D.C.: Public Health Service Publication No. 1836, 1968.
24. Pearlman, C., and Greenberg, R. Effect of REM Deprivation on Retention of Avoidance Learning in Rats. Paper read at APSS, Denver, 1968.
25. Pegram, G. V., Jr. Changes in EEG, temperature and behavior as a function of prolonged sleep deprivation. *Dissert. Abstracts* 29:1190-B, 1968.
26. Roffwarg, H. R., Muzio, J. N., and Dement, W. C. Ontogenetic development of the human sleep-dream cycle. *Science* 152: 604, 1966.
27. Rust, L. D. Changes in bar pressing performance and heart rate in sleep-deprived rats. *J. Comp. Physiol. Psychol.* 55:621, 1962.
28. Snyder, F. Toward an evolutionary theory of dreaming. *Amer. J. Psychiat.* 123:121, 1966.
29. Stern, W. C. Effects of REM Sleep Deprivation upon the Acquisition and Maintenance of Learned Behavior in the Rat. Paper read at APSS, Boston, 1969.
30. Stern, W. C. Effects of REM Sleep Deprivation, Drugs and Electroconvulsive Shock on Reactivity to Foot Shock and Shock Induced Aggression in Rats. Paper read at APSS, Boston, 1969.
31. Stern, W. C. Stress Effects of REM Sleep Deprivation in Rats: Adrenal Gland Hypertrophy. Paper read at APSS, Boston, 1969.
32. Stern, W. C. Stress Effects of REM Sleep Deprivation in Rats: Startle Response Habituation. Paper read at APSS, Boston, 1969.
33. Webb, W. B. Some effects of prolonged sleep deprivation on the hooded rat. *J. Comp. Physiol. Psychol.* 55:791, 1962.

Dreaming and Memory

RAMON GREENBERG

Several investigators [2, 4, 8, 15, 17, 29] have suggested that recent research on the neurophysiology of dreaming has provided evidence that dreaming (stage REM sleep) plays a role in the organization of memory. In this paper I would like to review some of the reasons for this hypothesis. The approach will be in terms of a beginning, quite simple hypothesis, with a gradual refining of the hypothesis as new experimental evidence is added.

Let us begin with the evidence that dreaming might have something to do with memory, defined as storage of new information. The first observation to be made is that a dream consists of perceptual events, e.g., things seen, heard, touched. Furthermore, the eye movements during stage REM sleep have been shown [27] to correlate with the actual visual imagery in the dream. Several studies show that these events are repetitious of recent awaking perceptions. This has been demonstrated in our study [12] of the dreams of quadriplegic and paraplegic patients. These patients revealed in their dreams an absence of those same tactile and kinesthetic perceptions which were unavailable in their waking lives. Blind patients who once had sight show a fading of visual imagery in their dreams and a reduction of rapid eye movements during sleep as their ability to have waking visual imagery fades [1]. Patients with lesions of visual association areas, causing an attention hemianopia, do not have eye movements during stage 1 sleep in the direction of the affected field of vision [10]. (Cats also show a loss of REM when the visual association areas are damaged [19].) Decorticate patients show an almost complete loss of REM with only rare, isolated movements and no clusters of eye movements [10, 20].

TRANSFER OF PERCEPTIONS

It seems clear then that dreams consist of perceptions which have been experienced by the patient during his recent waking life. If certain waking perceptions are unavailable, such perceptions do not appear in the dreams. Is there any meaning to this? Freud [7] raised the question of whether perceptions could be stored in the same area of the brain in which they are perceived. He reasoned that this could not be so, for then the perceptual areas would become full, like writing on a blackboard. We have taken this question, plus the observation of the perceptual events in the dream, and formulated the hypothesis [12] that dreaming serves to transfer recent perceptions from the perceptual areas, or short-term memory stores, to areas for long-term memory storage, clearing the perceptual areas so that they would be free for new perceptions.

This hypothesis is open to an important question. It is also open to experimental testing. The question involves the fact that the perceptual events in dreams are not replications of all the perceptions occurring during recent waking life. The perceptions that do appear are associated with strong emotional components in each person's life. We will return to this question in the process of refining the hypothesis.

In terms of experimental testing, the hypothesis suggests that an individual who is dream-deprived might have difficulty learning new material or recalling recently perceived information, since the perceptual areas would be saturated. We have studied this with subjects who were dream-deprived for 3 days. Some were given lists of nonsense syllables and others were given 100 paired word association lists [15]. In both cases dream deprivation showed no clear effect on the subjects' memory as tested by these kinds of tests.

DREAMING AND CORTICAL-LIMBIC PROCESSES

Thus it seems that dreaming is not involved in purely cognitive memory. However, the fact that the perceptions noted in dream material are related to emotionally meaningful events in a person's life might give a clue as to the kind of memory that is involved in dreaming. This might be called emotionally meaningful learning. Additional support for this line of thinking is provided by the finding [24, 25] of hippocampal activation during paradoxical sleep in cats. This activation is similar to what is seen when the cat is awake and excited. Furthermore, this kind of activation—hippocampal theta—has been related [23] to learning and memory processes in animals. It should be noted here that animal learning always involves cortical-limbic associations, whereas human learning may involve cortical-cortical (cognitive learning) connections or cortical-limbic connections [9].

I would suggest, therefore, that dreaming deals with processes involving cortical-limbic connections. One way to study this would be in patients who have lesions of the cortical-limbic circuits. Post-alcoholic Korsakoff patients provide such an opportunity, for they have lesions of the mammillary bodies disrupting the hippocampal-cortical pathway. Such patients also have serious memory difficulties. We studied [14] sleep patterns in a group of Korsakoff patients and found some interesting changes. The levels of stage REM in patients with recent Korsakoff's was significantly higher (30 percent of total sleep) than in those with chronic (more than 1 year) disability (20 percent). The high levels of stage REM in the more recent cases was also remarkable in that it was fragmented into many short periods.

We reasoned from these findings that the lesion producing a memory impairment was also impairing the normal function of the "dream mechanism." In the early stages of the illness, we reasoned, there is some attempt or pressure to rectify the memory difficulty and therefore increased pressure to dream. The process is ineffective, however, and eventually in the chronic stages a new equilibrium is developed. These changes in sleep patterns coincide with the typical clinical evolution of the illness. There is confusion, disorientation, and confabulation early in the disease, and relatively affectless resignation in later stages. We also found that the dream content, when remembered by these patients, was mundane and lacking in emotion. We concluded at this point that the memory function of dreaming involved the integration of internal emotions and experiences using the limbic system with recent external perceptions.

An interesting neurophysiological observation [23] can be brought into relation with this hypothesis of cortical-limbic integration. It has been noted during conditioning studies with monkeys that in the initial stages, when the conditioned stimulus is presented, hippocampal theta appears. When the conditioning is established there is no hippocampal theta. This has been explained as a difference between responding to new information (theta) versus responding to already stored information (no theta). In our study [13] of patients with electrodes implanted in the hippocampus and amygdala we found, in the one patient with a relatively normal sleep record, that the hippocampal theta during stage REM was not continuous as in the cat, but appeared in bursts. Could these bursts of theta represent the appearance in the dream of new information recently perceived, which is then integrated with past memories with cessation of the theta activity?

Because animal learning involves cortical-limbic connections, one might predict that animal learning would be particularly sensitive to dream deprivation. This has now been studied by several investigators. In one study [26] all rats who were dream deprived for 24 hours after a single experience with a shock failed to remember, while 70 percent of control rats showed clear evidence of remembering. Stern [30] demonstrated that several types of learning tasks, both active and passive, were significantly impaired by REM deprivation in rats. Fishbein [5] in a series of studies using mice again showed significant impairment of long-term memory registration following or preceded by REM deprivation. Thus all of these experiments confirm the crucial role of stage REM (dreaming) in the learning experience of an animal.

INTEGRATION OF EMOTIONAL EVENTS HELPED BY DREAMS

We reach a point then where the kind of memory storage (for humans) that seems involved has to do with emotionally meaningful events using limbic pathways. If this is so, then one would expect that emotionally significant events experienced and perceived during the day would appear in dreams; and furthermore, if a person experiencing an emotionally meaningful or stressful event is deprived of dreaming, he would show a failure to integrate or handle this event. Both of these suppositions have been borne out by experimental studies.

Several studies confirm the incorporation of stressful stimuli. First, and perhaps most clear, is Whitman's finding [31] that the experimental situation is frequently represented in the dreams of subjects in sleep experiments. Then Witkin and Lewis [32] found that subjects shown emotionally charged films revealed significant evidence of incorporating material from the films into their dreams. They found a clear difference between the dreams of subjects after emotionally charged films and after neutral films. Breger's group found that presurgical patients [22] and patients in group therapy [18] incorporated obviously stressful features of their experiences into their dreams. Finally, Collins, Davison, and Breger [3] found that subjects shown a stressful movie revealed evidence of incorporation of the material from the movie within the first minutes of the onset of stage REM. Thus there seems little question that a stressful experience will appear in a dream. Is there any significance to this?

In a study [16] to try to answer this question, we showed subjects a stressful movie in the evening and then repeated the same movie the next morning. Previous studies had shown that considerable adaptation in terms of lessened anxiety occurs on second viewing under normal circumstances. In this study some of the subjects were stage REM deprived, some were awakened a comparable number of times during NREM sleep, and some were allowed to sleep through the night between the viewings. The findings were that the REM deprived subjects showed less adaptation to the second viewing than either the control awakening or the uninterrupted sleep subjects. Put in another way, the dream deprived subjects acted more as if the second viewing were a first viewing.

If we now take this information and try to apply it to normal life experiences and dreaming we can further refine our hypothesis about dreaming and memory. We can assume that each person, in the course of his daily life, has experiences that are emotionally meaningful to him both in terms of the present and in terms of what such experiences might remind him of in regard to earlier life experiences. We could now phrase the hypothesis to say that the dreams of the night serve to make the new experiences of the day part of the memory system in association with earlier memories of similar emotional tone or meaning. Furthermore, these new experiences and the emotions they evoke would be dealt with in the same manner as the earlier memories, that is, the same kind of defense mechanisms would be brought to bear on them. For example, if the individual had previously used repression to deal with feelings about loss, he would now use repression to deal with his feelings about a current loss.

To test this hypothesis we did a study [15] to determine the kinds of psychological changes that occur in dream deprived subjects. We started with the assumption that whatever changes might occur would depend on the base-line personality of each subject rather than be the same for all subjects. Since earlier studies [21, 28] using checklist and question and answer types of tests failed to show consistent changes with dream deprivation, we used the Rorschach and Holzman projective tests. Subjects were tested under base-line conditions after 3 nights of dream deprivation and after 3 nights of control awakenings from NREM sleep. The psychologists were told which were the base-line tests and were asked to evaluate changes from base line in the other two tests for each subject, without being told under which conditions the later tests were administered. The findings were striking and quite pertinent to the hypothesis as now formulated: The greatest changes occurred following dream deprivation. These changes took a particular form. The typical defenses seen on base-line testing were not apparent after dream deprivation, and material which had been well defended against in base-line tests appeared, after dream deprivation, in a much more open fashion.* It is of great interest that Fiss and Kline [6] had similar findings in a somewhat different study. They eval-

* The findings after control awakenings were intermediate between these two. Since the control awakenings were always done after dream deprivation, these changes may have been due either to the nondream awakenings or to the fact that such material had already emerged with dream deprivation.

uated the base-line personality and conflicts of their subjects. They then allowed subjects only a limited amount of dreaming by awakening them early in the stage REM period. They collected the dream reports and found that as dream curtailment continued, the manifest content revealed more and more clearly conflictual material that had been well defended against under base-line conditions.

These findings can help to clarify our hypothesis. If we assume that in our daily life we have experiences which touch on and arouse memories involving conflict-laden experiences, then we must ask what happens to such aroused memories and their associated feelings. It would seem that under normal circumstances these aroused feelings are once again defended against, put to sleep, so to speak. Our suggestion is that this occurs primarily during dreaming. When a subject is deprived of dreaming, this cannot occur, and the result is that conflictual material is much less repressed.

Some corollaries to this must also be considered. First, we may have an explanation of why so much of what we dream is forgotten. If the function of a dream is to restore defenses against aroused conflictual material, then when this task is accomplished, the material —that is, the dream content—is no longer easily accessible to consciousness. Only when the dream is interrupted by awakening prior to completion of this task or when the task cannot be completed because the conflict is overwhelming, as in traumatic dreams, or when defenses are reduced, as during therapy or illness, can the dreams be remembered.

Another possible corollary is that the dream may serve the purpose of bringing new perceptions or new experiences into contact with old memories or patterns of behavior, thus leading to modified patterns of information storage which can allow growth or change. It is of interest that the addition of new information to the memory system can be associated with higher levels of stage REM. This was demonstrated in our study [11] of aphasic patients. We found that improving aphasics had significantly higher levels of stage REM than those who were not improving. Furthermore, Zimmerman et al. [33] found that subjects who began wearing prismed glasses creating inverted images had an increase in REM as compared to their own base lines.

SUMMARY

We have considered the evidence for the theory that dreaming is related to a specialized type of memory storage. This evidence included the kinds of events that occur in dreams, both psychological and physiological, and the relationships between them. Clearly dreams deal with an individual's recent experiences. These experiences are related to the emotional life of the individual. When a person is deprived of dreaming, these emotion-laden experiences are not dealt with in the usual manner. When we put this evidence together, we are led to the following hypothesis about a function of dreaming. The dream process serves to bring together perceptions of recent emotionally meaningful experiences with memories of past experiences of a similar nature. In this process the recent experiences become part of the memory system filed, so to speak, with material of a similar kind.* Furthermore, the new experiences can be dealt with in the same manner as the earlier experiences, or the new experience might indicate that the earlier experiences no longer need to be handled with the old, characteristic but outmoded methods of adaptation. This latter event can be seen as effecting a change in the memory system rather than just adding new information to it.

REFERENCES

1. Berger, R. J., Olley, P., and Oswald, I. The EEG, eye movements and dreams of the blind. *Quart. J. Exp. Psychol.* 14:183, 1962.
2. Breger, L. The function of dreams. *J. Abnorm. Psychol.* Monograph No. 641, 1967.
3. Collins, G., Davison, L., and Breger, L. The Function of Dreams in Adaptation to Threat. Paper read at Association for the Psychophysiological Study of Sleep (APSS), Santa Monica, Cal., 1967.
4. Dewan, E. The P (programming) hypothesis for REMs (abstract). *Psychophysiology* 4:365, 1968.

* The idea of filing according to emotional tone was originally presented to me by E. Dewan.

5. Fishbein, W. The Effects of Paradoxical Sleep Deprivation During the Retention Interval on Long-Term Memory. Paper read at APSS, Boston, 1969.
6. Fiss, H., Kline, G., Shollar, E., and Levine, B. Changes in dream content as a function of prolonged REM sleep interruption. *Psychophysiology* 5:217, 1968.
7. Freud, S. A Note Upon the Mystic Writing Pad. *Collected Papers,* Vol. 5. London: Hogarth Press, 1925.
8. Gaarder, K. A conceptual model of sleep. *Arch. Gen. Psychiat.* (Chicago) 14:253, 1966.
9. Geschwind, N. Disconnexion syndromes in man. *Brain* 88: 237, 1965.
10. Greenberg, R. Cerebral cortex lesions: The dream process and sleep spindles. *Cortex* 2:357, 1966.
11. Greenberg, R., and Dewan, E. Aphasia and Rapid Eye Movement Sleep. *Nature* 223:183, 1969.
12. Greenberg, R., and Leiderman, P. H. Perceptions, the dream process and memory. *Compr. Psychiat.* 7:507, 1966.
13. Greenberg, R., and Pearlman, C. Sleep patterns in temporal lobe epilepsy. *Compr. Psychiat.* 9:194, 1968.
14. Greenberg, R., Pearlman, C., Brooks, R., Mayer, R., and Hartmann, E. Dreaming and Korsakoff's psychosis. *Arch. Gen. Psychiat.* (Chicago) 18:203, 1968.
15. Greenberg, R., Pearlman, C., Fingar, R., Kantrowitz, J., and Kawliche, S. The Effects of Dream Deprivation. *Brit. J. Med. Psychol.* In press.
16. Greenberg, R., Pillard, R., and Pearlman, C. The effect of dream deprivation on adaptation to stress (abstract). *Psychophysiology* 5:238, 1968.
17. Hawkins, D. R. A review of psychoanalytic dream theory in the light of recent psycho-physiologic studies of sleep and dreaming. *Brit. J. Med. Psychol.* 39:85, 1966.
18. Hunter, I., and Breger, L. The Effect of Pre-sleep Group Therapy upon Subsequent Dream Content. Paper read at APSS, Santa Monica, Cal., 1967.
19. Jeannerod, M., Mouret, J., and Jouvet, M. Étude de la motricité oculaire au cours de la phase paradoxale du sommeil chez le chat. *Electroenceph. Clin. Neurophysiol.* 18:554, 1965.
20. Jouvet, M. Personal communication.
21. Kales, A., Hodemaker, F. S., Jacobson, A., and Lichtenstein, E. L. Dream deprivation: An experimental reappraisal. *Nature* (London) 204:1337, 1964.

22. Lane, R., and Breger, L. The Effect of Preoperative Stress on Dreams. Paper read at APSS, Santa Monica, Cal., 1967.
23. Meissner, W. Hippocampal functions in learning. *J. Psychiat. Res.* 4:235, 1966.
24. Parmeggiani, P., and Zannocco, G. A study on the bioelectric rhythms of cortical and subcortical structures during activated sleep. *Arch. Ital. Biol.* 101:385, 1963.
25. Passouant, P., and Cadhilhac, J. Les rythmes theta hippocampiques au cours du sommeil. In P. Passouant (Ed.), *Physiologie de l'hippocampe.* Paris: C.N.R.S., 1962. P. 331.
26. Pearlman, C., and Greenberg, R. Effect of REM Deprivation on Retention of Avoidance Learning in Rats. Paper read at APSS, Denver, 1968.
27. Roffwarg, H., Dement, W., Muzio, T., and Fisher, C. Dream imagery: Relationship to rapid eye movements of sleep. *Arch. Gen. Psychiat.* (Chicago) 7:235, 1962.
28. Sampson, H. Psychological effects of deprivation of dreaming sleep. *J. Nerv. Ment. Dis.* 143:305, 1966.
29. Shapiro, A. Dreaming and the physiology of sleep. *Exp. Neurol.* [Suppl.] 4:56, 1967.
30. Stern, W. Effects of REM Sleep Deprivation upon the Acquisition and Maintenance of Learned Behavior in the Rat. Paper read at APSS, Boston, 1969.
31. Whitman, R., Pierce, C., Mass, J., and Baldridge, B. The dreams of the experimental subject. *J. Nerv. Ment. Dis.* 134:431, 1962.
32. Witkin, H., and Lewis, H. The relation of experimentally induced presleep experiences to dreams: A report on method and preliminary findings. *J. Amer. Psychoanal. Assoc.* 13:819, 1965.
33. Zimmerman, J., Stoyva, J., and Metcalf, D. Distorted Visual Experience and Rapid Eye Movement Sleep. Paper read at APSS, Boston, 1969.

The Functions of Sleep

*What can one conclude from research so far as to the possible function of sleep as a whole? Of S-sleep (NREM sleep)? Of the D-state (REM sleep)?**

On the Functions of the Sleep Phases

HARMON S. EPHRON AND
PATRICIA CARRINGTON

In answering the question posed at the start of this chapter, we will extend the scope of a hypothesis of the function of REM sleep which we previously suggested [3, 4] and propose that wakefulness and sleep may be looked upon as wide swings of a pendulum which moves constantly between the poles of organismic activation and deactivation. The REM and NREM sleep phases will be seen as representing narrower swings between these two poles. In this manner, we suggest, relative equilibrium may be ensured between two organismic tendencies: a deactivating tendency which leads toward avoidance of overloading of the various adap-

* The reader interested in this question may wish to refer also to papers by Kahn (p. 25), Baekeland and Hartmann (p. 33), Hauri (p. 70), Globus (p. 78), Karacan and Williams (p. 93), Lewis (p. 199), Stern (p. 249), Greenberg (p. 258), Pearlman (p. 329), Jones (p. 335), Ephron and Carrington (p. 344), Kleitman (p. 352), Wilkinson (p. 369), and Hursch (p. 387).

tive systems, and an activating tendency which leads toward exercise of those functions necessary for the work required in maintaining animal existence. Marked skew in the direction of either tendency (that is, a pathologically hyperactivated or hypoactivated animal) would in this way be avoided under most conditions.

We might visualize sleeping and waking behavior as comprising three levels of operation which can be compared to the rhythmical waxing and waning of large bodies of water. The ocean swells and recedes on both a great and a small scale, and each type of motion can be studied separately by changing our observational set. We can, for example, measure the ebb and flow of the ocean tides, or we can observe the rhythmic rise and fall of the waves (whose shapes become correspondingly more meaningful as we calculate the influence of the underlying tidal pull upon them). If we are so inclined, we can also study the ripples on the surface of the waves (which again become more meaningful if we know the shape of the wave upon which they are superimposed). In watching the movements of the sea we observe both a regularity of motion, as large bodies of moving water obey the laws of gravity, and impressive individual variations within the overall pattern, as for example when gusts of wind speed up or (blowing in a counter direction) retard incoming waves and flatten ripples, or when the sea encounters internal obstacles such as reefs or beds of vegetation. Rhythmicity based on constant laws thus combines with incidental influences to produce both general and specific phenomena.

INTERRELATEDNESS OF SLEEP AND WAKING

Bearing in mind the limitations of an analogy between a living process and a purely physical one, we will use this comparison to illustrate the manner in which sleep, wakefulness, and the contrasting sleep phases may be interrelated. Sleep and wakefulness will be likened to the tides,* REM sleep and NREM sleep to the

* This poetic metaphor is not intended to imply that sleep and wakefulness are locked in phase with physical forces, as are the ocean tides.

waves, and momentary fluctuations in level of activation to the surface ripples.

In our previous publications on this subject, we suggested that NREM sleep involves a progressive loss of cerebral vigilance which nevertheless must somehow be maintained within adaptively appropriate limits, and a homeostatic interplay between the sleep phases was postulated. This involved two complementary tendencies, one tendency leading toward deepening NREM sleep and organismic rest which, when it reaches a preset level, triggers the release of another tendency leading toward REM sleep and organismic activation.

NREM sleep, looked upon as a state of *functional deafferentation,* was seen as occurring in response to overloading of sensory and memory systems with incoming data (i.e., *overafferentation*) in waking life, and the typical seesaw action of homeostatic mechanisms was identified in the interaction of NREM sleep, REM sleep, and the waking state.

It was suggested that REM sleep performs its homeostatic function by increasing cortical "tonus" or a readiness for adaptive responses, following loss of such tonus in NREM sleep. This restorative effect of REM sleep on cortical functioning was viewed in turn as brought about by a process of *endogenous afferentation* (internally generated sensory "input") peculiar to this state and reflected, in man, in the vivid dreaming of this period.

RELATION OF SLEEP PHASES AND SLEEP

Enlarging this concept to account for data from all states of consciousness, let us turn to the analogy of the sea and consider how the waves of deactivation and activation, represented by the NREM and REM phases, may be related to the tidal deactivation of sleep itself, to whose overriding influence both sleep phases are presumably subordinate.

The REM state might be considered as providing the neocortex with an arousal substitute which, paradoxically, permits sleep to continue. Although about 85 percent of REM periods in man are interrupted or followed by brief awakenings of a few seconds in duration (with similar awakenings occurring in lower animals), these token arousals are normally followed by a return to NREM sleep. Sleep therefore is generally maintained despite the cortical activation of REM sleep, and certain features of the REM period seem to support this continuance of sleep. The blocking of motor impulses at the periphery which typically occurs in REM sleep effectively prevents the arousing effects of gross motor behavior, and the fact that REM dreams frequently assimilate intrusions from external stimuli without responding to them by awakening [2] are among the data which suggest that the organism is resistant during REM sleep to any distinct or prolonged interference with sleep.

The prevailing tides of activation and deactivation are abnormally skewed, however, during human sleep, apparently because of man's 15 to 17 hours of enforced wakefulness. At day's end man may be *overafferented* in a manner not characteristic of any of the lower animals (nor of the human infant), who regularly punctuate their waking life by naps. Heavy concentrations of NREM sleep in the early portion of the night and compensatory heavy concentrations of REM sleep in the morning hours appear the result of man's artificially extended daytime wakefulness.

Considering the skewed sleep pattern of human beings, we might expect REM or NREM periods to be more or less effective as activating or deactivating influences according to the stage of the deactivation cycle in which they occur; that is, we might expect them to be modified by the overall tidal drift. If an REM period were triggered in response to loss of cortical tonus when the tide was moving toward quiescence and NREM sleep, the REM sleep activating tendency might be evidenced only in a short and feeble REM period or, if the prevailing tidal pull were strong enough, be reduced to no more than an abortive attempt at REM sleep. Such attenuated REM periods are, in fact, typical of the early stages of the night.

If, on the other hand, an REM period were triggered when the tide was once again moving toward activation (as appears the case in the morning hours), the REM period would be in harmony with the tidal drift and, according to the present theory, would increase the tidal momentum by supplying large quantities of endogenous afferentation to the brain.

In a similar manner, NREM sleep appears to be influenced by the prevailing drift of the tides. Early in the night when the tidal pull is toward quiescence, NREM sleep tends to be "deepest," showing more stage 3 and 4 sleep, higher arousal thresholds, and fewer spontaneous awakenings than at any other time of the night. By contrast, when the tidal pull is toward activation in the morning hours, NREM sleep becomes "shallower" (i.e., shows a preponderance of stage 2 sleep), and awakenings from NREM sleep at this time elicit reports of mental activity which becomes progressively more vivid and perceptual ("dreamlike") as the night proceeds [5]. The nature of this morning NREM mentation suggests that cortical tonus has now been sufficiently raised by large concentrations of REM sleep (and possibly other manifestations of homeostatic activating trends) during the night to ensure that cortical efficiency will remain relatively high during *all* stages of morning sleep. Presumably cortical centers deafferented in the early part of the night are now rested and in readiness for such a progressive buildup of tonicity.

Further evidence suggests that an advancing tide of activation in the morning hours maintains its forward course after awakening occurs. A tendency toward activation may predominate until a turning point is reached some time in the afternoon when requirements for attenuation of cortical stimulation lead the organism once again gradually to lessen its responsiveness to sensory input. Thus we find, for example, that on numerous measures of performance, speed and accuracy are typically poor during the morning postawakening period, with efficiency gradually increasing to a peak in midafternoon, and thereafter slowly diminishing to a low by bedtime [6].

The notion of a continuing tide of activation in the late morning also appears consistent with findings indicating that subjects returning to sleep at 9 A.M. after being awake for two hours [9] and subjects permitted to sleep uninterruptedly into the late morning hours [8] maintain high concentrations of REM sleep and a predominance of stage 2 NREM sleep. The prepotent organismic requirement at this time therefore appears to be for toning up of the cortex through afferentation (either through REM sleep if asleep, or through external stimulation if awake). This direction appears reversed only as a state of overafferentation develops in the afternoon.

As might be expected if the concept of a tidal turning point in the afternoon is correct, subjects napping at 1:30 P.M. show REM latencies and REM percentages which lie approximately midway between those of late morning and those of evening sleep [7]. Presumably 1:30 P.M. may lie near the hypothetical turning point, so that activating and deactivating tendencies may be in almost balanced relationship, and the skewed distribution of sleep phases seen at other times may thus not be evident.

The notion of a tidal drift toward activation in the morning does not, however, imply that homeostatic interplay between NREM sleep and REM sleep ceases at this time. The ocean waves are not leveled by the movements of the tide, but persist in rhythmic alternation even though their size and direction may be partially determined by underlying tidal currents. Thus in Verdone's sleepers [8], late morning REM sleep was found to be essentially proportional to NREM sleep, with the length of the NREM periods showing a positive correlation with the length of subsequent REM periods.

ADJUSTMENTS IN LEVELS OF ACTIVATION

Let us return to our analogy of the sea and consider the ripples on the ocean's surface, which we have likened to minute fluctuations in level of activation. It is well known that momentary activating tendencies may be evidenced throughout NREM sleep in the form of spontaneous K-complexes and skin potential changes, isolated bursts of faster eye movements, brief "lightenings" of the

EEG pattern, and other manifestations of increased alertness or temporary engagement of the sensory motor systems. Similarly, *deactivating* tendencies are often noted during REM sleep in the form of occasional sleep spindles or even delta waves which may intrude on the low voltage, fast activity of the EEG during this sleep phase. Possibly the quiescent intervals which separate the phasic events of REM sleep also represent relative deactivation within REM sleep. Waking life seems likewise sporadically interrupted by the intrusion of deactivating tendencies in the form of EEG alpha rhythms or even isolated delta waves ("microsleeps"). These counter tendencies often make precise distinctions between different stages of alertness quite difficult.

We suggest that these intrusions of one state of consciousness upon its opposite may reflect immediate adjustments in the level of activation which operate under continuous feedback controls, setting in force trends in opposition to the prevailing one. Typical of servomechanisms, these adjustment mechanisms would be highly responsive to momentary imbalances and would bring about relatively rapid adjustments. As Dell [1] points out, such rapid adjustments may be superimposed, at any one moment, on more slowly developing changes. He suggests that the former are often neural, whereas the slower, more cyclical changes are likely to be humorally mediated. The slower homeostatic changes will also tend to be more unavoidable, and hence prepotent, while the rapid adjustments which are transmitted neurally pass through relays which have filters and gain controls and can therefore more easily be preferentially suppressed or intensified.

We suggest that these relatively rapid fluctuations in level of activation regulate the degree of cortical tonus around some optimal level or "set point" (which may vary slightly for the different behavioral states). While necessary for homeostatic purposes, such rapid adjustments would not be capable of instituting long-lasting changes in level of activation such as are also presumably necessary if deafferentation, endogenous afferentation, and waking behavior are to be sustained. For the latter task, homeostatic mechanisms capable of maintaining a state of activation over a longer period of time would be required. We have suggested that such slower acting mechanisms may operate in the alternation of NREM sleep, REM sleep, and the waking state.

TENDENCIES TO ACTIVATION AND DEACTIVATION

With regard to the theoretical implications of the position we have outlined, it would seem that the various sleeping and waking states might be viewed less as discrete entities than as evidence of a temporary preponderance of one or the other tendency (i.e., of activation or deactivation). Such a notion has certain implications for research seeking to determine the function of the various sleep stages through measuring the effects of selective sleep stage deprivation. If, for example, the two basic tendencies just described were to be considered the pertinent variables, instead of the configuration or patterning of such tendencies in a restricted sleep "stage," then we would have to ask whether depriving an organism of a particular stage of sleep effectively blocks the *tendency* which predominates in that stage. If it does *not,* then conclusions based on the sleep stage–deprivation model could prove misleading. In this respect, adoption of a unifying concept of cortical homeostasis to account for sleep–wakefulness phenomena might alter the questions we ask of our data.

REFERENCES

1. Dell, P. Reticular Homeostasis and Critical Reactivity. In G. Moruzzi, A. Fessard, and H. H. Jaspers (Eds.), *Brain Mechanisms.* New York: Elsevier, 1963. Pp. 82–104.
2. Dement, W. C., and Wolpert, E. A. The relationship of eye movement, body motility, and external stimuli to dream content. *J. Exp. Psychol.* 55:543, 1958.
3. Ephron, H. S., and Carrington, P. Rapid eye movement sleep and cortical homeostasis. *Psychol. Rev.* 73:500, 1966.
4. Ephron, H. S., and Carrington, P. Ego Functioning in Rapid Eye Movement Sleep: Implications for Dream Theory. In J.

Masserman (Ed.), *Science and Psychoanalysis,* Vol. XI. New York: Grune & Stratton, 1967. Pp. 75–102.
5. Foulkes, D. *The Psychology of Sleep.* New York: Scribner's, 1966.
6. Kleitman, N. *Sleep and Wakefulness.* Chicago: University of Chicago Press, 1963.
7. Maron, L., Rechtschaffen, A., and Wolpert, E. A. Sleep cycle during napping. *Arch. Gen. Psychiat.* (Chicago) 11:503, 1964.
8. Verdone, P. Sleep satiation: Extended sleep in normal subjects. *Electroenceph. Clin. Neurophysiol.* 24:417, 1968.
9. Webb, W. B., Agnew, H. W., Jr., and Sternthal, H. Sleep during the early morning. *Psychonomic Science* 6:277, 1966.

REM Sleep and Mechanisms of Oculomotor Control

RALPH J. BERGER

Until the discovery of rapid eye movement sleep [4], the function of sleep had generally been taken for granted: that it constituted a period of necessary organismic rest [48]. However, there was little concrete physiological evidence to support this interpretation. The observations of the periodic appearance of the activated physiological patterns of REM sleep also necessitated revision of the traditional conception of sleep as a uniform state of general quiescence which varied only along a continuum of depth. The enigmatic nature of REM sleep in this context resulted in the focusing of attention in recent years on its functions rather than on those of the more orthodox NREM sleep, which are still generally considered to be self-evident.

I have recently formulated a hypothesis [9] concerning a possible function of REM sleep, which draws to some extent from earlier theories [18, 56] but attempts to explain a larger body of data than those and other theories [19, 59]. However, the hypothesis is primarily concerned with the function of REM sleep in relation to eye movement and does not deal directly with other psychophysiological variables such as penile erections [23, 32], middle ear muscle contractions [17], and dreaming [16].

The hypothesis is that REM sleep provides a mechanism for the establishment of the neuromuscular pathways serving voluntary conjugate eye movement in phylogenesis and ontogenesis and maintains their integrity during extended periods of sleep throughout the life of the individual.

The degree of fine neuromuscular coordination involved in the execution of voluntary conjugate eye movements in the higher mammals exceeds that of any other system of muscles in the body. During NREM sleep the eyes adopt an upward divergent resting position [49]. Sometimes occasional disconjugate rolling eye movements are also present. Electromyographic (EMG) activity of the eye muscles is almost entirely absent [11, 37]. During NREM sleep innervation of the oculomotor system is therefore at a minimum. It has been well established that lack of afferent input can lead to degeneration of neural processes [53]. Similarly, it is proposed that without the periodic innervation of the oculomotor system provided by REM sleep, the integrity of the central neural processes involved in the coordination of eye movement would be temporarily lost after extended periods of sleep.

REM SLEEP AND THE EVOLUTION OF BINOCULARLY COORDINATED EYE MOVEMENT

Spontaneous binocularly coordinated eye movement first evolved in the mammal in conjunction with partial decussation of the optic nerve fibers at the optic chiasma and provided the mechanism for stereopsis [62]. The amount of partial decussation can serve as an index of the degree of spontaneous coordinated mobility of the eyes [63]. That REM sleep evolved by establishing and maintaining the neural processes serving coordinated eye movements in vertebrates is supported by the high correlation between the amount of partial decussation at the optic chiasma and the percentage of total sleep time (TST) spent in REM sleep, normalized for the different TSTs of each species (REM/TST^2, Fig. 1). It was

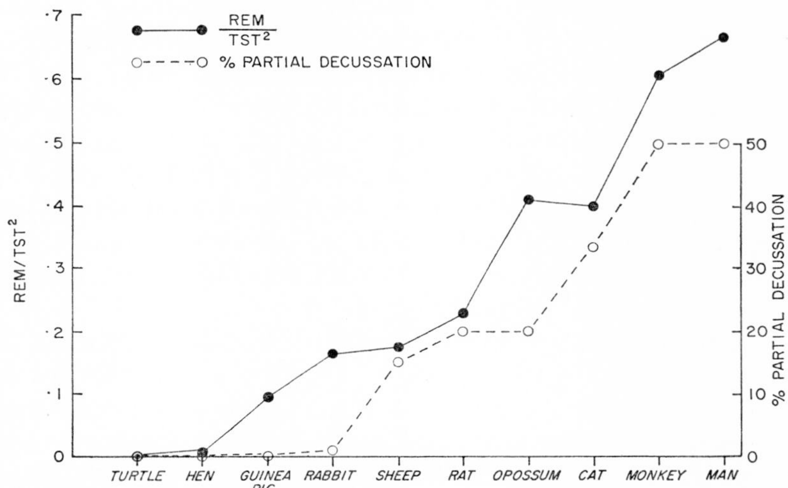

FIGURE 1. *Percentage of total sleep time (TST) spent in REM sleep normalized for the different TSTs of each species, REM/TST^2, and percentage of partial decussation plotted for each species*

originally thought that all mammals exhibited REM sleep; however, the absence of REM sleep in the spiny anteater (echidna, *Tachyglossus aculeatus*) was recently reported [1]. The significance of the absence of REM sleep in this primitive mammal may lie in the fact that it also does not exhibit any waking eye movements.

Qualitative evidence is also provided by the sleep characteristics of an animal such as the guinea pig which is transitional between animals displaying total decussation of their optic nerves and those having considerable numbers of uncrossed fibers. The guinea pig exhibits a unique two-stage pattern of onset of REM sleep. An approximately 30-second period during which the EEG changes from a high voltage slow wave pattern to a low voltage pattern with dominant theta rhythms always precedes the decrease in EMG activity and appearance of REMs [9, 30, 45]. In addition, the EMG rarely becomes isoelectric as in other mammals during REM sleep.

The lowest order of primate, the tree shrew (*Tupaia glis*), has only 3 percent of its optic fibers uncrossed, compared with the higher primates who have almost 50 percent uncrossed. Preliminary studies of sleep in the tree shrew in our laboratory have revealed peculiarities in its physiological patterns unlike those of other primates. The most striking characteristic is the increase in EMG activity at the onset of REM sleep (Fig. 2). During NREM sleep phases preceding REM sleep periods, the EMG is invariably isoelectric. In addition, the EEG pattern during REM sleep is not one of continuous low voltage, mixed frequency as in other mammals, but is interspersed with rhythmic sinusoidal bursts of 7 to 8 cycles per second (cps) activity (Fig. 2).

Electrophysiological changes resembling mammalian NREM or REM sleep have not been seen in fish [47], reptiles [33, 52] or amphibia [25]. Birds such as the hen and pigeon show rudimentary phases of REM sleep which last only a few seconds and occupy 0.5 percent of total sleep time [34]. Conjugate REMs, a low voltage desynchronized EEG, and lowered EMG activity are present during these brief periods. During preliminary studies on burrowing owls, whose eyes are immobile, we have not seen REM sleep similar to that of the hen or pigeon. Brief periods of behavioral sleep accompanied by a low voltage desynchronized EEG pattern occurred following typical phases of EEG high voltage slow wave sleep, but without change in levels of EMG activity (Fig. 3). Innervation of the eye muscles accompanied head movements and eye blinks, and the desynchronized EEG periods were frequently preceded by eye blinks or closure of the eyes; but eye blinks were also frequent during episodes of high voltage slow wave sleep as well as during wakefulness. The prediction made from the present hypothesis—that owls, differing from other birds in having immobile eyes, would fail to exhibit typical characteristics of REM sleep—was confirmed. However, a similar prediction with regard to the virtually blind mole has not been confirmed in a recent report [2],

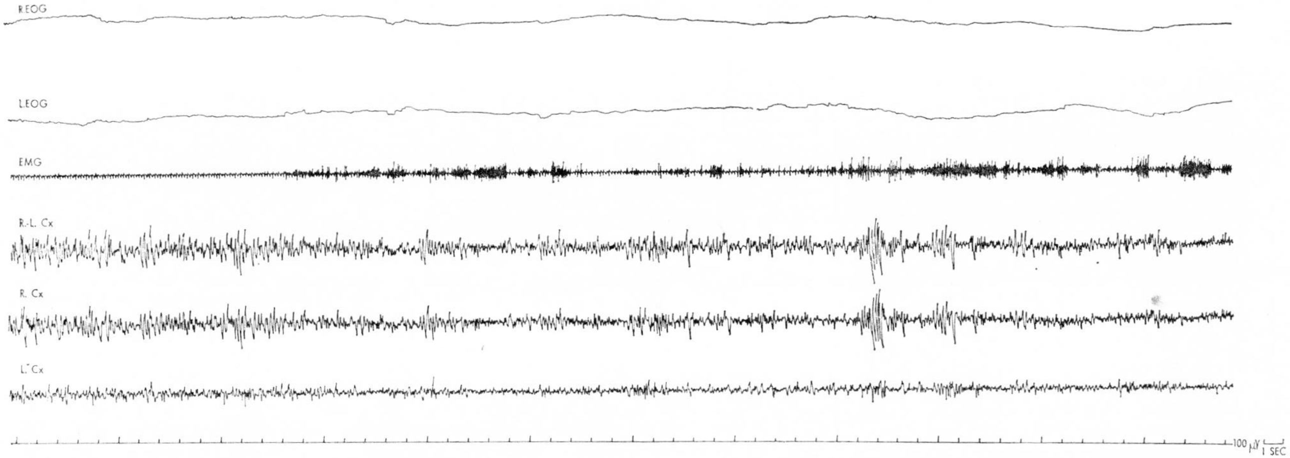

FIGURE 2. *An example of the onset of REM sleep in the tree shrew* (Tupaia glis). *Note the increase in neck EMG activity and the rhythmic sinusoidal bursts of 7 to 8 cps activity in the EEG.* (*R.= right; L. = left;* Cx *= cortex*)

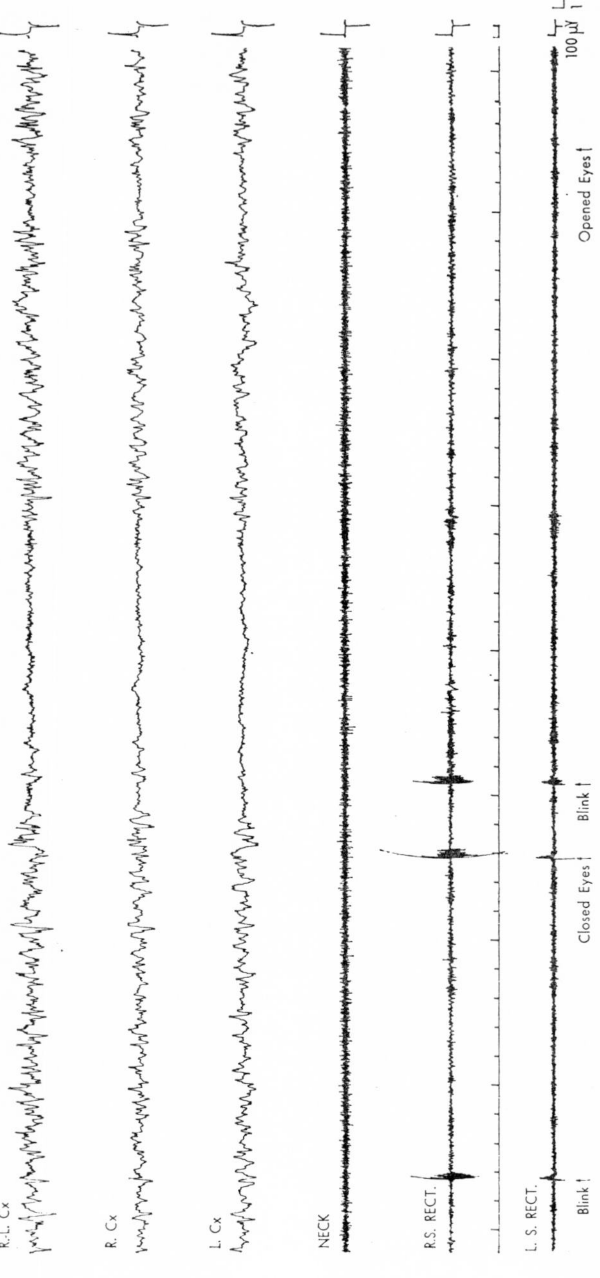

FIGURE 3. *Examples of brief periods of low voltage desynchronized EEG sleep in the burrowing owl. Note the unchanging level of tonic neck and eye muscle EMG activity throughout the record. Phasic increases in eye muscle EMG activity accompany eyelid movements. Closure of the eyes frequently precedes the onset of the low voltage desynchronized EEG sleep periods. (R. = right; L. = left; Cx = cortex; S. Rect. = superior rectus muscle)*

in which phases typical of mammalian REM sleep, except for the absence of REMs, were described. This result in the mole might possibly be reconciled with the present hypothesis if the mole's evolutionary ancestors exhibited coordinated binocular eye movements prior to going underground. The eye of the placental mole is a degenerated organ [62].

ONTOGENY OF REM SLEEP AND CONJUGATE EYE MOVEMENT

That "ontogeny recapitulates phylogeny" is frequently stated. It is proposed that this statement can be applied to REM sleep processes.

The mechanisms whereby conjugate eye movement is developed in ontogeny have not been elucidated. It is often assumed that these mechanisms are dependent upon the prior development of visual perception, whereby adjustments of the eyes occur in response to diplopia caused by a lack of oculomotor coordination. However, this explanation, which implies that oculomotor responses succeed the development of visual perceptual processes, is inconsistent with the view that the development of visual perception must necessarily occur in the absence of diplopia, thereby requiring the prior development of oculomotor processes. It is more reasonable that REM sleep provides an intrinsic mechanism whereby the neural pathways serving coordinated eye movement are initially laid down so that fused perceptions automatically result during development. In support of this interpretation are recent observations [5] demonstrating that for any given angle of convergence of the eyes, the distances of various objects in the visual field determine the selective responses of different sets of neurons in the visual cortex. Which particular sets of neurons are activated is dependent upon the retinal disparities projected by the points in the visual field. It appears that coordination of the eyes may be intrinsically present without occurring in response to diplopic perceptions.

The large amounts of REM sleep seen in infancy and the decline of these amounts with age [56] thus represent a change in the functional role of REM sleep—from that of establishing neural pathways serving coordinated eye movement in the developing organism to that of merely maintaining the integrity of those pathways during extended sleep. That REM sleep more frequently occurs following periods of wakefulness than following periods of NREM sleep in the newborn [35] but invariably follows NREM sleep in the adult [56] is consistent with this viewpoint. The adult human, who has learned by choice to stay awake for long periods during the day, unlike other mammals, does not exhibit a constant cycling of the two sleep phases. Instead he shows an increase in frequency of the sleep cycle throughout the night, and the REM episodes early in the night are usually very short [20, 31]. These characteristics are consistent with a change in function of REM sleep from an initiating mechanism for coordinated eye movement in infancy, to a periodic facilitatory function for coordinated eye movement during sleep in adulthood.

Of further interest to this discussion is the fact that the REMs in the newborn human infant are always conjugate [51, 54], whereas the waking eye movements are partly uncoordinated in the horizontal plane, but well coordinated in the vertical plane [64]. It is therefore significant that vertical REMs predominate over horizontal REMs at birth [40, 54], while the reverse is true in the adult [55]. The greater innervation of vertical oculomotor processes during REM sleep results in the earlier appearance of waking vertical conjugate eye movements, according to the present hypothesis.

CHARACTERISTICS OF THE REMS

The characteristics of the REMs were described in considerable detail by Dement [15]. Recent work has revealed the remarkable constancies of the patterns, frequencies, velocities, and interval distributions of the REMs in the cat [26], monkey [10, 24], and man [3, 60]. These fixed characteristics indicate that the REM-generating processes are not random but highly organized. Other peripheral manifestations of REM sleep do not appear to show equivalent degrees of independent organization, although they have yet to be studied as closely as the REMs.

If REM sleep serves the function of maintaining facilitation of oculomotor neural processes during sleep, it might be expected that the amount of innervation of such processes would be reciprocally related to that which had occurred during wakefulness preceding the onset of sleep. That such a reciprocal relationship does indeed exist was shown serendipitously in a recent experiment [7] from which arose the present hypothesis. Monkeys were conditioned to move their eyes at high and low rates during wakefulness, using two different schedules of reinforcement, with the horizontal electrooculogram as the operant [8]. The subjects were then run for six successive sessions on each schedule prior to falling asleep. The rate of REM and total number of REMs were significantly higher and the REM sleep periods significantly longer following low rates of waking eye movement than following high rates. These results could not be explained by conventional learning mechanisms but were interpreted within the framework of the present hypothesis. Thus the larger amounts of wakeful innervation of the oculomotor system during sessions in which the monkeys moved their eyes at high rates may have produced a relatively reduced "need" for innervation during subsequent sleep, resulting in lower rates of REM and shorter REM periods, compared with sessions in which they moved their eyes at low rates.

PLASTICITY OF THE OCULOMOTOR SYSTEM

It has been established that plastic changes in afferent neural processes can result from sensory deprivation [53] and that psychological processes can be influenced by relatively short periods of sensory restriction [58]. It is likely that similar reversible changes can and do occur in central efferent systems if they are not periodically innervated.

Voluntary binocularly coordinated eye movements evolved by coming under increased control of the cerebral cortex. Their cortical representation is larger than that of any other muscles of the body, despite their small mass [46]. An increase in corticalization of motor function results in greater plasticity in muscular control, so that new motor patterns can be learned. But in order to be preserved, such learned movements must be repeatedly practiced.

If REM sleep periodically innervates the oculomotor system and thereby maintains its integrity throughout sleep, one should be able to detect degenerative changes in oculomotor coordination either during wakefulness when normal innervation is disrupted, or during episodes of NREM sleep when innervation is at its lowest levels.

Suggestive evidence of such degenerative processes during wakefulness is provided by a study in which ocular imbalances were probably produced over extensive periods of time [61]. Marked deterioration in accuracy of depth perception was found to occur in subjects who experienced alternating monocular occlusion of each eye every 2 or 3 hours for a period of 24 hours. Monocular occlusion eliminates the binocular fixation reflex so that the occluded eye deviates from its position relative to the other eye, producing a mild heterophoria. The deteriorations in depth perception may well have been caused by a temporary lack of binocular coordination following this period of monocular occlusion. It may be more than coincidental that the period required for recovery was about twenty minutes, equal to the mean duration of REM periods throughout a night of sleep.

As predicted from the hypothesis, Thomas Scott and I recently found that accuracy of binocular depth perception was significantly better at the end of REM periods than at their onset ($p < .01$, one-tailed t test) while monocular depth perception showed no systematic variation (Table 1). That the monocular depth perception task was a sensitive one was shown by the associated finding that accuracy of monocular depth perception was significantly worse after final awakening in the morning than prior to falling asleep initially ($p < .05$, two-tailed t test) while binocular depth percep-

TABLE 1. *Mean error in binocular and monocular depth perception tasks at the onsets and endings of REM periods during 4 nights of sleep for each subject*

	Mean Error			
	Monocular Task (mm.)		Binocular Task (1/16 in.)	
Subject	Onsets	Endings	Onsets	Endings
1	57.4	44.0	8.2	8.5
2	55.5	59.3	10.7	8.2
3	41.9	25.9	12.0	9.0
4	91.0	51.7	10.7	7.0
5	36.1	26.2	13.7	10.4
6	41.5	58.2	10.1	8.4
7	22.0	27.9	10.4	8.6
8	40.4	36.5	14.7	11.6
Means	48.2	41.2	11.8	9.0

tion showed a significant increase in accuracy from evening to the following morning ($p < .05$, two-tailed t test). These results were predicted from the assumption that if binocular coordination of the eyes is impaired following extensive periods of NREM sleep, then binocular depth perception should be dependently affected. Preliminary data we have since obtained show that the eyes are poorly coordinated during oculomotor tracking tasks performed following awakenings at the onset of REM periods while binocular coordination is intact at the end of REM periods.

NEUROPHYSIOLOGY OF REM SLEEP

It appears significant in the present context that the most distinctive changes in electrical activity of the brain during REM sleep should be confined to structures involved in vision. The REMs are accompanied by bilaterally synchronous monophasic waves in the pontile reticular formation, oculomotor nuclei, lateral geniculate nuclei, and visual cortex [13, 39, 44]. Similar electrical waves also accompany waking eye movements [6, 12, 21]. During

REM sleep each burst of EMG activity in the ocular muscles is synchronized with these monophasic waves [36]. It has been pointed out earlier how constant the REM characteristics are from one REM period to another. A similar constancy exists in the frequency of monophasic waves from one REM episode to another, so that their number totals 12,000 to 13,000 a day in the cat [28]. The rigid organization of the oculomotor system during REM sleep is reflected in these constancies of REM and electrical patterns of activity.

Especially interesting is the recent finding that cats, deprived of monophasic wave activity by repeated arousals at the occurrence of monophasic waves during NREM sleep, showed larger compensatory increases in REM sleep on recovery than cats who had been deprived of REM sleep in the conventional manner by awakening them at the onset of EMG hypotonia [22]. Furthermore, when a sufficient number of monophasic waves were allowed to occur in NREM sleep while depriving the cats of REM sleep, no compensatory increases in REM sleep were seen. These results indicate that innervation of the oculomotor and visual system alone in the absence of the tonic aspects of REM sleep eliminates the REM deprivation-compensation phenomenon.

It is interesting that splitting of the brainstem eliminates REM sleep but releases synchronous bilateral isolated monophasic waves in lateral geniculate and visual cortex during wakefulness and NREM sleep [38]. This result has been difficult to understand, since the pontile reticular nuclei necessary for the integrity of REM sleep [14, 27] remained intact on each side of the medial lesion. The significance of the split-brain preparation, therefore, probably lies in the interruption of decussating fibers in the brain stem. This is consistent with the present hypothesis which emphasizes the involvement of these decussating fibers in the generation of conjugate REMs during REM sleep.

On the other hand, the presence of the REMs is not necessary for the continuation of the other manifestations of activated sleep. Morrison and Pompeiano [42, 43] have reported disappearance of the REMs, bursts of monophasic waves, phasic pyramidal discharges and associated myoclonic twitches, phasic depression of spinal reflexes, and pupillary dilations following bilateral lesions of the medial and descending vestibular nuclei [41, 50].

The tonic aspects of EEG desynchronization and EMG suppression have been eliminated by lesions of the nucleus locus coeruleus in the pons [29]; however, this result has been disputed by others [14]. Because the vestibular nuclei are involved in the generation of the REMs as well as in the control of the skeletal muscular system, one can see why a mechanism for tonic suppression of nonocular musculature should have developed. If all muscle systems were activated in conjunction with each REM, sleep would be disturbed by the massive afferent input thereby generated. Large movements of an animal's extremities during sleep would also be likely to attract the attention of foraging predators. The safety and sleep of the animal would therefore be preserved by inhibition of nonocular musculature during REM sleep. The internuncial network of the pontile reticular formation is probably the center of integration of these tonic and phasic influences during REM sleep.

SUMMARY AND CONCLUSIONS

It has been proposed that REM sleep provides a mechanism for the establishment of the neuromuscular pathways involved in voluntary conjugate eye movement in phylogenesis and ontogenesis and maintains their integrity during extended periods of sleep throughout the life of the individual.

The hypothesis has been considered in the light of the phylogenetic and ontogenetic characteristics of sleep and its underlying neurophysiological mechanisms. Data from studies of monocular and binocular depth perception during sleep are consistent with those predicted from the hypothesis.

It has not been the intention in this discussion to convey the impression that the function of REM sleep as proposed is an exclusive one. It is possible that REM sleep serves a variety of functions including those that have already been proposed by others

[18, 19, 56, 59]. Respiration could be presented as an analogous example of a physiological process that can serve the function of oxygenating the body as well as the function of speech. It is felt that one attraction of the present hypothesis is that it readily generates well-formulated experimental predictions which are currently being tested [9].

REFERENCES

1. Allison, T., and Goff, W. R. Sleep in a primitive mammal, the spiny anteater. *Psychophysiology* 5:200, 1968.
2. Allison, T., and Van Twyver, H. Notes from underground: Sleep in the moles, *Scalopus aquaticus* and *Condylura cristata*. *Psychophysiology* 6:229, 1969.
3. Aserinsky, E., and Cady, W. W. Quantitative aspects of rapid eye movements (REM) in sleep of normal men. *Fed. Proc.* 26: 327, 1967.
4. Aserinsky, E., and Kleitman, N. Regularly occurring periods of eye motility and concomitant phenomena during sleep. *Science* 118:273, 1953.
5. Barlow, H. B., Blakemore, C., and Pettigrew, J. D. The neural mechanism of binocular depth discrimination. *J. Physiol.* 193: 327, 1967.
6. Berger, R. J. When is a dream is a dream is a dream? In C. D. Clemente (Ed.), Physiological Correlates of Dreaming. *Exp. Neurol.* [Suppl.] 4:15, 1967.
7. Berger, R. J. Characteristics of REM sleep following different conditioned rates of waking eye movement in the monkey. *Percept. Motor Skills* 27:99, 1968.
8. Berger, R. J. Operant conditioning of eye movement in the monkey (*Macaca nemestrina*). *J. Exp. Anal. Behav.* 11:311, 1968.
9. Berger, R. J. Oculomotor control: A possible function of REM sleep. *Psychol. Rev.* 76:144, 1969.
10. Berger, R. J., and Meier, G. W. Eye movement during sleep and waking in infant monkeys (*Macaca mulatta*) deprived of patterned vision. *Develop. Psychobiol.* 1:266, 1968.
11. Breinin, G. M. The position of rest during anesthesia and sleep: Electromyographic observations. *Arch. Ophthal.* (Chicago) 57:323, 1957.

12. Brooks, D. C. Waves associated with eye movement in the awake and sleeping cat. *Electroenceph. Clin. Neurophysiol.* 24:532, 1968.
13. Brooks, D. C., and Bizzi, E. Brain stem electrical activity during deep sleep. *Arch. Ital. Biol.* 101:648, 1963.
14. Carli, G., and Zanchetti, A. A study of pontine lesions suppressing deep sleep in the cat. *Arch. Ital. Biol.* 103:751, 1965.
15. Dement, W. C. Eye Movements During Sleep. In M. B. Bender (Ed.), *The Oculomotor System.* New York: Harper & Row, 1964.
16. Dement, W. C., and Kleitman, N. The relation of eye movements during sleep to dream activity: An objective method for the study of dreaming. *J. Exp. Psychol.* 53:339, 1957.
17. Dewson, J. H., Dement, W. C., and Simmons, F. B. Middle ear muscle activity in cats during sleep. *Exp. Neurol.* 12:1, 1965.
18. Ephron, H. S., and Carrington, P. Rapid eye movement sleep and cortical homeostasis. *Psychol. Rev.* 73:500, 1966.
19. Feinberg, I., and Evarts, E. V. Changing Concepts of the Function of Sleep. Paper presented to the Society for Biological Psychiatry, Washington, D.C., 1968.
20. Feinberg, I., Koresko, R. L., and Heller, N. EEG sleep patterns as a function of normal and pathological aging in man. *J. Psychiat. Res.* 5:107, 1967.
21. Feldman, M., and Cohen, B. Electrical activity in the lateral geniculate body of the alert monkey associated with eye movements. *J. Neurophysiol.* 31:455, 1968.
22. Ferguson, J., Henriksen, S., McGarr, K., Belenky, G., Mitchell, G., Gonda, W., Cohen, H., and Dement, W. Phasic event deprivation in the cat. *Psychophysiology* 5:238, 1968.
23. Fisher, C., Gross, J., and Zuch, J. Cycle of penile erection synchronous with dreaming (REM) sleep. *Arch. Gen. Psychiat.* (Chicago) 12:29, 1965.
24. Fuchs, A. F., and Ron, S. An analysis of rapid eye movements of sleep in the monkey. *Electroenceph. Clin. Neurophysiol.* 25:244, 1968.
25. Hobson, J. A. Electrographic correlates of behavior in the frog with special reference to sleep. *Electroenceph. Clin. Neurophysiol.* 22:113, 1967.
26. Jeannerod, M., Mouret, J., and Jouvet, M. Étude de la motricité oculaire au cours de la phase paradoxale du sommeil chez le chat. *Electroenceph. Clin. Neurophysiol.* 18:554, 1965.

27. Jouvet, M. Recherches sur les structures nerveuses et les mécanismes responsables de différentes phases du sommeil physiologique. *Arch. Ital. Biol.* 100:125, 1962.
28. Jouvet, M. Mechanisms of the State of Sleep: A Neuropharmacological Approach. In S. S. Kety, E. V. Evarts, and H. L. Williams (Eds.), *Sleep and Altered States of Consciousness.* New York: Williams & Wilkins, 1967.
29. Jouvet, M., and Delorme, F. Locus coeruleus et sommeil paradoxale. *Comptes Rendus des Séances de la Société de Biologie* (Paris) 159:895, 1965.
30. Jouvet-Mounier, D., and Astic, L. Étude du sommeil chez le cobaye adulte et nouveau-né. *C. R. Soc. Biol.* (Paris) 160:1453, 1966.
31. Kales, A., Wilson, T., Kales, J. D., Jacobson, A., Paulson, M. J., Kollar, E., and Walter, R. D. Measurements of all-night sleep in normal elderly persons: Effects of aging. *J. Amer. Geriat. Soc.* 15:405, 1967.
32. Karacan, I., Goodenough, D. R., Shapiro, A., and Starker, S. Erection cycle during sleep in relation to dream anxiety. *Arch. Gen. Psychiat.* (Chicago) 15:183, 1966.
33. Klein, M. Étude polygraphique et phylogénétique des différents états de sommeil. Thèse de Médecine, Lyon: Bosc. Edition, 1963.
34. Klein, M., Michel, F., and Jouvet, M. Étude polygraphique du sommeil chez les oiseaux. *C. R. Soc. Biol.* (Paris) 158:99, 1964.
35. Meier, G. W., and Berger, R. J. Development of sleep and wakefulness patterns in the infant rhesus monkey. *Exp. Neurol.* 12:257, 1965.
36. Michel, F., Jeannerod, M., Mouret, J., Rechtschaffen, A., and Jouvet, M. Sur les mécanismes de l'activité des pointes au niveau du système visuel au cours de la phase paradoxale du sommeil. *C. R. Soc. Biol.* (Paris) 158:103, 1964.
37. Michel, F., Rechtschaffen, A., and Vimont-Vicary, P. Activité électrique des muscles oculaires extrinsèques au cours du cycle veille-sommeil. *C. R. Soc. Biol.* (Paris) 158:106, 1964.
38. Michel, F., and Roffwarg, H. P. Chronic split brain stem preparation: Effect on the sleep-waking cycle. *Experientia* 23: 126, 1967.
39. Mikiten, T. H., Niebyl, P. H., and Hendley, C. D. EEG desynchronization during behavioral sleep associated with spike discharges from the thalamus of the cat. *Fed. Proc.* 20:327, 1961.

40. Monod, N., and Pajot, N. Le sommeil du nouveau-né et du prématuré. I. Analyse des études polygraphiques (movements oculaires, respiration et EEG) chez le nouveau-né à terme. *Biol. Neonat.* 8:281, 1965.
41. Morrison, A. R., and Pompeiano, O. Vestibular influences on vegetative functions during the rapid eye movement periods of desynchronized sleep. *Experientia* 21:667, 1965.
42. Morrison, A. R., and Pompeiano, O. Vestibular influences during sleep. II. Effects of vestibular lesions on the pyramidal discharge during desynchronized sleep. *Arch. Ital. Biol.* 104: 214, 1966.
43. Morrison, A. R., and Pompeiano, O. Vestibular influences during sleep. IV. Functional relations between vestibular nuclei and lateral geniculate nucleus during desynchronized sleep. *Arch. Ital. Biol.* 104:425, 1966.
44. Mouret, J., Jeannerod, M., and Jouvet, M. L'activité électrique du système visuel au cours de la phase paradoxale du sommeil chez le chat. *J. Physiol.* (Paris) 55:305, 1963.
45. Pellet, J. Étude électropolygraphique et comportementale des états de veille et de sommeil chez le cobaye (*Cavia porcellus*). *C. R. Soc. Biol.* (Paris) 7:1476, 1966.
46. Penfield, W., and Rasmussen, T. *The Cerebral Cortex of Man: A Clinical Study of Localization of Function.* New York: Macmillan, 1950.
47. Peyrethon, J., and Dusan-Peyrethon, D. Étude polygraphique du cycle veille-sommeil d'un Téléostéen (*Tinca tinca*). *C. R. Soc. Biol.* (Paris) 161:2533, 1967.
48. Piéron, H. *Le problème physiologique du sommeil.* Paris: Masson, 1913.
49. Pietrusky, F. Das Verhalten der Augen im Schlafe. *Klin. Mbl. Augenheilk.* 68:355, 1922.
50. Pompeiano, O., and Morrison, A. R. Vestibular influences during sleep. III. Dissociation of the tonic and phasic inhibition of spinal reflexes during desynchronized sleep following vestibular lesions. *Arch. Ital. Biol.* 104:231, 1966.
51. Prechtl, H. F. R., and Lenard, H. G. A study of eye movements in sleeping newborn infants. *Brain Res.* 5:477, 1967.
52. Rechtschaffen, A., Bassan, M., and Ledecky-Janecek, S. Activity patterns in Caiman Sclerops (Crocodilia). *Psychophysiology* 5:201, 1968.
53. Riesen, A. H. Sensory Deprivation. In E. Stellar and J. Sprague (Eds.), *Progress in Physiological Psychology.* New York: Academic, 1967.

54. Roffwarg, H. P., Dement, W. C., and Fisher, C. Preliminary Observations of the Sleep-Dream Pattern of Neonates, Infants, Children, and Adults. In E. Harms (Ed.), *Problems of Sleep and Dream in Children*. Monographs on Child Psychiatry, No. 2. New York: Pergamon, 1964.
55. Roffwarg, H. P., Dement, W. C., Muzio, J. N., and Fisher, C. Dream imagery: Relationship to rapid eye movements of sleep. *Arch. Gen. Psychiat.* (Chicago) 7:235, 1962.
56. Roffwarg, H. P., Muzio, J. N., and Dement, W. C. Ontogenetic development of the human sleep-dream cycle. *Science* 152:604, 1966.
57. Roussel, B., Buguet, A., Bobillier, P., and Jouvet, M. Locus coeruleus, sommeil paradoxal, et noradrénaline cérébrale. *C. R. Soc. Biol.* (Paris) 161:2537, 1967.
58. Schultz, D. P. *Sensory Restriction: Effects on Behavior*. New York: Academic, 1965.
59. Snyder, F. Toward an evolutionary theory of dreaming. *Amer. J. Psychiat.* 123:121, 1966.
60. Spreng, L. F., Johnson, L. C., and Lubin, A. Autonomic correlates of eye movement bursts during stage REM sleep. *Psychophysiology* 4:311, 1968.
61. Wallach, H., and Karsh, E. B. Why the modification of stereoscopic depth-perception is so rapid. *Amer. J. Psychol.* 76:413, 1963.
62. Walls, G. L. *The Vertebrate Eye and Its Adaptive Radiation*. Bloomfield Hills, Mich.: Cranbrook Press, 1942.
63. Walls, G. L. The evolutionary history of eye movements. *Vision Res.* 2:69, 1962.
64. Worth, C. *Squint: Its Causes, Pathology and Treatment*. Philadelphia: Blakiston, 1903.

The Programing (P) Hypothesis for REM Sleep

EDMOND M. DEWAN

THE USE OF THEORY IN SLEEP RESEARCH

At the present stage of development of sleep and REM research enough facts have accumulated to make it inconvenient for anyone to memorize them all. Whenever this happens in a particular discipline, conceptual schemes are usually developed which, at least in a limited way, make "sense" out of these facts by providing a background or context in which these facts fit together coherently. When such schemes are successful, one can *deduce* the facts from a small number of basic hypotheses and can thus "remember" what is known. These conceptual schemes, of course, are called models or theories and, if they are to be taken really seriously, they must also give rise to new experimental predictions. Inevitably, theories must be modified in the light of new experiments, but their helpfulness consists not in their "correctness" but in their ability to direct experimental investigation. Theory can thus be regarded as a convenient tool to help recall facts and also to guide experiments.

In this paper a hypothesis is advanced which has already shown itself useful in these respects. In the attempt to learn its limitations we have learned some startling facts. It is almost certain at the outset that this hypothesis has limitations and must be modified accordingly, but this is totally irrelevant. The strength of the hypothesis is entirely in its "vulnerability" to test and to the large number of tests it suggests. Space limitations allow the discussion of only a few of the total number of possible experimental predictions and questions, but these will suffice to illustrate the technique.

The Heuristic Development of the P (Programing) Hypothesis

We begin by pointing out some general observations which lead to the suggestion that REM sleep is related to a process of setting up functional structures (programs) in the brain.

First there is the observation that biological phenomena ranging from adaptation, evolution, and homeostasis to learning behavior all exhibit the "error correction" or "optimization" effects so common in any control system. In other words the concept of feedback in its various forms is one of the most intrinsic phenomena to living processes. This sort of observation is especially pertinent to the ability of higher animals to learn and to adapt to changing situations throughout their lifetimes. The further, reasonable postulate that nature is "economical" or nearly "optimal" implies that brains of such animals would be set up to perform functions relevant to the *current needs* of the animal. The information which is no longer needed by it would presumably be stored more economically at the price of accessibility, and so on. In short, we hypothesize that the brains of higher animals are in a state of constant alteration in the sense that their functional structure is constantly being revised for current situations and needs. This is analogous to programing and reprograming in the computer. In my opinion there is no question that it takes place. The question is only of when and how it happens. One's first guess might be that sleep plays an important role since the animal disconnects in some sense from the environment in that condition, and this would be necessary if reprograming must be done "off line," as they say in the computer business.

Two of the most indicative observations about REM sleep (D-state) are (1) the phylogenetic development [19] which increases from zero percent in the lowest and least adaptable (fixed programed) animals to about 25 percent of sleep on the average for the mammals, and (2) the ontogenetic development [31] which decreases from birth and childhood (when the animal is most plastic and able to learn) to adulthood and senility when learning and memory recall for new memories are at their lower values. In this connection it has been estimated that at about 24 to 30 weeks gestational age in the human fetus, 100 percent of sleep is in REM sleep [27]. This is especially interesting from our point of view since presumably the *initial* programing of the brain occurs at a maximum rate during earlier stages of the embryo's development.

The most theoretically compelling of early observations about REM sleep, in the context of the above remarks, are these: (1) REM sleep is associated with dreams [8], and (2) percent of REM sleep rebounds [7] after suppression, implying that it does *something* of importance to or for the organism.

Thus we are led to make the guess or hypothesis that REM sleep plays an important role in programing the brain. But this general statement lacks the precision or vulnerability necessary to suggest experiments to directly test (i.e., disprove) it. In the following, therefore, we prefer to consider what limitations and qualifications must be made to the statement that "REM sleep is necessary and sufficient for P." In this way we hope eventually to arrive at the simplest theory possible—but we must of necessity begin with one *simpler* than possible.

The organization of the remainder of this paper is as follows: (1) the examination of six aspects of P (programing), (2) the discussion of some known facts in this context, and (3) the deduction of experimental predictions and important experimental questions from the hypothesis.

THE CONCEPT OF P IN THE COMPUTER AND THE BRAIN

In modern computers there are two methods employed to set up programs or functional structures. The first is to connect various computing components with an arrangement of wires which can be plugged or unplugged from a "patch panel." The other is to store instructions in the form of coded numbers in the computer memory ("memory stored control"). During computer operation these instructions are called forth in sequence. Changing the program consists of replacing instructions in the memory device. In either type of programing one has an alterable functional structure, and we are hypothesizing that in the brain the functional structure ("pathways") can also be altered. Some computers can automatically reprogram themselves in some sense; however, a human programmer is responsible for most of the significant changes and the creation of new programs. In this paper we hypothesize that the brain has a method of reprograming itself spontaneously and automatically.

The six categories of P to be considered (involving experiments from several disciplines) are these: (1) physical or structural aspects, (2) memory aspects, (3) input-output (I-O) programs having to do with perception, sensory motor coordination, motor skills, and attention phenomena, (4) organization of P by emotion and drive, (5) homeostatic and biorhythmic aspects of P, and (6) P-system breakdown.

DETAILED DESCRIPTIONS, EXPERIMENTAL PREDICTIONS, QUESTIONS, AND RESULTS

Physical Aspects of P

The P needed for the following tasks is included in this category: (1) establishing new functional pathways as neurons die with age and are not replaced (at the rate of 1000 to 10,000 per day) [33], (2) initial programing of the embryo brain, and (3) establishing new functional pathways after brain damage. This aspect of P is in some ways analogous to wound healing, metamorphosis, morphogenesis, and regeneration, in that macroscopic structures are organized in an adaptive manner. There is an especially great similarity between the brain and a developing embryo since in both cases (presumably) macromolecules in some way control the development of global structures, and vice versa. For this reason a better understanding of morphogenesis may have relevance to neurophysiology in connection with the P process.

These notions raise interesting questions: 1. Does long-term deprivation of REM sleep cause permanent physical damage? (We'd expect the answer to be yes because of the neuron deaths.) 2. Does REM deprivation in the embryo (e.g., by drugs) cause it to be malformed or inhibit the natural anatomical growth of the brain? (Prediction: yes.) Do embryos of even the lower forms show high amounts of REM sleep at some early stage? (Prediction: yes.) Adametz's observation [1] that a lesion which is made in two steps is dramatically less damaging functionally than if made all at once is quite suggestive of P processes. A prediction is that if REM deprivation is carried out during the interval of time between making the lesions there would be almost as much damage as when the lesions were made all at once. If this is true, it would be an impressive confirmation of the model.

Another approach to testing this phenomenon is to measure percent of REM sleep in aphasics who are rapidly improving and compare this to percent of REM sleep in those who are not improving. It has been shown [14] that there is a (statistically significant) higher amount of REM sleep in the subjects who were improving, as the hypothesis predicts. The next experiment would be to see if REM deprivation temporarily cuts down improvement in those subjects.

Memory P

In a computer, the use of memory devices is organized according to a hierarchical principle [26]: the less frequently used material is stored in progressively slower but more economical memories. Memories can be shifted to different devices as priorities change. There is an analogy to the brain's memory in that as information is used less often it can become no longer recallable but still recognizable—and so on until the memory manifests itself only in a savings in relearning time. In both cases the accessibility of information is optimized with respect to the memory structures available and to priority.

One special form of early learning, imprinting, also falls into the category of the memory type of P and we would expect high amounts of REM sleep during critical periods. We shall assume in the following that REM sleep has to do with consolidation of memory into the best configuration for the organism's needs (cf. later section on Organization of P by Drives and Goals).

According to the P hypothesis one can deduce the following predictions: (1) The Korsakoff patients, who show practically no ability to recall, should have no REM sleep. (2) Electroconvulsive therapy (ECT), which causes amnesia, should decrease REM pressure. (3) Lower animals (e.g., birds) when being subjected to a regimen of high amounts of learning (e.g., during operant conditioning experiments) would show more REM sleep. The first prediction was tested [16] and it was found that there was REM sleep in Korsakoff patients but that it was physiologically abnormal, suggesting that "abnormal REM" can occur *without* evidence of P. The prediction about ECT is true [5, 6] in the sense that REM deprivation will not give an REM rebound on a successive night if ECT intervenes. The third prediction is as yet unexplored.

Many other investigators have examined the memory aspect of "P." Greenberg [13], Pearlman [28], Fishbein [10], Feldman [9], and others have obtained evidence that REM sleep plays a role in memory processes. Briefly, their work suggests that REM sleep may involve both a necessary *preparation* for learning (a form of "metaprograming") and also a form of consolidation of information (for long-term memory). In addition it has been substantiated that chicks have large amounts of REM sleep shortly after hatching, i.e., during the critical imprinting time [15]. Further work with REM suppressing drugs (predicted to block imprinting) remains to be done, and it would also be of interest to see if nitrous oxide can cause imprinting to occur (on the basis [17] that nitrous oxide can bring on a state similar to REM sleep). Another important imprinting experiment would be to see if there is an REM sleep increase in ungulates during adult imprinting. If this came out positively it would suggest that some animals (i.e., those that exhibit "imprinting" in a dramatic way) are "reflex programers" and therefore show a low percent of REM sleep most of the time, and others are "spontaneous programmers"—i.e., have REM sleep even when not crucially needed. It would further substantiate the connection between REM sleep and P, since observations to date on REM sleep in chicks may also be explained merely by the ontological development, and not necessarily by the P hypothesis.

Input-Output (I-O) P

Perhaps the least explored area of research on REM sleep concerns the I-O programs of the brain. These consist of the programs having to do with the organization of perception, coordination of motor activity (acquisition of motor skills), coordination of sensorimotor relations, coordination of motor activity directly controlling perception (especially eye motion in visual perception), and finally attention programs which automatically filter the sense modalities and present the brain with the most relevant incoming information. These programs are assumed to be optimized in some sense to the organism's current needs (cf. the next section).

The first and only experiment to date that has been performed involved the adaptation to visual field rotation (180°) [35]. Originally Kohler [24] and Held [21] noted that subjects could adapt to visual rotation and distortion provided they exercised *willed* motor activity over a certain interval of time. This of course is P, therefore the prediction is that visual field inversion, and so on, should enhance REM sleep time and REM intensity (provided there was willed motor activity). Both were in fact observed [35]. This result, if substantiated by more extensive controlled tests, opens up an entirely new area for REM experimentation. Consider the new question raised: "Does ECT hamper adaptation to visual distortion in view of the fact that it decreases REM pressure? Do REM suppressing drugs delay adaptation? Can Korsakoff patients with their "abnormal REM" adapt? Do children (with higher REM sleep time) adapt faster than adults? Can lower forms ever adapt (with no REM sleep)? What happens if imprinting animals have their visual fields inverted during the critical period? What happens to REM sleep in schizophrenics if they have visual inversion? Is there an absence of the increased REM effect if the subject has visual inversion but performs no "willed motor activity" of consequence? This list can easily be extended by the reader, and the predictions of the model are obvious.

Numerous other forms of sensorimotor experiments suggest themselves involving percent of REM sleep and REM deprivation effects relative to learning to cope with conditions of weightlessness, sensorimotor time delay (using video tape recording for the visual delay), "human amplification situations"—e.g., having a man learn how to operate a vehicle or "construction equipment," and so on—all of which involve the development and incorporation of sensorimotor programs. In all of the above, dream content should be examined for relevance. One should also investigate REM effects and dream content in athletes preparing for a contest.

The attention P aspects of REM sleep might be examined, for example, by measuring contingent negative variation (CNV) patterns in a student pilot training in a cockpit simulator: REM sleep should be more intense during a concentrated training regimen, REM deprivation should cut down learning, and the CNV patterns, which theoretically should reflect the patterns of anticipated events for attention, would not become efficient as quickly, and so on.

Organization of P by Drives and Goals

It will be assumed that the intensity of an emotion is directly related to ability or inability to "cope," i.e., to the *need for P*. According to Simonov [32], a surplus amount of "ability to cope" gives rise to a pleasurable emotion and vice versa. It is also related to the strength of the associated drive. Thus, taking these two facts together it is an ideal measure for the priority of areas that need P [30]. Assuming this, the amount of emotionality experienced by a subject should affect REM pressure. An increase in emotion should lead to an increase in amount or intensity of REM sleep and vice versa. This may explain why some tranquilizers which decrease emotionality also reduce REM pressure [23, 25]. From this one would also expect REM deprivation to increase emotionality, given that the subject needed to cope with a new situation for which he was not prepared. These considerations also have obvious implications for dream content. Some experiments with stressful moving pictures support this prediction [2, 18].

We shall assume that emotion plays an additional role in programing, namely that it is used for tagging or labeling memories and programs for the purpose of consolidation during the P process. This could only be possible if the variety of emotional nuances or feelings were as great as the variety found in perception. This will be assumed here in spite of the lack of variety of verbal representation for these feelings. As Plutchik [29] has shown, there is evidence that emotional feelings are internally perceived and processed in a manner abstractly resembling color perception. Associated with each goal or drive would be a certain set of feelings which would then tag the perceptions and experiences occurring at any given time. We then hypothesize that during the P process all memories, programs, and so forth which are relevant to a current important need can be brought together and "filed" in one place by making use of these tags. This is analogous to the computer technique known as "associative memory" in which the address number of each memory location includes a coded numerical tag to identify the type of information stored there.

This scheme is suggested partly by Freud's description of dream content: displacement, condensation and symbolism, "primary process logic," and the organization of material by drive, wish, and instinctive needs. It can be shown that these aspects of dream content resemble a clever way to scan experience and organize information according to needs by the use of "feeling nuances" as tags. This will be described in detail elsewhere; however, a great deal of independent work, which should be consulted, has also been done by Breger [3] along similar lines.

The phenomenon of state dependent memory is entirely consistent with this viewpoint. The "state" can be regarded as a constellation of feelings. The model suggests that the available P's of all the types—I-O, perceptual and behavioral, as well as memory—should be state dependent. For example, the question is now raised:

"Can adaptation to distorted vision be state dependent?" In addition, this hypothetical mode of operation of the P system suggests certain causes of breakdown (discussed in the later section on that subject).

REM Periods, Homeostasis, and Biological Rhythms

Sleep and REM periods are both "gated" by biological rhythms (of approximate periods of 24 hours and 90 minutes, respectively). In this model, P (in all its aspects) is regarded as a form of complicated homeostasis which involves not only the animal's "ability to cope" but its mental processes and the entire range of physical bodily processes in support of this. Since REM sleep is locked in step to the bodily rhythms, it is tempting to conjecture that the hypothetical P processes they represent can in turn affect those rhythms. For example, the observations of Stroebel [22] suggest that the body can be programed for a certain type of emotionality as a function of time of day. More specifically, if an animal is repeatedly stressed at one time of day for several days, this tendency for stress will continue to appear at the time with circadian regularity and will not easily be extinguished unless it is deconditioned at that time of day (the time of day thus representing a "state" in a state dependent learning response). This suggests that P can program the hormone releases, and other somatic and homeostatic anticipatory activity to prepare the animal to "cope." REM deprivation should tend to prevent this; hence, an important experiment would be to repeat Stroebel's work but with REM deprivation. Other questions raised are these: (1) Does a large phase change of the circadian rhythms increase REM sleep? (Prediction: Possibly yes). (2) Can the length of the circadian rhythm (free running) depend on "need for P"—i.e., increase in length due to a greater need for P? In other words, do emotionally disturbed people or people with a large need for P for one reason or other need more sleep and tend to wake up later in the morning and go to bed late? Theoretically there would be a delayed phase due to a longer free running period. The therapeutic value of circadian desynchronization noted by Stroebel may also be explainable by this model.

Breakdown of the P System

The P process, involving as it does a very complex form of feedback and optimization, is at least as prone to breakdown as any other control process, be it homeostasis in biology or feedback control engineering. In the former, the breakdown can result in fever, and so on, and in the latter it shows up in forms ranging from oscillations to total self-destruction. Both the control engineers and physicians spend most of their time correcting for instability and in attempting to avoid breakdown.

The analogy between fever and schizophrenia was noted by S. Cobb [4], who pointed out that there are at least seven different classes of conditions which generally precede the schizophrenic reaction. He therefore regarded it as a common form of breakdown, like fever, and suggested that we do not need to regard it as a disease entity. In our model we regard schizophrenia as well as many other types of psychoses as forms of breakdown of the P system. For example, Freud's analogy [12] between dream state thought content and the thought disturbances of an awake psychotic might be explained by saying that the brain is "stuck in the P mode of operation." This would also explain the lack of REM rebound [34] in the schizophrenic as well as the lack of affect. Also the high percent of REM sleep observed in states of transition to psychosis [11] would represent the unsuccessful "last stand" of the P system before it flipped into an abnormal form of stable but more or less nonfunctional operation.

CONCLUSION

Various forms of programing assumed to take place in the brain have been discussed. P or programing ability to cope was related specifically to REM sleep, and the consequences of this hypothesis regarding experimental tests and predictions were investigated. The large number of experimental questions raised by this model suggests that it may serve a useful function in sleep research.

REFERENCES

1. Adametz, J. H. Rate of recovery of functioning in cats with rostral reticular lesions. *J. Neurosurg.* 16:85, 1959.
2. Baekeland, F., and Koulack, D. Effects of a Stressful Presleep Experience on EEG Recorded Sleep. Paper read at APSS, 1967.
3. Breger, L. The function of dreams. *J. Abnorm. Psychol.* Monograph.
4. Cobb, S. Thoughts on schizophrenia. *Amer. J. Psychiat.* 120: 707, 1964. See also L. Bellack, *Schizophrenia*. New York: Logos Press, 1958.
5. Cohen, H., and Dement, W. Sleep: Suppression of rapid eye movement phase in the cat after electroconvulsive shock. *Science* 154:396, 1966.
6. Cohen, H., Duncan II, R. F., and Dement, W. Sleep: The effect of electroconvulsive shock in cats deprived of REM sleep. *Science* 156:1646, 1967.
7. Dement, W. The effect of dream deprivation. *Science* 131: 1705, 1960.
8. Dement, W., and Kleitman, N. The relation of eye movements during sleep to dream activity. *J. Exp. Psychol.* 53:339, 1957.
9. Feldman, R., and Dement, W. Possible relationships between REM sleep and memory consolidation. *Psychophysiology* 5:243, 1968.
10. Fishbein, W. Paradoxical Sleep: A Periodic Mechanism for Securing and Maintaining Information for Long-Term Memory. University of Colorado Ph.D. Thesis, 1969.
11. Fisher, C., and Dement, W. C. Studies on the psychopathology of sleep and dreams. *Amer. J. Psychiat.* 119:1160, 1963.
12. Freud, S. The Interpretation of Dreams. In *The Standard Edition of the Complete Psychological Works of Sigmund Freud,* tr. and ed. by J. Strachey with others. London: Hogarth and the Institute of Psycho-Analysis, 1964. Vol. IV, p. 92.
13. Greenberg, R., and Leiderman, P. Perceptions, the dream process and memory. *Compr. Psychiat.* 7:517, 1966.
14. Greenberg, R., and Dewan, E. Aphasia and rapid eye movement sleep. *Nature* (London) 223:183, 1969.
15. Greenberg, R., Kelty, M., and Dewan, E. Sleep Patterns in the Newly Hatched Chick. Paper read at APSS, 1969.
16. Greenberg, R., Mayer, R., Brook, R., and Pearlman, C. Dreaming in patients with post alcoholic Korsakoff's disease. Paper read at APSS, 1967.

17. Greenberg, R., Pearlman, C., and Mahler, D. Nitrous Oxide and Dreaming. Paper read at APSS, 1967.
18. Greenberg, R., Pillard, R., and Pearlman, C. Dream deprivation and adaptation to stress. *Psychophysiology* 5:238, 1968.
19. Hartmann, E. L. The D-state: A review and discussion of studies on the physiologic state concomitant with dreaming. *Int. J. Psychiat.* 2:11, 1966.
20. Hartmann, E. Longitudinal studies of sleep and dream patterns in manic-depressive patients. *Arch. Gen. Psychiat.* (Chicago) 19:312, 1968.
21. Held, R. Plasticity in human sensory motor control. *Science* 142:455, 1963.
22. The Importance of Biological Clocks in Mental Health. (Contains a Summary.) In *Mental Health Program Reports,* No. 2. Washington, D.C.: Dept. of Health, Education, and Welfare, 1968. P. 323.
23. Jouvet, M. Private communication, April 1966.
24. Kohler, I. *The Formation and Transformation of the Perceptual World. Psychol. Issues* 3, Monograph 12, 1964.
25. Kramer, M., Whitman, R., Baldridge, W., and Ornstein, P. In G. Martin and B. Kisch (Eds.), *Enzymes in Mental Health.* Philadelphia: Lippincott, 1966. Pp. 102–116.
26. Neumann, J. von. *The Computer and the Brain.* New Haven, Conn.: Yale University Press, 1958.
27. Parmelee, A. H., et al. Activated Sleep in Premature Infants. Paper read at APSS, 1964.
28. Pearlman, C. Effect of REM Deprivation on Retention of Avoidance Learning in Rats. Paper read at APSS, 1968.
29. Plutchik, R. *The Emotions: Facts, Theories, and a New Model.* New York: Random House, 1962.
30. Rapaport, D. *Emotion and Memory.* New York: Science Editions, 1961.
31. Roffwarg, H. P., Muzio, J. N., and Dement, W. C. Ontogenetic development of the human sleep-dream cycle. *Science* 152:604, 1966.
32. Simonov, P. V. Studies of Emotional Behavior of Humans and Animals by Soviet Physiologists. (Consulting Ed., E. Toboch.) *Ann. N.Y. Acad. Sci.* 159:1112, 1969.
33. Talland, G. Private communication.
34. Zarcone, V., Gulevich, G., and Dement, W. Schizophrenia and Partial REM Sleep Deprivation. Paper read at APSS, 1967.
35. Zimmerman, J., Stoyva, J., and Metcalf, D. Distorted Visual Experience and REMS. Paper read at APSS, 1969.

The D-State and Norepinephrine-dependent Systems

ERNEST HARTMANN

Since the D-state (REM sleep) appears to be one of the basic organismic states of the body it may well prove difficult to find a single satisfactory function for it; as I have suggested previously it may, like waking or S-sleep (NREM sleep), have multiple functions in the body's economy which could certainly include functions at the biochemical, the neurophysiological, and the psychological-behavioral level [35]. However, given the orderliness of nature, which always emerges eventually if at times painfully slowly, it is most improbable that, even if there are many functions of the D-state, these should be totally unrelated functions. I wish to propose here a function of the D-state at the neurochemical level, to explore its psychological implications, and also to show how this function could integrate most of the other functions of the D-state for which evidence has been presented in the last few years.

It is probable a priori that sleep has some sort of restorative function, and that one of its two distinct states, the D-state, has some homeostatic or restorative function as well; and in fact most hypotheses have assigned it a function of this kind. It has been postulated that it may restore altered chemical patterns by allowing the discharge of some accumulated substance or "toxin" [13], that it may restore "cortical tonus" [18], "vigilance" [86], motor coordination in the extraocular muscles [2], or the ability to learn and to register new information [5, 14, 28, 29]. Something is probably being restored, but it is not clear exactly what. I believe that in the present state of knowledge these restorations can best be explained and connected at the neurochemical level. I wish to propose, in line with previous suggestions I have made [40–42], that the D-state functions to restore synaptically active brain norepinephrine (NE) and maintain the functioning of NE-dependent brain systems.* Needless to say, this involves speculation; there is no direct evidence at present for such a hypothesis.

I shall first present evidence that has led me to connect the D-state and norepinephrine in the manner just stated, then discuss what "NE-dependent brain systems" may consist of and what behaviors they control, and then present independent evidence that the D-state may have an effect on these same systems and behaviors.

D-TIME AND NE: A RECIPROCAL RELATIONSHIP

First of all, I have been struck by and have investigated an interesting inverse relationship between D-time or D-pressure and "active brain norepinephrine." Situations or agents associated with or which produce an increase in active or available norepinephrine are apparently associated with a decrease in D-time and D-pressure, i.e., a reduction in D-time without an immediate rebound recovery. Mania in human patients is such a situation, in which studies point to a probable increase in central available norepinephrine [76, 96] and in which we have shown D-time to be extremely low—far outside the normal range—without apparent rebound [40]. MAO (monoamine oxidase) inhibitors produce an increase in available norepinephrine (as well as other biogenic amines) and produce a clear fall in D-time in animals [52] as well as humans [11, 103] with absent or delayed rebound. Other antidepressant drugs, imipramine and amitriptyline, are also thought to increase synaptically available norepinephrine, probably by reducing cellular reuptake [79]. These compounds likewise reduce D-time and D-pressure [38, 39, 75]. Electroconvulsive shock has been shown to increase norepinephrine turn-

* "Restoring synaptically active brain NE" could be accomplished by increasing NE synthesis, decreasing its catabolism, shifting its location appropriately (e.g., affecting reuptake), or, finally, increasing in some way the sensitivity of postsynaptic neurons to NE.

I use the cumbersome expression "NE-dependent brain systems" to include networks and systems depending on NE levels or activity in certain portions of the brain. This implies noradrenergic synapses presumably *at some stage,* but does not imply that the systems are totally noradrenergic.

over by the normetanephrine pathway, indicating the presence of more synaptically available norepinephrine [53]. It also reduces D-pressure in animals [9]; human results are unclear so far since of course only severely ill patients receiving ECT can be studied.

Conversely, agents and conditions probably associated with decreased available norepinephrine are characterized by increased D-time or D-pressure. Severely depressed patients are thought to have less available central norepinephrine [76, 77] and are usually characterized by increased D-pressure [88]: when sleep time is relatively normal, as it is in some manic-depressives in their depressed phase, these patients actually show increased D-time [40]. When sleep time is severely compromised as it is in many psychotic depressions, D-time is not high, but short D-latencies, long first D-periods, and high eye movement densities in the D-periods attest to the increased pressure [40, 88, 89]. Reserpine is a well-known clinical drug which appears to act by interfering with the storage of biogenic amines and thus producing a markedly reduced level of norepinephrine (as well as of other amines). Our laboratory and others [34, 46, 102] have shown that reserpine has the almost unique property of being able to produce an increased D-time in man lasting several days. A selective way of reducing brain norepinephrine without altering levels of other amines is to prevent its synthesis by administering AMPT (alpha-methyl-para-tyrosine), an inhibitor of tyrosine hydroxylase, the rate-limiting step in norepinephrine synthesis [59, 90]. A single dose of 50 to 100 mg./kg. reduces brain norepinephrine levels in the rat by at least 50 percent for 6 to 12 hours. Preliminary results on sleep patterns are somewhat conflicting, depending greatly on dosage and route of administration [48, 55, 60, 100]; the drug can apparently cause severe renal damage and peritoneal irritation. In our studies to date AMPT in a single *oral* dose of 50, 75, or 100 mg. per kilogram significantly increased D-time in the rat, and the effect lasted about 12 hours [45]. It should be emphasized that it is extremely easy to reduce D-time in man and in animals—we have performed or reviewed studies of 50 to 60 drugs of very different groups, all of which produce a decreased D-time when first given [35, 42]; pharmacologically produced increases in D-time are very rare. In fact, in the experience of our laboratory, reserpine and AMPT are almost the only drugs that can clearly produce this effect. One other drug which has been reported to increase D-time is LSD [37, 64], whose mechanism of action is far from clear, but which does somewhat increase brain serotonin levels and decrease brain norepinephrine levels [25, 26].

Amphetamines, which apparently act by releasing brain norepinephrine as well as interfering with its cellular reuptake [8, 27, 33], have been shown markedly to reduce D-time in man [73] and animals [49, 54, 84]. The effects of amphetamines on norepinephrine last a relatively short time, only a few hours, whereas some effects of the antidepressant drugs may last for days or longer. The same is true of the effects of these substances on sleep: the decrease in D-time produced by amphetamine is dramatic but short-lasting and is followed by an immediate rebound [73]. The decrease produced by the antidepressants lasts several days [38, 75, 103] and a rebound, if it occurs at all, is greatly delayed.

A preliminary report indicates that small amounts of norepinephrine injected by cannula directly into the ventricular system of monkeys completely eliminate D-time for a period of 12 to 24 hours [12]. Such studies are difficult to evaluate, but the authors injected saline controls and a number of other substances including serotonin without obtaining this elimination of D-time.

On the basis of all this admittedly indirect evidence, we suggest that there may be a mechanism by which high norepinephrine levels "shut off" or "turn down" the D-state and low levels "turn on" the D-state. It appears as if NE can somehow functionally replace D-time. This is a reasonable arrangement only if there is negative feedback such that D-time in some way restores norepinephrine or its potential for activity. Thus when less norepinephrine is available, more D-time is "needed," which when it occurs restores the norepinephrine level or its activity.

(I should emphasize, of course, that this suggested reciprocal feedback mechanism involving D-time and norepinephrine, though it involves an important possible *function* of D, represents only one aspect of the *neurochemistry* of the D-state. Brain serotonin levels, for instance, play an important role in controlling total sleep time [50, 51], the length of the sleep-dream cycle [36, 37], and possibly also relative amounts of S- and D-sleep.)

THE NE-DEPENDENT SYSTEMS

What functions and behaviors does naturally occurring norepinephrine govern in the brain? Again, there is little certain proof. Evidence is based on effects of altering norepinephrine levels by inhibitors of synthesis, especially AMPT, effects of releasers such as reserpine alone and in combination with inhibitors or precursors, and effects of the amphetamines which, according to the weight of present evidence, act by releasing naturally occurring norepinephrine [8, 27, 33] and by diminishing its cellular reuptake [27] rather than by a direct amphetamine effect.

I can only summarize my current impressions of such norepinephrine functions without giving adequate space to evidence for or against each proposition. First there is evidence, already referred to, that active brain norepinephrine* is involved in human depression. Lowered norepinephrine levels are thought to characterize depression, while an increase of norepinephrine levels counteracts depression. Human depressive illness is a very complex phenomenon, however, and it is my impression that the effects of raising norepinephrine levels in depressed patients can be seen more specifically as *reversing lethargy* or *increasing energetic behavior*—this can be seen in animal as well as human studies—and has something to do with increasing *motivation* as well as with *improving mood.*

* I speak here, as in the past section, of "active brain norepinephrine" or simply "brain NE" as a kind of shorthand. In some of the studies what is actually involved is total brain catecholamines, in some studies brain NE, or NE in specific brain areas, in some studies NE metabolized through the normetanephrine pathways—chiefly an extracellular process and thus thought to indicate "released" or "synaptically active" NE—and in some studies there is evidence that "newly synthesized" NE may form a separate pool, responsible for drug (amphetamine) effects [97]. Thus while most evidence points to NE for the effects I am discussing, it is admitted on the one hand that dopamine may play a role as well on NE, and on the other hand that only a certain perhaps "newly synthesized" fraction of NE may be involved.

There is a good deal of evidence from inhibitor and releaser studies in animals that catecholamine levels positively influence *motor behavior,* usually studied in previously learned tasks [15, 56, 62, 63, 68, 71, 72, 80, 81, 97]. Higher levels are associated with increased performance and vice versa. One study, for instance, showed that reserpine plus AMPT, each in a dose far too small to affect performance when given alone, seriously disrupted learned behavior [72]. Human studies suggest that amphetamines and related compounds in some circumstances produce increased *motor coordination* and *psychomotor performance* (most easily seen after, but not restricted to, conditions of sleep deprivation or other states of reduced function) [3, 47, 57, 65, 82, 99]. Catecholamine levels also appear to facilitate *new learning* or *short-term memory* in a number of reward and avoidance tasks [16, 56, 58, 91]. In one study, catecholamine levels in several strains of mice were directly correlated with ability to learn avoidance tasks [83]. One review [66] concludes with the statement that norepinephrine is probably involved especially in *registration of information* and *short-term memory,* as well as *passage from short-term to long-term memory.*

The well-known effects of amphetamines make it probable that norepinephrine is involved in functions such as *vigilance* or *directed attention,* as well as *arousal* or *counteracting of fatigue* [82, 99]. These are clearly functions involving the reticular activating system. Callaway [6, 7] some years ago presented a series of studies suggesting that central sympathomimetic systems produced "*narrowed attention.*" I have suggested that the so-called paradoxical effect of amphetamines in man (stimulants in adults, they can quiet hyperactive children) are not truly paradoxical. If amphetamines act by increasing *directed attention, task-oriented attention,* or *secondary process at the expense of primary process,* this will appear as stimulation—increased ability to concentrate, increased motivated learning, and so on—in an adult already involved in secondary process activities, but it will help to quiet a child whose overactivity is based on distraction by primary process intrusion. Along these lines, my observations indicate that the effects of moderate doses of amphetamines in adults seem to include *directed at-*

tention and also *strengthening of the subject's usual defensive patterns.*

Stein in a number of papers [91, 92] has presented evidence that norepinephrine is involved in a *reward system* occupying chiefly the medial forebrain bundle; this is derived principally from studies on self-stimulation in rats. The "reward system" is shown to be involved not only in positive reinforcement learning but in certain aspects of avoidance learning as well, so that *motivation* or *reinforcement* may be considered attributes of this system as well as "reward." Possibly related to this in man is *euphoria* and an increased motivation: amphetamine effects in man have been summarized as producing, in addition to and more prominently than an actual increased achievement on certain tasks, an increase in *"need to achieve"* [19].

Attempting to summarize briefly, there may be several separate but closely interrelated affects and behaviors subserved by brain norepinephrine: a tendency to *euphoric mood* or *antidepression,* closely related to *increased "energy"* and *motivation; motor coordination; new learning* or *short-term memory*—especially *reward systems* and *motivated learning; vigilance, attention, task-orientation, secondary process;* perhaps *strengthened defensive patterns;* and *need to achieve.*

THE D-STATE AND THE NE-DEPENDENT SYSTEMS

Is there any evidence that the D-state might have a role in maintaining or restoring the functioning of these systems? There is, although a great deal of evidence so far comes from experiments on D-deprivation in animals and in man, and these must be interpreted cautiously since it is not easy to control adequately for the nonspecific stressful effects of the various D-deprivation procedures.

Several experiments suggest that D-deprivation may have a detrimental effect both on *new learning* and on *retention of previous learning* [1, 23, 24, 67, 93, 95]. To my mind the evidence for the former effect is more convincing than for the latter. One study by

Stern [94] especially relevant to the present hypothesis found a decrease in learning of both active and passive avoidance tasks after D-deprivation by the rat-on-an-island technique, and then demonstrated that chemical agents expected to increase active brain catecholamine levels (MAO inhibitors, imipramine) were able to reverse this behavioral deficit. We are currently continuing and extending these studies, using other behavioral tasks and other techniques of D-deprivation.

D-time may be related to human learning or intelligence in a more general way, but studies are only suggestive so far. Feinberg [20, 21] has shown that in certain extreme groups—aged persons with and without "chronic brain syndrome," and certain mentally deficient persons—there is a positive correlation between *intellectual functioning* and D-time. Zimmerman et al. [104] have shown that intense *new learning,* in human subjects adapting to the wearing of inverting prisms, is associated with increased D-time at night. These are fascinating early studies with many implications for better psychological understanding of the functions of the D-state; they do suggest, tentatively, that something in the systems involved in new learning may be related to D-time, in the sense that more or better learning is associated with more D-time.

It is well recognized that amphetamines are useful in temporarily reversing subjective and objective effects of sleep deprivation *(counteracting fatigue).* It is not yet clear whether the effects of D-deprivation specifically are counteracted; but the fatigue-countering effect may well be due to the released catecholamines temporarily replacing D-time or performing the function which the D-time of the night would normally have performed. "Good sleepers" who subjectively feel they sleep well, report little fatigue, and *feel well* in the morning, have significantly more D-time than "poor sleepers" [61]. Preliminary results suggest that within subjects too, nights with more D-time are followed by better *mood* in the morning [43].

It has been shown in the rat that after 4 days of D-deprivation the lethality of d-amphetamine is reduced [22]. This is a striking finding since these D-deprived rats are under severe stress and have usually lost at least 10 percent of their weight; severe stress usually greatly increases the lethality of amphetamine. The effect could be explained in terms of our hypothesis: The releasing of norepinephrine will be less toxic if the relevant central areas are deficient in norepinephrine or if receptors are less sensitive to released norepinephrine.

Wilkinson's data [101] (also see pp. 369–381) from his long and painstaking experiments on the behavioral effects of varying amounts of sleep deprivation in man have led him to suggest that deprivation of deep slow wave sleep affects physical *ability to perform* on long vigilance tasks, while D-deprivation interferes with the *motivation to perform.* This suggests that the D-state has a function in maintaining *motivation,* one of the functions closely associated with the NE-dependent systems.

We have studied a group of short sleepers—human subjects who normally get along on less than 6 hours of sleep per night. These subjects show considerably less D-time than average sleepers, whereas their slow wave sleep time is normal; they appear in other words to require less D-time than most persons. In our psychological studies of these subjects, we found that they were *energetic,* highly *task-oriented* and *motivated,* very social with a high *"need to achieve,"* and frequently *euphoric* or *hypomanic* [44] (also see pp. 33–43). They seem somewhat like persons who have taken a small dose of amphetamines; perhaps they are persons who somehow have an elevated functioning of what we have called the NE-dependent systems. We are planning to study catecholamine excretion in these subjects.

A recent report indicates that *hyperactive children* have unusually high D-times and high REM density within D-periods [85]. This is of interest because these are the children mentioned previously who appear deficient in *attention, task-orientation, secondary process,* who are often greatly improved by amphetamines [4, 10]. We might speculate that the chemical problem producing the distractibility and hyperactivity, and the possibility of improvement by amphetamines, is a relative lack or unavailability of central norepinephrine, or decreased receptor sensitivity to norepinephrine, which "turns up" the D-state regulator. This chemical defect would be similar to that postulated in adult depressed patients; and in fact, some psychiatrists have suggested on clinical grounds that these children may be depressed.

Although the psychological effects of D-deprivation are still controversial, several studies suggest changes in the direction of *loosening of the subject's usual defensive patterns* and a tendency for emergence of primary process material [13, 30]. Total sleep deprivation, of course, also may show such effects, which we could attribute to the deficient functioning (exhaustion) of NE-dependent systems.

CONTRADICTORY EVIDENCE

There are at least two pieces of experimental evidence which appear contradictory to the present hypothesis or at least very difficult to reconcile with it. One is the fact that alpha-methyl-dopa in the cat apparently greatly reduces D-time [17]. This finding by the Lyon group has led them [50] to postulate that norepinephrine produces or triggers D-periods, which is the direct opposite of what is being proposed here. Aside from questions of dosage and route, one problem is that alpha-methyl-dopa is known to produce alpha-methyl-norepinephrine (a "false transmitter") in considerable quantities in addition to blocking synthesis of normal norepinephrine. If the effect reported for alpha-methyl-dopa is indeed due directly to its interference with norepinephrine levels, this would be in contradiction to our hypothesis. However, if the alpha-methyl-norepinephrine formed perhaps has a similar action on the D-state mechanism as that which we have proposed for norepinephrine, then the results would be entirely consistent with our hypothesis. For the moment it is not possible to separate these possibilities.

The other finding is more tangentially related to the present thesis. Vogel [98] has presented fascinating results indicating that D-deprivation may produce improvement in depressed patients. This result, which needs to be confirmed, is in the direction opposite to what would have been predicted on the basis of the present hypothesis. Further studies in these areas are obviously needed.

CONCLUSIONS: THE FUNCTIONS OF THE D-STATE

The function or interrelated scheme of functions I have proposed for the D-state will no doubt need modification, at the very least, but it has already suggested numerous experiments both on the biochemical level and on the behavioral level.

Some attempts at direct neurochemical studies are in progress, but these may not be definitive; for instance if manipulation of the D-state, such as D-deprivation, in carefully stress-controlled studies, does result in alterations of norepinephrine synthesis or catabolism, this will be significant (so far preliminary studies [69, 78] are contradictory), but a failure to find clear changes in norepinephrine turnover would still leave the possibility of altered receptor sensitivity difficult to investigate at present. I believe our studies in progress on behavioral systems affected by D-deprivation or other sleep changes and the effect of altering norepinephrine on these same systems will also be useful in supporting, clarifying, or perhaps demolishing the present hypothesis.

I would like to conclude by proposing, in line with my suggestion at the beginning, that this hypothesis, far from contradicting other proposed functions of the D-state, can actually integrate and help to explain many of them.

First the biochemical or "toxin" theory is directly incorporated in the present hypothesis, except that the "toxin" (never taken entirely literally) in this view is now not an excess of some substance which builds up during W or S states, or both, and is discharged during D-time, but more or less the reverse: a relative lack of active norepinephrine (or insensitivity of receptors to norepinephrine) "builds up" during W and/or S and is then "restored" during D-time.

The hypothesis that the D-state functions to improve coordination of the extraocular musculature [2] can be included in our scheme if indeed *motor coordination* is among the NE-dependent functions. The delicate nature of oculomotor muscular coordination insures that if motor coordination is involved it will probably be best demonstrable in these muscles.

The view that the D-state serves a vigilance function [86] is implied in the function of restoration of norepinephrine systems since these certainly involve vigilance. My view, however, would emphasize the gradual improvement of vigilance by restoration of the NE-dependent systems during each D-period and over a series of D-periods, rather than the view that each D-period produces a vigilance-serving quasi-arousal.

The hypothesis that the D-state functions to stimulate the development of the cortex of the young animal and the fetus in utero [74] is attractive as an explanation for the very high D-times found early in life. I would agree with a developmental function of this kind, adding that perhaps it is the NE-dependent systems which are particularly developed in this way. Obviously the functions we have discussed—e.g., *motor coordination, new learning, directed attention*—develop rapidly early in life. In the human the age of 5 or 6 is the time at which D-time has fallen close to adult levels and is also approximately the time when secondary process functioning becomes established as the dominant way of life.

The hypothesis that the D-state functions in memory storage and new learning [5, 14, 28] is certainly part of the present hypothesis: The norepinephrine systems we suggest are restored during D-time almost certainly serve *new learning* (especially *motivated learning*), which we would expect to be improved after D-time and to be worse after D-deprivation. My hypothesis cannot speak to the specific mechanisms that might be involved in this restoration: the suggested mechanisms of programing or some form of reorganization of memory and learning systems are certainly compatible with the hypothesis, which would suggest in addition that the reprograming affects especially the behaviors mentioned as NE-dependent.

This brings up a final psychological aspect of the hypothesis. I have previously described the D-state as an information-handling system with a high activity level, as in waking, but with very rough feedback control, unlike the fine control during waking activity [35]. The rough control, allowing relatively great swings of pulse, blood pressure, and so on during D-time is shown especially in the work of Guazzi et al. [31, 32] in the cat. Human studies [87] of autonomic variables are also suggestive of this rough feedback, and in fact psychic content in the experienced dream can be seen in this light as well: A strong emotion may be set off by a minor element, or by a (latent content) association to a manifest dream element; this emotion grows more intense, possibly until the sleeper awakens, and is apparently unchecked or poorly checked by testing against further cognitive content, as would occur in the nonpsychotic waking person.

Possibly, in engineering terms, this "rough feedback state" of the nervous system is what results when the sensitive NE-dependent systems are "uncoupled" while being restored or reprogramed during D, leaving a more primitive adjustment perhaps under the control of serotonin. Or perhaps a certain amount of nightly primitive "drive-organization of memories" [70] is somehow needed to restore normal waking "conceptual organization of memories."

A rough-adjustment system with gross affect swings and so on is another way of describing primary process [70], which is thus associated once again with the D-state. It appears that a certain amount of this rough-adjustment primary process activity is required every night, and our hypothesis suggests that one function of the primary process–dominated D-state is to restore and maintain proper secondary process functioning during subsequent waking.

REFERENCES

1. Adelman, S., and Hartmann, E. Psychological Effects of Amitriptyline-induced Dream-Deprivation. Paper read at the Association for the Psychophysiological Study of Sleep (APSS), Denver, 1968; abstract in *Psychophysiology* 5:240, 1968.
2. Berger, R. Oculomotor control: A possible function of REM-sleep. *Psychol. Rev.* 76:144, 1969.

3. Blum, B., Stern, N., and Melville, K. A comparative evaluation of the action of depressant and stimulant drugs on human performance. *Psychopharmacologia* (Berlin) 6:173, 1964.
4. Bradley, C. The behavior of children receiving benzedrine. *Amer. J. Psychiat.* 94:577, 1937.
5. Breger, L. The Function of Dreams. *J. Abnorm. Psychol.* Monograph 641, 1967.
6. Callaway, E., and Dembo, D. Narrowed attention. *A.M.A. Arch. Neurol. Psychiat.* 79:74, 1958.
7. Callaway, E., and Thompson, S. Sympathetic activity and perception. *Psychosom. Med.* 15:443, 1953.
8. Carr, L., and Moore, K. Norepinephrine: Release from brain by d-amphetamine in vivo. *Science* 164:322, 1969.
9. Cohen, H., and Dement, W. Sleep: Suppression of rapid eye movement phase in the cat after electroconvulsive shock. *Science* 154:396, 1966.
10. Cole, J. The amphetamines in child psychiatry: A review. *Seminars Psychiat.* 1:174, 1969.
11. Cramer, H., and Kuhlo, W. Effets des inhibiteurs de la monoaminoxydase sur le sommeil et l'electroencephalogramme chez l'homme. *Acta Neurol. Belg.* 67:658, 1967.
12. Crowley, T., Smith, E., and Lewis, O. The Biogenic Amines and Sleep in the Monkey: A Preliminary Report. Paper read at APSS, Denver, 1968.
13. Dement, W. Experimental Dream Studies. In J. Masserman (Ed.), *Science and Psychoanalysis: Scientific Proceedings of the Academy of Psychoanalysis.* New York: Grune & Stratton, 1964.
14. Dewan, E. The P (programming) hypothesis for REMS (abstract). *Psychophysiology* 4:365, 1968.
15. Dominic, J., and Moore, K. Acute effects of alpha-methyltyrosine on brain catecholamine levels and on spontaneous and amphetamine-stimulated motor activity in mice. *Arch. Int. Pharmacodyn.* 178:166, 1969.
16. Doty, B., and Doty, L. Facilitation effects of amphetamine on avoidance conditioning in relation to age and problem difficulty. *Psychopharmacologia* (Berlin) 9:234, 1966.
17. Dusan-Peyrethon, D., Peyrethon, J., and Jouvet, M. Suppression elective du sommeil paradoxal chez le chat par a-methyl-dopa. *C. R. Soc. Biol.* (Paris) 162:116, 1968.
18. Ephron, H., and Carrington, P. Rapid eye movement sleep and cortical homeostasis. *Psychol. Rev.* 73:500, 1966.

19. Evans, W., and Smith, R. Some effects of morphine and amphetamine on intellectual functions and mood. *Psychopharmacologia* (Berlin) 6:49, 1964.
20. Feinberg, I., Braun, M., and Shulman, E. Relationship of Age and Intellectual Function of Sleep Variables in Mentally Retarded Subjects. Paper read at APSS, Denver, 1968.
21. Feinberg, I., Koresko, R. L., and Heller, N. EEG sleep patterns as a function of normal and pathological aging in man. *J. Psychiat. Res.* 5:107, 1967.
22. Ferguson, J., and Dement, W. The Effect of REM Sleep Deprivation on the Lethality of D-Amphetamine Sulfate in Grouped Rats. Paper read at APSS, Santa Monica, Cal., 1967; abstract in *Psychophysiology* 4:380, 1968.
23. Fishbein, W. The Effects of Paradoxical Sleep Deprivation During the Retention Interval on Long-Term Memory. Paper read at APSS, Boston, 1969; abstract in *Psychophysiology* 6:225, 1969.
24. Fishbein, W. The Effects of Paradoxical Sleep Deprivation Prior to Initial Learning on Long-Term Memory. Paper read at APSS, Boston, 1969; abstract in *Psychophysiology* 6:225–226, 1969.
25. Freedman, D. Psychotomimetic drugs and brain biogenic amines. *Amer. J. Psychiat.* 119:843, 1963.
26. Freedman, D., and Giarman, N. Brain Amines, Electrical Activity, and Behavior. In G. Glasser (Ed.), *EEG and Behavior.* New York: Basic Books, 1963.
27. Glowinski, J., and Axelrod, J. Effects of drugs on the uptake, release, and metabolism of H^3NE in rat brain. *J. Pharmacol. Exp. Ther.* 149:43, 1965.
28. Greenberg, R., and Dewan, E. Aphasia and dreaming: A test of the P-hypothesis (abstract). *Psychophysiology* 5:203, 1968.
29. Greenberg, R., and Leiderman, P. Perceptions, the dream process and memory. *Compr. Psychiat.* 7:517, 1966.
30. Greenberg, R., Pearlman, C., Fingar, R., and Kantrowitz, J. The Effects of Dream Deprivation. Report to the American Psychiatric Association, Boston, 1968.
31. Guazzi, M., Baccelli, G., and Zanchetti, A. Carotid body chemoceptors: Physiological role in buffering fall in blood pressure during sleep. *Science* 153:206, 1966.
32. Guazzi, M., Bacelli, G., and Zanchetti, A. Reflex chemoceptive regulation of arterial pressure during natural sleep in the cat. *Amer. J. Physiol.* 214:969, 1968.

33. Hanson, L. Evidence that the central action of amphetamine is mediated via catecholamines. *Psychopharmacologia* (Berlin) 10:289, 1967.
34. Hartmann, E. Reserpine: Its effect on the sleep-dream cycle in man. *Psychopharmacologia* (Berlin) 9:242, 1966.
35. Hartmann, E. *The Biology of Dreaming.* Springfield, Ill.: Thomas, 1967.
36. Hartmann, E. The effect of tryptophane on the sleep-dream cycle in man. *Psychonomic Science* 8:479, 1967.
37. Hartmann, E. The sleep-dream cycle and brain serotonin. *Psychonomic Science* 8:295, 1967.
38. Hartmann, E. Amitriptyline and Imipramine: Effects on Human Sleep. Paper read at APSS, Denver, 1968; abstract in *Psychophysiology.* 5:207, 1968.
39. Hartmann, E. The effect of four drugs on sleep patterns in man. *Psychopharmacologia* (Berlin) 12:346, 1968.
40. Hartmann, E. Longitudinal studies of sleep and dream patterns in manic-depressive patients. *Arch. Gen. Psychiat.* (Chicago) 19:312, 1968.
41. Hartmann, E. Monoamines and Need for D. Paper read at APSS, Denver, 1968; abstract in *Psychophysiology* 5:211, 1968.
42. Hartmann, E. Pharmacological studies of sleep and dreaming: Chemical and clinical relationships. *Biol. Psychiat.* 1:243–258, 1969.
43. Hartmann, E. What Is Good Sleep? In E. Hartmann (Ed.), *Sleep and Dreaming.* Boston: Little, Brown, 1970.
44. Hartmann, E., Baekeland, F., Zwilling, G., and Hoy, P. Long and Short Sleepers: Preliminary Results. Paper read at APSS, Boston, 1969; abstract in *Psychophysiology* 6:255–256, 1969.
45. Hartmann, E., and Bridwell, T. Unpublished studies, 1969.
46. Hoffman, J., and Domino, E. Effects of Reserpine on the Sleep Cycle in Man and Cat. Paper read at APSS, Santa Monica, Cal., 1967.
47. Holliday, A. The effects of d-amphetamine on errors and correct responses of human beings performing a simple intellectual task. *Clin. Pharmacol. Ther.* 7:312, 1966.
48. Iskander, T., and Kaebling, R. Catecholamine Depletion by 1-alpha-methyl-para-tyrosine (AMPT) and Paradoxical Sleep. Paper read at APSS, Boston, 1969; abstract in *Psychophysiology* 6:219–220, 1969.
49. Jewett, R., and Norton, S. Effects of some stimulant and depressant drugs on sleep cycles of cats. *Exp. Neurol.* 15:463, 1966.

50. Jouvet, M. Biogenic amines and the states of sleep. *Science* 163:32, 1969.
51. Jouvet, M., Bobillier, P., Pujol, J., and Renault, J. Effets des lesions du systeme du raphe sur le sommeil et la serotonine cerebrale. *C. R. Soc. Biol.* (Paris) 160:2343, 1966.
52. Jouvet, M., Vimont, P., and Delorme, F. Suppression elective du sommeil paradoxal chez le chat par les inhibiteurs de la monoamineoxidase. *C. R. Soc. Biol.* (Paris) 159:1595, 1965.
53. Kety, S., Javoy, F., Thierry, A., Julou, L., and Glowinski, J. A sustained effect of electroconvulsive shock on the turnover of norepinephrine on the central nervous system of the rat. *Proc. Nat. Acad. Sci. U.S.A.*, No. 58, p. 1249, 1967.
54. Khazan, N., and Sawyer, C. Mechanisms of paradoxical sleep as revealed by neurophysiologic and pharmacologic approaches in the rabbit. *Psychopharmacologia* (Berlin) 5:457, 1964.
55. King, C., and Jewett, R. Enhancement of Slow Wave Sleep and REM Sleep in the Cat by L-alpha-methyl-p-tyrosine. Paper read at APSS, Boston, 1969; abstract in *Psychophysiology* 6:220, 1969.
56. Kulkanni, A. Facilitation of instrumental avoidance learning by amphetamine: An analysis. *Psychopharmacologia* (Berlin) 13:418, 1968.
57. Laties, V., and Weiss, B. Performance Enhancement by the Amphetamines: A New Approach. In H. Brill, J. Cole, P. Deniker, H. Hippius, and P. Bradley (Eds.), *Proceedings of the Fifth International Congress of Neuropsychopharmacology*. Amsterdam: Excerpta Medica Foundation, 1967.
58. Latz, A., Goldman, M., and Kornetzky, C. Maze learning after the administration of antidepressant drugs. *J. Pharmacol. Exp. Ther.* 156:76, 1966.
59. Levitt, M., Spector, S., Sjoerdsma, A., and Udenfriend, S. Elucidation of the rate-limiting step in norepinephrine biosynthesis in the perfused guinea pig heart. *J. Pharmacol. Exp. Ther.* 148:1, 1965.
60. Marantz, R., and Rechtschaffen, A. The effect of alphamethyltyrosine on sleep in the rat. *Percept. Motor Skills* 25:805, 1967.
61. Monroe, L. Psychological and physiological differences between good and poor sleepers. *J. Abnorm. Psychol.* 72:255, 1967.
62. Moore, K. Effects of alpha methyltyrosine on brain catechol-

amines and conditioned behavior in guinea pigs. *Life Sci.* 5:55, 1966.

63. Moore, K., and Rech, R. Antagonism by monoamine oxidase inhibitors of alpha-methyltyrosine induced catecholamine depletion and behavioral depression. *J. Pharmacol. Exp. Ther.* 156:70, 1967.
64. Muzio, J., Roffwarg, H., and Kaufman, E. Alterations in the nocturnal sleep cycle resulting from LSD. *Electroenceph. Clin. Neurophysiol.* 21:313, 1966.
65. Nash, H. Psychologic effects of amphetamines and barbiturates. *J. Nerv. Ment. Dis.* 134:203, 1962.
66. Oliverio, A. Neurohumoral Systems and Learning. In L. Goodman and A. Gilman (Eds.), *Psychopharmacology: A Review of Progress 1957–1967* (3d ed.). New York: Macmillan, 1965.
67. Pearlman, C., and Greenberg, R. Effect of REM Deprivation on Retention of Avoidance Learning in Rats. Paper read at APSS, Denver, 1968.
68. Pirch, J., and Rech, R. Behavioral recovery in rats during chronic reserpine treatment. *Psychopharmacologia* (Berlin) 12:115, 1968.
69. Pujol, J., Jouvet, M., Mouret, J., and Glowinski, J. Increased turnover of cerebral norepinephrine during rebound of paradoxical sleep in the rat. *Science* 159:112, 1968.
70. Rapaport, D. Toward a Theory of Thinking. In D. Rapaport (Ed.), *Organization and Pathology of Thought.* New York: Columbia University Press, 1951.
71. Rech, R., Borys, H., and Moore, K. Alterations in behavior and brain catecholamine levels in rats treated with alphamethyltyrosine. *J. Pharmacol. Exp. Ther.* 153:412, 1966.
72. Rech, R., Carr, L., and Moore, K. Behavioral effects of alpha-methyltyrosine after prior depletion of brain catecholamines. *J. Pharmacol. Exp. Ther.* 160:326, 1968.
73. Rechtschaffen, A., and Maron, L. The effect of amphetamine on the sleep cycle. *Electroenceph. Clin. Neurophysiol.* 16: 438, 1964.
74. Roffwarg, H., Muzio, J., and Dement, W. Ontogenetic development of the human sleep-dream cycle. *Science* 154:604, 1966.
75. Ryba, P., Shapiro, A., and Freedman, N. The Effects of Imipramine on Sleep Patterns of Psychiatric Patients. Paper read at APSS, Gainesville, Fla., 1966.

76. Schildkraut, J. The catecholamine hypothesis of affective disorders: A review of supporting evidence. *Amer. J. Psychiat.* 122:509, 1965.
77. Schildkraut, J., Davis, J., and Klerman, G. Biochemistry of Depressions. In D. Efron (Ed.), *Psychopharmacology: A Review of Progress 1957–1967* (3d ed.). New York: Macmillan, 1965.
78. Schildkraut, J., and Hartmann, E. 72 Hours on an Island: Effects on the Turnover and Metabolism of Norepinephrine in Rat Brain. Paper read at APSS, Boston, 1969; abstract in *Psychophysiology* 6:220, 1969.
79. Schildkraut, J., Schanberg, S., Breese, G., and Kopin, I. Norepinephrine metabolism and drugs used in the affective disorders: A possible mechanism of action. *Amer. J. Psychiat.* 124:600, 1967.
80. Schoenfeld, R., and Seiden, L. Alpha-methyltyrosine: Effects on fixed ration schedules of reinforcement. *J. Pharm. Pharmacol.* 19:771, 1967.
81. Schoenfeld, R., and Seiden, L. Effect of alpha-methyltyrosine on operant behavior and brain catecholamine levels. *J. Pharmacol. Exp. Ther.* 167:319, 1969.
82. Seashore, R., and Ivy, A. Effects of amphetamine drugs in relieving fatigue. *Psychol. Monogr.* 67:1, 1953.
83. Seiden, L., and Peterson, D. Reversal of the reserpine-induced suppression of the conditioned avoidance response by L-dopa: Correlation of behavioral and biochemical differences in two strains of mice. *J. Pharmacol. Exp. Ther.* 159: 422, 1968.
84. Shimizu, A., and Himwich, H. The effects of amphetamine on the sleep-wakefulness cycle of developing kittens. *Psychopharmacologia* (Berlin) 13:161, 1968.
85. Small, A., and Feinberg, I. The Effects of Dextro-amphetamine on the EEG Sleep Patterns of Hyperactive Children. Paper read at APSS, Boston, 1969; abstract in *Psychophysiology* 6:257–258, 1969.
86. Snyder, F. Toward an evolutionary theory of dreaming. *Amer. J. Psychiat.* 123:121, 1966.
87. Snyder, F., Hobson, J., Morrison, D., and Goldfrank, F. Changes in respiration, heart rate, and systolic blood pressure in human sleep. *J. Appl. Physiol.* 19:417, 1964.
88. Snyder, F., Scott, J., Karacan, I., and Anderson, D. Presumptive evidence of REMS deprivation in depressive illness. *Psychophysiology* 4:382, 1968.

89. Snyder, F., Verdone, P., Weinberg, A., Bunney, W., Durell, J., and Schildkraut, J. Longitudinal Studies of Sleep Patterns in Depressed Patients. Paper read at APSS, Washington, D.C., 1965.
90. Spector, S., Sjoerdsma, A., and Udenfriend, S. Blockade of endogenous norepinephrine synthesis by alpha-methyl-tyrosine, an inhibitor of tyrosine hydroxylase. *J. Pharmacol. Exp. Ther.* 147:86, 1965.
91. Stein, L. Chemistry of Reward and Punishment. In D. Efron (Ed.), *Psychopharmacology: A Review of Progress 1957–1967.* New York: Macmillan, 1965.
92. Stein, L. Noradrenergic Substrates of Positive Reinforcement: Site of Motivational Action of Amphetamine and Chlorpromazine. In H. Brill, J. Cole, P. Deniker, H. Hippius, and P. Bradley (Eds.), *Proceedings Fifth Congress Collegium Internationale Neuro-Psycho-Pharmacologicum; Washington, D.C., 1966.* International Congress Series, No. 129. Amsterdam: Excerpta Medica Foundation, 1967. P. 765.
93. Stern, W. Effects of REM Sleep Deprivation upon the Acquisition and Maintenance of Learned Behavior in the Rat. Paper read at APSS, Boston, 1969.
94. Stern, W. Pharmacological Modifications of the Effects of REM Sleep Deprivation upon Active and Passive Avoidance in the Rat. Paper read at APSS, Boston, 1969; abstract in *Psychophysiology* 6:224, 1969.
95. Stern, W. Behavioral and Biochemical Aspects of Rapid Eye Movement Deprivation in the Rat. University of Indiana Ph.D. Dissertation, 1969.
96. Strom-Olsen, R., and Weil-Malherbe, H. Humoral changes in manic-depressive psychosis with particular reference to the excretion of catecholamines in urine. *J. Ment. Sci.* 104:696, 1958.
97. Sulser, F., Owens, M., Norwich, M., and Dingell, J. The relative role of storage and synthesis of brain norepinephrine in the psychomotor stimulation evoked by amphetamine or by Desipramine and Tetrabenazine. *Psychopharmacologia* (Berlin) 12:322, 1968.
98. Vogel, G., Traub, A., Ben-Horin, P., and Meyer, G. REM deprivation. II. The effects on depressed patients. *Arch. Gen. Psychiat.* (Chicago) 18:301, 1968.
99. Weiss, B., and Laties, V. Enhancement of human performance by caffeine and the amphetamines. *Pharmacol. Rev.* 14:1, 1962.

100. Weitzman, E., McGregor, P., Moore, C., and Jacoby, J. The Effect of Alpha-methyl-para-tyrosine on Sleep Patterns of the Monkey: A Preliminary Report. Paper read at APSS, Denver, 1968; abstract in *Psychophysiology* 5:210, 1968.
101. Wilkinson, R. The effects of sleep loss on performance. *Med. Res. Counc. Appl. Psychol. Res. Unit,* Report No. 323, 1958.
102. Williams, H., Lester, B., and Coulter, J. Monoamines and the EEG Stages of Sleep. Paper read at APSS, Denver, 1968.
103. Wyatt, R., Engleman, K., Kupfer, D., Scott, J., Sjoerdsma, A., and Snyder, F. Effects of MAO Inhibitors and Parachlorophenylalanine in Longitudinal Sleep Studies. Paper read at APSS, Denver, 1968; abstract in *Psychophysiology* 5:209, 1968.
104. Zimmerman, J., Stoyva, J., and Metcalf, D. Distorted Visual Experience and Rapid Eye Movement Sleep. Paper read at APSS, Boston, 1969.

The Functions of Dreaming

*What is the function of dreaming? Does dreaming have a function aside from the functions of the D-state?**

The Adaptive Function of Dreaming

CHESTER A. PEARLMAN, JR.

Several characteristics of stage REM sleep, reviewed by Hartmann [9], suggest that it has an important adaptive function. Most current theoretical speculations have emphasized biological processes that might be involved. This paper discusses psychological aspects of dreaming that may play a role in adaptation.

The brilliant ingenuity of Freud's theory of wish fulfillment as a key to the understanding of dreams has obscured the fact that his more general hypothesis—that dreams serve to discharge instinctual tensions which would otherwise disturb sleep—was not well founded (cf. Jones [13]). Even without current knowledge of

* The reader interested in this question may wish to refer also to papers by Baekeland (p. 49), Witkin (p. 154), Foulkes (p. 165), Van de Castle (p. 171), Skinner (p. 213), Hawkins (p. 233), Zetzel (p. 240), Greenberg (p. 258), Ephron and Carrington (p. 269), Dewan (p. 295), Hartmann (p. 308), and Hursch (p. 387).

the biological rhythmicity of the stages of sleep, one could question the necessity of nocturnal hallucinatory gratification of infantile wishes just to remain asleep. The fact that such wishes are more apparent during dreaming does not mean that they have greater impetus than during waking life. Many analysts have indicated the limitations of this hypothesis as a total theory of dreaming. Most of them have claimed that the phenomena of dreams could be more completely understood as an attempt at resolution of the dreamer's current emotional conflicts, of which the infantile wish element was only one part.

Maeder [16] was the first to formulate this idea clearly. Jung, Adler, Silberer, and Ferenczi said essentially the same thing within their own frames of reference. More recently, the idea has been expressed by Hall, Miller, Saul, and Ullman. Garma [5], Wolff [20], Jones [12], and French and Fromm [4] have each collected considerable clinical material to support this conceptualization. Jones [12] and Hawkins [10] have reviewed the various theoretical presentations.

Freud was aware of this adaptive interpretation of dreaming, but he contended that it was unimportant because the mental operations involved in attempted resolution of emotional conflicts during dreaming seemed to be identical with those utilized during waking life, i.e., examples of secondary process as distinct from the presumably more meaningful primary process operations. Despite its superficial plausibility, if this assumption were literally correct, it would be very difficult to account for the "dreamlike" quality of dreams. An alternative interpretation would be that although the mental operations are similar, a different process is occurring. The distinction between intellectual and emotional insight is familiar to all psychotherapists. It refers to the difference between knowing the solution to a problem and making it a part of oneself, i.e., adaptation. It may be the latter process which occurs during stage REM sleep.

It is universally accepted that adaptation requires time. Why sleeping on a problem should make such a difference is not so clear. A vast experience since Ebbinghaus with a wide range of learning experiments in both humans and animals has suggested that learning occurs within a short period after exposure to the material to be learned and the material is then gradually forgotten. Another class of learning tasks, however—those which involve a significant degree of habituation or emotional adaptation to the situation—do not follow the Ebbinghaus type of forgetting curve. Retention in these situations may even tend to improve with time. This apparently paradoxical effect has stimulated much conflicting theoretical interpretation. Many experiments have excluded one or another variable which might be involved, but the possible effect of the diurnal cycle was ignored until recently.

Stage REM sleep has many properties of a hypothetically ideal memory fixation mechanism: intense cerebral activity with exclusion of extraneous sensory input and motor output, limbic-cortical interaction, and so forth. Thus it is hardly surprising that several writers [1, 2, 6, 7, 17] have suggested that stage REM is involved in formation of memory traces, reprograming of the brain, integration of new experiences with existing personality, and so on. These proposals were made on the basis of various lines of suggestive evidence.

Recently some directly relevant data have been obtained. Greenberg, Pillard, and Pearlman [8] found that a night of dream deprivation interfered with adaptation to viewing of an anxiety-provoking movie. Dream-deprived subjects reacted with as much anxiety to the second viewing of the film as to the first viewing, instead of showing a normal tendency to habituation.

Passive avoidance learning is a good example of the kind of task which primarily involves emotional adaptation to the learning situation. The subject has only to recognize the place where an unpleasant experience has occurred and to do something (usually nothing, i.e., inhibition of normal exploratory behavior) in an effort to avoid a recurrence of the experience. The more complex cognitive operations involved in most other types of learning are not required in this situation. In rats, Pearlman and Greenberg [18] found that 24 hours of REM deprivation completely abolished retention of an incompletely learned passive avoidance response. Fishbein [3] found a similar effect upon passive avoidance with 3 days of stage REM deprivation in mice. He also discovered that retention could be restored by allowing the mice a night of undisturbed sleep before retention testing. Interpolation of an electroconvulsion between REM deprivation and recovery night blocked restoration of retention. Thus Fishbein concluded that stage REM sleep is necessary for long-term fixation of the memory trace, and REM deprivation keeps the trace in a labile form which is susceptible to interference by an electroconvulsion.

Closer examination of what is involved in emotional adaptation may clarify both the time factor and the connection with dreaming. From a psychoanalytic viewpoint, Joffe and Sandler [11] characterize adaptation as a process whereby the ego creates new organizations of the ideal state of the self to preserve the feeling of safety and to avoid the experience of being traumatically overwhelmed. Successful adaptation involves the continual relinquishing of ideals (wishes) which are no longer appropriate to present reality. Joffe and Sandler note that previous ideal states of the self are not always readily abandoned and will often show their influence in the content of new goals. All the elements of this description of adaptation are convincingly demonstrated in Jones's epigenetic approach [12] to dream analysis. The question thus arises: When does the creation of new ego organizations actually occur? One could postulate the existence of processes of adaptation during waking life, perhaps connected to the preconscious stream [14], analogous to physiological homeostatic processes. This hypothesis is attractively simple, but no evidence for it has ever been presented. There is some evidence suggesting that it is incorrect. Garma [5] shows that the usual initial reaction of the ego to new experience which requires some adaptive change is repression. This reaction appears to be necessary for the individual to continue functioning. If it is not effective, the ego becomes traumatically overwhelmed and the person experiences more or less incapacitating anxiety. Garma notes that the repressed experience is manifested in the dreams of the following night. This would seem to be a much more appropriate time to review the situation and effect any changes which seem to be necessary. The posttraumatic nightmare is a vivid example of unsuccessful functioning of the adaptive mechanism (cf. also Leveton [15]).

This characterization of the adaptive process could provide another explanation of why most dreams are forgotten [19]. The material would be conscious only when it is "under consideration" during the state of stage REM sleep. It would then become unavailable to consciousness unless the subject were awakened during the REM period or under the influence of psychedelic drugs or circumstances, like the psychoanalytic situation, which strive to create conditions similar to that of stage REM sleep in order to favor the emergence of repressed material for further consideration.

Thus we may conclude that dreaming with its richness of symbolic pictorialization is the human form of a general mammalian process of emotional adaptation which occurs during stage REM sleep.

REFERENCES

1. Breger, L. Function of dreams. *J. Abnorm. Psychol.*, Monograph No. 641, 1967.
2. Dewan, E. Sleep as a Programming Process and REM as a Coding Procedure. Paper read at Association for the Psychophysiological Study of Sleep (APSS), Santa Monica, Cal., 1967.
3. Fishbein, W. Paradoxical Sleep: A Periodic Mechanism for Securing and Maintaining Information for Long-Term Memory. University of Colorado Ph.D. Dissertation, 1968.
4. French, T. M., and Fromm, E. *Dream Interpretation: A New Approach.* New York: Basic Books, 1964.
5. Garma, A. *The Psychoanalysis of Dreams.* New York: Dell, 1966.
6. Greenberg, R., and Leiderman, P. H. Perceptions, the dream process and memory: An up-to-date version of notes on a mystic writing pad. *Compr. Psychiat.* 7:517, 1966.
7. Greenberg, R., Pearlman, C., Kawlische, S., Kantrowitz, J., and Fingar, R. The Psychological Effect of Dream Deprivation. Presented to the American Psychoanalytic Association, Boston, 1968.

8. Greenberg, R., Pillard, R., and Pearlman, C. Dream Deprivation and Adaptation to Stress. Paper read at APSS, Denver, 1968.
9. Hartmann, E. *The Biology of Dreaming.* Springfield, Ill.: Thomas, 1967.
10. Hawkins, D. R. A review of psychoanalytic dream theory in the light of recent psycho-physiological studies of sleep and dreaming. *Brit. J. Med. Psychol.* 39:85, 1966.
11. Joffe, W. G., and Sandler, J. Comments on the psychoanalytic psychology of adaptation. *Int. J. Psychoanal.* 49:445, 1968.
12. Jones, R. M. *Ego Synthesis in Dreams.* Cambridge, Mass.: Schenkman, 1962.
13. Jones, R. M. The psychoanalytic theory of dreaming—1968. *J. Nerv. Ment. Dis.* 147:587, 1968.
14. Kubie, L. S. A reconsideration of thinking, the dream process, and "the dream." *Psychoanal. Quart.* 35:191, 1966.
15. Leveton, A. F. The night residue. *Int. J. Psychoanal.* 42:506, 1961.
16. Maeder, A. E. The dream problem. *J. Nerv. Ment. Dis.* Monograph No. 22, 1916.
17. Pearlman, C., and Greenberg, R. The Relation of Dreaming to Formation of the Memory Trace. Paper read at APSS, Washington, D.C., 1965.
18. Pearlman, C., and Greenberg, R. Effect of REM Deprivation upon Retention of Avoidance Learning in the Rat. Paper read at APSS, Denver, 1968.
19. Whitman, R. M. Remembering and forgetting dreams in psychoanalysis. *J. Amer. Psychoanal. Ass.* 11:752, 1963.
20. Wolff, W. *The Dream-Mirror of Conscience.* New York: Grune & Stratton, 1952.

Possible Functions of Dreaming

RICHARD M. JONES

Since nothing can be said with precision to the questions posed at the beginning of this chapter, nothing can be lost by seeking to address them from as comprehensive a point of view as possible. This may best be done by raising the entirely speculative possibility that a relationship of isomorphism exists between the biological functions of REM sleep and the psychological functions of dreaming. At this writing five different biological functions have been hypothetically ascribed [2, 5, 14, 17, 18, 20] to REM sleep (the D-state): (1) a *neutralizing* function, in counteractive relation to some noxious by-product of mammalian metabolism; (2) a *stimulating* function, in compensatory relation to the periodic sensory deprivations of sleep; (3) a *reorganizing* function, in response to the disorganizing effects of sleep on the mammalian central nervous system; (4) a *vigilance* function, in preparation for mammalian fight and flight patterns; and (5) an *innervating* function, in the specific service of mammalian depth perception.

Let us now suppose that as REM sleep (D-state) may neutralize this or that cerebral toxin, dreaming may neutralize this or that noxious impulse or memory. Similarly, as REM sleep may stimulate the cortex in this or that state of efferent deprivation, dreaming may stimulate emotion or memory in this or that state of experiential deprivation. Similarly, as REM sleep may reorganize firing patterns in the central nervous system in response to the disorganizing effects of sleep, dreaming may serve to reorganize patterns of ego defense and ego synthesis in response to the disorganizing effects of waking life. Similarly, as REM sleep may serve an alerting function in respect to potential threats to physical integrity, dreaming may serve an alerting function in respect to potential threats to psychosocial integrity. Finally, as REM sleep may help to establish and maintain depth perception, dreaming may help to establish and maintain, if you will, "perceptiveness in depth." Each of these suppositions will serve as a point of focus around which to review what we are able to hypothesize at this writing regarding the psychological functions of dreaming.

NEUTRALIZATION

Nothing in the modern researches into the psychophysiology of sleep and dreaming has called into question Freud's original hypothesis that dreams serve as periodic "safety valves" in respect to the periodic psychonoxious effects of repressed infantile wishes. The hypothesis stands, as capable as ever of ordering accumulated observations that dream contents regularly include hypermnesic infantile images and perceptions. Nor has it been shaken by my own reading of REM sleep research, which suggests that the fulfillment in dreams of repressed infantile wishes is best conceived as a consequence rather than the cause of dreaming [11].

STIMULATION

The views of Schactel [15] and Silberer [16] combine to suggest that dreaming may serve a stimulating or restitutive function in response to recurrent psychological impoverishments imposed by certain external and internal conditions which are integral to human life.

Schactel's theory of repression suggests that a consequence of dreaming is the repeated utilization of those symbolic forms which in the dreamer's society are relatively useless or irrelevant and therefore not available to consciousness in ordinary waking life. In most literate societies it is the primary process which is most often found to be useless or irrelevant. Thus dreaming, which tends to be governed by the primary process, may be seen as a recuperative response to the unavoidable conventionalizing influences of everyday life in literate societies—thus routinely reminding man of his capacity for the unconventional, the creative response.

Similarly, dreaming may be seen as a recuperative response to the necessarily recurrent intrapsychic conditions of apperceptive deficiency and apperceptive insufficiency, as defined by Silberer—the one stemming from recurrent situations of reduced psychic power (of which sleep itself is one), the other stemming from inevitable situations of growth and development. Actually, one major category of the day residue, as Freud defined it ("What has not been dealt with owing to the insufficiency of our intellectual power—what is unresolved" [8]) is but another way of referring to the condition of apperceptive insufficiency.

These views have received recent support from the independent and refreshingly literate thinking of Koestler [13] on the subject of dreaming in his epic work, *The Act of Creation:*

> . . . the fact that art and discovery draw on unconscious sources indicates that one aspect of all creative activity is a regression to ontogenetically or phylogenetically earlier levels, an escape from the restraints of the conscious mind, with the subsequent release of creative potentials—a process paralled on lower levels by the liberation from restraint of genetic potentials or neural equipotentiality in the regeneration of structures and functions. The scientist, traumatized by discordant facts, the artist by the pressures of sensibility, and the rat by surgical intervention, share, on different levels, the same super-flexibility enabling them to perform "adaptations of a second order" rarely found in the ordinary routines of life.

REORGANIZATION

The idea that dreaming affords special opportunities for reorganization of ego functions has been most explicitly advanced by French and Fromm [7], Jones [10], Breger [3], and Dewan [6]. Two specific principles of ego reorganization are considered by French and Fromm to be frequent aspects of the dream work: *increased cognitive grasp,* in which previously unnoticed facets of a recent focal conflict or its historical background are brought into view, usually by way of analogy; and *prophylactic defense,* in which the ego seeks to achieve an optimal degree of commitment to the focal conflict, again usually by way of analogy. The implication in both instances is that increased mastery of the analogous materials may be transferred to subsequent encounters with the focal conflict in reality.

In a previous monograph [10] I proposed the hypothesis that dreaming may serve ego synthesis functions as well as the reorganization of ego defense functions. It seemed to me that this hypothesis could best be studied by subjecting manifest dreams to an analytic method derived from a theory of adaptive human development. And I chose for that purpose what I believe is our most viable such theory: the epigenetic dimension of psychoanalytic theory, as originally formulated by Erik Erikson. The hypothesis was systematically stated as follows:

> . . . a manifest dream is the product of a confluence of psychodynamic forces: (1) a motivating repressed wish of infantile origin; (2) the defense ego, which so discharges the energy of the repressed wish as to maintain a healthy state of sleep; and (3) the synthesis ego, which so governs the setting, style, and rhythm of the dream's formation as to support a subsequently adaptive state of wakefulness.

I described this third process as involving the preconscious redifferentiation and reintegration of previous epigenetic successes and failures in the context and under the pressure of contemporary development crises.

Breger [3] refers the question of the function of dreaming to an interesting admixture of psychoanalytic theory and information theory:

> . . . *dreams are one output of particular memory systems operating under the guidance of programs that are peculiar to sleep.* These programs stem from certain early modes of psychological operation and, hence, dreams may be said to be regressive, though not exactly the way that Freud used the term. Certain memory systems have been activated during the period prior to sleep and have set into operation emotional reactions that feed back and keep these particular systems active or "ready." Such activation may have been initiated by a specific event—for example, a rejection by an important person—or by a train of thought or fantasy. But the involve-

ment of emotional reactions serves to potentiate these systems as opposed to the many others that are in operation during the pre-sleep period.

A fourth view of dreaming as a reorganizational process has been proposed by Dewan [6]. It is very similar to Breger's view except that Dewan takes the further step of referring the question of dream function to the analogy of information processing devices. Dewan asks us to view the brain as a computer and then to consider the hypothesis that the purpose of sleep is to program or reprogram the brain. The function of dreaming is then hypothetically seen to be that of "sorting" (or "addressing") memories as well as motor and perceptual "sub-routines" with respect to drives and goals by using labels provided by associated feelings or emotional nuances.

VIGILANCE

Much electronic sleep monitoring evidence supports Ullman's hypothesis [19] that the function of dreaming is not the preservation of sleep but the maintenance of an optimal state of vigilance. The human organism, notes Ullman, shares with lower forms of life a need for vigilance.

Unique in the human, however, are the manner and form of vigilance operations. Behavior, consciously directed in the waking state, is geared toward the maintenance of relatedness to the social environment. Potential threats arise out of the context of social existence, and the diffuse ramifications of the threats extend to experiences that expose the flaws, gaps, inadequacies, and misconceptions of consciousness. Such threats now extend to any experience that challenges value systems, social status, or psychologic mechanisms of defense. In the everyday experience of the human being, threats of this nature overshadow direct threats to physical existence. While he is awake, vigilance is tempered by adequate conceptualization, communication, and behavior. . . .

The problem of vigilance comes into focus more sharply in connection with the sleep-wakefulness cycle: the necessities which confront the human organism in connection with sleep are of a two-fold nature. With the inception of the sleeping state there

> arises the need to affect a radical transformation in the activity of the individual. Social orientation and relatedness to the external environment give way to a form of activity governed primarily by physiological needs and hence occurring at an involuntary level.
>
> Similarly, the transition from sleep to wakefulness in response to any stimulus of sufficient strength impinging upon the organism is characterized not simply by the process of awakening, but more significantly by the resumption of consciousness of one's social existence. In the human being these significant stimuli now include symbolic as well as direct sensory effects. The state of vigilance during sleep has shifted from one involving danger to the organism at an animal level, viz., in terms of physical attack, to one involving danger to the organism in its relatedness to society.

The nice compatibility of Snyder's hypothesis [17] of the function of REM sleep and Ullman's hypothesis of the function of dreaming merits emphasis. Snyder's focus is on the vigilance function of REM sleep, its adaptive value in mammalian evolution, in which readiness to flee, attack, or hide is at a premium. Ullman's focus is on the vigilance function of dreaming, its adaptive value in *human* evolution, in which adaptation by way of social organization is at a premium. Since man is a product of mammalian evolution we are not called upon to try to see these two views as competitive. Rather, there emerges from their conjoinment perhaps our first truly psychobiological hypothesis regarding the functions of the D-state—with good support at the levels of both phylogenetic and ontogenetic considerations. Moreover, as we move to considerations of individual human development it is reassuring to note how immediately Ullman's discussions of vigilance to problems of relatedness in respect to social environments, changes in value systems, and psychological patterns of defense suggest the views of French and Jones.

"PERCEPTIVENESS IN DEPTH"

We were obviously engaged in a play on words when we supposed that the cultivation in dreaming of "perceptiveness in depth" might be the counterpart to what Berger has proposed may be the role of REM sleep in the development and maintenance of human depth perception. Let us therefore first remove the quotation marks from around "perceptiveness in depth" by specifying what we mean by the term. We mean perceptiveness of *self,* awareness of diversity within self, self-insight in the senses that modern psychology has come to associate with psychological health and the optimal development of self-actualizing personality patterns.

The views of Jung, Angyal, and Piaget can be combined to suggest that dreaming may serve to cultivate human perceptiveness in depth defined in these ways:

Jung's approach [12] to dream interpretation was based on the assumption that the human psyche is a self-regulative system in which unconscious processes function in a compensatory relation to conscious processes, seeking, as it were, to check conscious excesses and to challenge conscious attitudes of false complacency when either of these tendencies threaten to compromise an individual's capacities to develop his particular potentials to their fullest.

From Angyal's theory [1] of personality I have derived the hypothesis [9] that a consequence of dreaming is the exposure to consciousness of shifts in the balances of power which take place from night to night between an individual's two potential systems for organizing his total personality—the health system and the neurotic system—under the conditions of freedom from the constraints of social expedience which are characteristic of sleep.

Castle [4] has drawn attention to Piaget's view of dreaming as a highly egocentric form of thought, experienced as action, a function of which is that of "giving form to affective schemas and thus generating ideas on the level of 'individual truth'."

While the evidence does not exist to support a choice between any of these hypotheses at either the biological or psychological levels, I should like to state my own biases of the moment for what they may be worth: I think Snyder's sentinel hypothesis is the most commendable of those which seek to understand the purposes served by REM sleep in phylogenesis, because it is both sufficiently specific to explain the apparently exclusive role of REM sleep in the evolution of mammals and sufficiently general to take cognizance of its variations in duration and intensity from species to species within the genus. Thus it provides ample conceptual space for including the various proposed developmental functions of REM sleep if any or all of these prove to be valid.

Among the various companion hypotheses regarding the psychological function of human dreaming, I think Ullman's vigilance hypothesis is the most promising. It commends itself as our best leading hypothesis, first for the reason that it follows most naturally from Snyder's evolutionary theory, and second for the reason that it has similar properties: it is sufficiently *psychophysiological* to promise an eventual understanding of how it is that dreaming may be an augmentative human response to the D-state, and it is at the same time sufficiently *psychological* to provide a framework within which to understand the functions of dreaming from the point of view of species adaptation *and* from the point of view of individual adaptation. The point of view of species adaptation requires that we show dreaming to be functionally relevant to man's three distinguishing adaptive achievements, which have made him the naturally selective rather than the naturally selected mammal: technology, social organization, and language. The point of view of individual adaptation requires that we show dreaming to be functionally relevant to the capacities of individual humans to utilize both the constraints and the liberties to which these species adaptations have committed all of us, in the service of perpetuating the only kinds of mutations that can now help us, in that they require particular technologies, particular forms of social organization, and particular languages to be adap*tive* rather than adapt*ed*; namely, new ideas.

In other words, it may be that once nature committed man to his point of no return, his capacity to make his own culture—as she committed the tiger to his tooth, the elephant to his trunk, and the baboon to his troop—she then equipped him with the means to make the most of it. This, by making it not possible but *necessary* that he dream—every night—about every ninety minutes.

REFERENCES

1. Angyal, A. *Neurosis and Treatment.* New York: Wiley, 1965.
2. Berger, R. Oculo-motor control: A possible function of REM sleep. *Psychol. Rev.* In press.
3. Breger, L. Function of Dreams. *J. Abnorm. Psychol.* Monograph No. 641, 1967. P. 19.
4. Castle, P. Unpublished manuscript.
5. Dement, W. Experimental Dream Studies. In J. Masserman (Ed.), *Science and Psychoanalysis: Scientific Proceedings of the Academy of Psychoanalysis.* New York: Grune & Stratton, 1964. Vol. 7, pp. 129–162.
6. Dewan, E. Sleep as a Programming Process and Dreaming ("D-State") as an Addressing Procedure. Paper read at Association for the Psychophysiological Study of Sleep, Santa Monica, Cal., 1967.
7. French, T., and Fromm, E. *Dream Interpretation.* New York: Basic Books, 1964.
8. Freud, S. *The Interpretation of Dreams* (1900). In *The Standard Edition of the Complete Psychological Works of Sigmund Freud,* tr. and ed. by J. Strachey with others. London: Hogarth and the Institute of Psycho-Analysis, 1953. Vol. IV–V, p. 554.
9. Jones, R. M. Unpublished manuscript.
10. Jones, R. M. *Ego Synthesis in Dreams.* Cambridge, Mass.: Schenkman, 1962. P. 43.
11. Jones, R. M. The psychoanalytic theory of dreaming—1968. *J. Nerv. Ment. Dis.* 147:587, 1968.
12. Jung, C. G. *Modern Man in Search of a Soul.* New York: Harcourt, Brace & World, 1933.
13. Koestler, A. *The Act of Creation.* New York: Dell, 1964. P. 462.
14. Roffwarg, H., Muzio, J., and Dement, W. Ontogenetic development of the human sleep-dream cycle. *Science* 152:604, 1966.
15. Schactel, E. G. On memory and childhood amnesia. *Psychiatry* 10:1, 1947.
16. Silberer, H. The dream: Introduction to the psychology of dreams. *Psychoanal. Rev.* 42:361, 1955.
17. Snyder, F. Speculations About the Contribution of the Rapid Eye Movement State to Mammalian Survival. Paper read at symposium "Activité Onirique et Conscience," Lyon, France, 1965.

18. Snyder, F. Toward an evolutionary theory of dreaming. *Amer. J. Psychiat.* 123:121, 1966.
19. Ullman, M. Dreaming, altered states of consciousness and the problem of vigilance. *J. Nerv. Ment. Dis.* 133:529, 1961.
20. Weiss, T. Discussion of "The D-state" by E. Hartmann. *Int. J. Psychiat.* 2:32, 1966.

The Dream as "Guardian of Sleep": Indications for Further Research

HARMON S. EPHRON AND
PATRICIA CARRINGTON

Since the vivid dreams associated with the REM state appear dependent upon the presence of that state and seemingly cannot be independently elicited as responses to stimuli, the freudian hypothesis [3] of the dream as the "guardian of sleep" has fallen into increasing disfavor with sleep researchers. Little attention is now devoted to the possibility that dreaming *among other things* may represent an attempt to cope with concurrent stimuli so as to preserve sleep in a generalized sense, despite occasional brief awakenings or returns of alpha rhythm on the EEG. The pendulum may, however, be overdue for a swing back toward investigation of the role of concurrent stimuli in actively shaping the dream experience, as opposed to mere passive incorporation of a single stimulus in a single portion of a dream.

STIMULI AND REM SLEEP

Numerous studies show the regular cyclic alternation of the sleep phases to be fairly constant in terms of smoothed curves, but from the first, experimenters have noted that this overall consistency is subject to marked individual variations. Latency to sleep onset or to REM sleep, duration of sleep phases, number and extent of accompanying body movements, degree of intrusion of alpha waves during sleep, variations in the intensity and spacing of phasic events during REM sleep and NREM sleep, and numerous other sleep parameters vary between different individuals, within the same individual from night to night, and from cycle to cycle during the same night in the same individual.

From a statistical point of view, such incidental differences may be treated as random fluctuations about a mean and described by measures of variability. Such a summative procedure, while useful for identifying general trends, does not, however, answer questions posed by these very fluctuations. The concept of *random,* as employed in statistical operations, is no more than a convenient method for handling data, the cause or causes of which remain unknown. It should not deter the researcher from exploring the reasons for the observed variations.

Since the variations on the central themes REM and NREM are numerous, complex, and as yet unexplained, it might prove useful to approach the question of the influence of concurrent stimuli on the sleep-dream cycle from a somewhat different standpoint than that formerly used. There is, to be sure, no evidence that applied stimuli can trigger a full-blown REM state in an organism which is not already in readiness for and requiring REM sleep. The apparent intraorganismic regulation of the cyclic alternation of sleep phases has, in fact, given rise to the authors' proposed homeostatic hypothesis [2] (also see p. 271 of this issue). Despite this seeming central regulation of sleep phases, however, situational factors occurring on a given night might conceivably influence the precise onset or quality, or both, of REM sleep. That is to say, environmental factors might be effective in influencing REM onset during a period of general readiness or preparedness of the organism for REM sleep to take place, but *not at any other time.* If so, a specific REM period might be a sleep response made by the organism to stimuli which call for alerting and orienting behavior during sleep.

The similarity of many of the manifestations of the REM state to those of the well-known orienting response is at least suggestive of such a possibility.

Both the REM state and the orienting reaction have in common EEG changes toward increased arousal characterized by faster, lower amplitude activity. Both show a number of autonomic reactions which suggest preparation of the body for emergency action, and in the orienting reaction there is an increase in sensitivity of sense organs, while during REM sleep there is increased activation of sensorimotor centers. Dement [1] notes that in humans the onset of REM sleep is often accompanied by a sudden respiratory apnea which suggests an orienting response. It should also be noted that the orienting reaction is typically accompanied by behavior which seeks to determine the source of the stimulus as, for example, a turning of the head toward the stimulus, quick darting movements of the eyes, sniffing. Is it possible that such searching responses are partially reflected in the rapid searching eye movements of REM sleep? In cats with ablation of the nucleus locus coeruleus, the center which has been experimentally demonstrated [4] to be responsible for the atonia of REM sleep, some animals may, in fact, turn their heads, as though in an orienting reaction, at the commencement of an REM period.

While it is thus at least possible that REM sleep may be a modified form of orienting response occurring during sleep, sensitivity of the REM timing mechanisms to concurrent stimuli might be masked quite effectively by the overall regularity of the sleep cycle and by the obvious limits on the time interval during which REM sleep might theoretically occur as a response to noxious or alerting stimuli. Only further investigation can determine whether such is the case.

In brief, then, we suggest that superimposed on a basic homeostatic process which leads to more or less regular alternation of activated (REM) and deactivated (NREM) sleep, there may occur temporary increases of sensitivity of the REM sleep triggering mechanisms to disruptive stimuli, such increases occurring during a brief critical interval when there exists a sufficient degree of organismic readiness for REM sleep. In addition, there may be a responsiveness of phasic components of REM sleep to stimuli perceived *during* the REM state. This concept of REM sleep as being (in part) a response to concurrent stimuli might serve to explain some of the variations within and among individuals in the REM state's occurrence, duration, and intensity. Further research may even, in time, reveal that the REM-NREM cycle is significantly influenced by regularly recurring sleep-connected stimuli of a physiologic or external nature, or both, which today are barely suspected.

STIMULI AND DREAMING

Let us now turn to the dream. In order to conceptualize the dream as being in certain respects a response to stimuli perceived during sleep, we need not return to prefreudian reductionist views where dreaming is seen in totality as a mere reflection of disturbing stimuli. The dream can best be understood as behavior, and with respect to stimuli during sleep, dream behavior might be viewed as an attempt to deal with a given stimulus so as to reduce its unpleasant effects. Such behavior would in turn reveal the characteristic coping techniques, personality traits, and current or pervasive emotional concerns of the sleeper.

The theoretical effect of a concurrent stimulus on dream content might be likened to the effect of a Rorschach inkblot on an examinee. Rorschach cards have been shown to have certain intrinsic stimulus properties, but since these are relatively amorphous, a subject responds to each card in an idiosyncratic manner, structuring the stimulus material according to his unique personality and experience. While the response is usually *related* to the inkblot, it does not passively mirror the stimulus, except under unusual pathological circumstances. Even more markedly, a dreaming response to a concurrent stimulus might be a springboard for a rich elaboration of personality attributes.

Negative Representation of Stimulus

There would be an essential difference, however, between the dreamer's task, as we see it, and that of the subject responding to a projective test in waking life. During dreaming, the less efficient sleeping cortex does not seem to have access to full cognizance of the precise nature of either external or internal stimuli. What is more, when a pull to continued sleep leads to an effort not to recognize the necessity to awake, this may result in a negative, rather than positive, representation of the stimulus. That is, it may simply bring about persistent efforts to blot our awareness of the stimulus or to escape from it.

An interesting example of apparent negative representation was noted by one of us (H. S. E.) after awakening from a rather lengthy afternoon nap in a chair. During this nap his feet had been resting on another chair, placed opposite to him, and he awoke to an intense and persistent pain in his left heel and discovered that the heel had been pressing against the chair opposite, carrying undue weight on it. He then recalled a lengthy and vivid (seemingly REM-like) dream which he had had during the nap. The dream depicted a series of attempts to escape from some rowdy dream characters who looked like Bowery derelicts. In the opening scene these two ruffians were standing together in front of a neighboring house, away from the dreamer (just as his two feet were situated "away from him" on a neighboring chair?). The derelict on the right was vaguely perceived, while the one on the left appeared to be much more vivid and more active.

The dreamer then attempted, by one ingenious ruse after another, to escape from and to outwit these unpleasant characters. He found himself persistently fleeing from them, first by trying to circle around them in a wide arc to the left, later by fleeing to the right. While this elaborate series of escape maneuvers richly revealed varying levels of personality conflict, emotional concern, and the dreamer's characteristic methods of coping with problems, the dream imagery appears to have been largely determined by an attempt to escape from perception of the painful left heel. Interestingly, with typically reduced acumen of the dreaming psyche, *both* feet, instead of one, were perceived as inimical characters (though some identification of the precise source of stimulation may have been evidenced in the greater vividness and activity accorded to the *left-hand* ruffian in the dream).

Despite the apparently clear negative representation of the stimulus in this dream through intense efforts to escape from it, the usual laboratory study would have concluded that no incorporation of the painful stimulus had taken place. It could thus easily have been overlooked that the apparent "aim" of the dream was not to recognize but to ignore the causative stimulus with its annoying, arousing aspects.

The theoretical drawbacks implicit in the search for *direct* incorporation of stimuli in dreams must be recognized if we are to understand the reason why the sleep preserving function of the dream has been so readily discounted. If we assume, for example, that a successful dream from the standpoint of sleep preservation is one which copes with the annoying stimulus in such an efficient fashion that it never intrudes upon the consciousness of the dreamer, then we have a far more subtle process to study than may hitherto have been recognized.

Study of Dreaming Responses to Stimuli

The methodological problems involved in the study of indirect, disguised responses to concurrent stimuli are appreciated. We believe, however, that if investigators were to aim specifically at exploring the behavioral or "coping" hypothesis of dreaming, appropriate experimental designs might be devised. One might, for example, seek to correlate a subject's typical waking methods of coping with threatening stimuli, with his dreams occurring concurrently with certain unwelcome stimuli. If a subject should tend during waking life to meet threat with heightened aggression, will heightened aggression occur in his dream concurrent with persistent annoying stimuli? Similarly, if his response to waking threat is to escape the field, to indulge in placating behavior, or any number of other coping techniques, will these motifs become more prevalent in his dreams during the presentation of a noxious stimulus?

In such studies one would face an additional problem. If we entertain the notion that every dream may be in part a response to concurrent stimuli, then we have an exceedingly complex task, for many forms of stimuli impinging on the sleeping organism are more or less continuous in their manifestations. States of heat or cold, hypostatic congestive conditions, immobilization of limbs by body weight, problems of balance, bladder pressures, nasal congestion, digestive difficulties, daylight penetrating the eyelids, hunger, thirst, sexual tension, room sounds, weight or constriction of blankets, oppressive atmospheric conditions, or any number of other stimuli may be persistently registered by a sleeping organism minimally alert, for obvious adaptive purposes, to its environment. An important attribute of most of these conditions is that they might be expected to result in a gradual, rather than an abrupt, increase of tension as the night proceeds.

When the organism is "primed" for REM sleep by reason, we suggest, of homeostatic regulation of cortical tonus around some optimal level [2], it seems possible that such persistent nighttime stimuli may serve either as facilitators of the REM sleep triggering mechanism or, if the stimuli are sufficiently urgent (or the organism unusually alert), they may serve to counteract REM sleep by leading directly to awakening. When the organism is not primed for REM sleep (at other points in the sleep cycle) the same stimuli, if they reach threshold level, may serve to trigger brief lightenings of the EEG patterns, K-complexes, body movements, NREM dreamlets, or other manifestations of increased activation which may occur in NREM sleep.

If such a hypothesis is valid, then the experimental introduction of any stimulus during sleep would usually be superimposed on existing stimuli to which the organism is already responding. This factor could make identification of the response to the laboratory stimulus somewhat difficult.

Unpleasant stimuli which can prevail throughout the sleeping period, such as heated blankets applied to subjects to raise body temperature [5] or other continuous conditions which lead to a relatively slow buildup of tension, may provide a model for dream responsiveness which more closely approximates the normal sleep state than does the introduction of punctate stimuli (the usual experimental method). While there are obvious difficulties in the path of replicating in the laboratory the natural processes typical of nighttime stimulation, there is no inherent reason why slowly accumulating noxious conditions could not be experimentally devised and manipulated, and response to them measured in terms of specific coping tendencies of the sleeper. Since such coping devices may be expected to be as varied as the personality of each individual sleeper, however, precise and delicate personality measurement would seem to be an essential ingredient in predicting, or postdicting, from the dreaming response to the concurrent stimuli.

REFERENCES

1. Dement, W. C. Possible physiological determinants of a possible dream-intensity cycle. *Exp. Neurol.* [Suppl.] 4:38, 1967.
2. Ephron, H. S., and Carrington, P. Rapid eye movement sleep and cortical homeostasis. *Psychol. Rev.* 73:500, 1966.
3. Freud, S. The Interpretation of Dreams (1900). In *The Standard Edition of the Complete Psychological Works of Sigmund Freud,* tr. and ed. by J. Strachey with others. London: Hogarth and the Institute of Psycho-Analysis, 1953. Vols. IV–V.
4. Jouvet, M. Mechanisms of the States of Sleep: A Neuropharmacological Approach. In S. Kety, E. Evarts, and H. Williams (Eds.), *Sleep and Altered States of Consciousness.* New York: Grune & Stratton, 1967. Pp. 86–126.
5. Williams, R. L., Karacan, I., and Hursch, C. J. The Effects of Environmental Hyperthermia on Sleep Patterns. Paper read at Association for the Psychophysiological Study of Sleep, Boston, 1969.

Does Dreaming Have a Function?

NATHANIEL KLEITMAN

The term *function*—when applied to a process, rather than to a tissue, organ, or system of organs—describes the contribution of that process to the survival, well-being, or reproduction of an organism. There is a tendency to seek a teleological explanation of the process, to look for a purpose it might serve. Yet some processes clearly serve no useful purpose. Thus motion sickness, expressed as nausea and vomiting, in response to unusual translational or rotational stimulation of the vestibular apparatus, cannot be said to be of use to the organism. Motion sickness results from the spread of excitation from the vestibular centers in the medulla to the nearby vomiting center. This *causative* explanation of motion sickness is generally accepted and can even be used for diagnostic purposes, as in testing the proper performance of the vestibular system; no *purposive* explanation need be invoked.

Dreaming, as a phenomenon, occurs predominantly during the activity phase of the basic rest-activity cycle (BRAC) of sleep, characterized, among other features, by a low voltage, fast activity of the EEG, and by changes in the heart rate and respiration. This does not mean that dreaming is a *function* of the activity phase. To use a crude analogy, vocal speech is usually carried on during the expiratory phases of repetitive respiratory cycles. If a person is strangled while speaking, he stops speaking and dies. Nobody will say that this person died of "speech deprivation," but the titles of early reports on the effects of repeated deprivation or curtailment of the activity phase of the BRAC during sleep referred to "dream deprivation" [1, 2].

As indicated elsewhere [3], dreaming, as a hallucinatory experience, involves

> the analysis of incoming, or locally generated, impulses, in the light of the animal's or person's previous experience (learning and

memory), and the elaboration of appropriate reactions—although actual innervation of peripheral effector structures may be blocked. In other words, dreaming is a manifestation of critical reactivity, or consciousness, operating at a much lower level than that prevailing during alert wakefulness. The low-grade critical reactivity shows itself both in the analysis of sensations (acceptance of certain impossible situations as real) and in the integration of the response, particularly with respect to projection of events into the future—the highest form of cortical activity, often expressed as an act of inhibition rather than execution. The level of consciousness during dreaming may be likened to that of the very young child, the senile person, or the normal adult under the influence of a large dose of alcohol.

The short memory span of a dream experience resembles the inability to recall events that occur during alcoholic intoxication. The commission of antisocial acts during dreaming likewise parallels the behavior of some drunken persons.

Dream-content reports may be of diagnostic and therapeutic value to a psychoanalyst, but dreaming, as a process, is as inevitable in the activity phases of the BRACs during sleep as thinking is in wakefulness. In ontogenetic development, the appearance of dreaming in a child's sleep is probably synchronous with the manifestation of critical reactivity during wakefulness. The same criterion applies, in phylogenetic development, to the occurrence of dreaming in an animal's sleep.

REFERENCES

1. Dement, W. C. The effects of dream deprivation. *Science* 131: 1507, 1960.
2. Kales, A., Hoedemaker, F. S., Jacobson, A., and Lichtenstein, E. L. Dream deprivation: An experimental reappraisal. *Nature* (London) 204:1337, 1964.
3. Kleitman, N. The basic rest-activity cycle and physiological correlates of dreaming. *Exp. Neurol.* [Suppl.] 4:2, 1967.

Approaches to Mind-Body Problems

---

*Can sleep-dream research teach us anything basic about mind-body relationships? Can sleep-dream research be used as a paradigm for other research in psychophysiological relationships?**

The Public (Scientific) Study of Private Events

JOHANN M. STOYVA

We think that electrophysiological studies of dreaming can be used as a paradigm for other research in psychophysiological relationships, and that the recent studies of dreaming have something special to offer in this respect.

Admittedly some doubts have been expressed as to whether electrophysiological studies of dreaming have really added anything of significance to what we know about *dream content.* A great deal has certainly been learned about the physiology of sleep and dreaming, but has the discovery that there are physiological correlates of

* The reader interested in this question may wish to refer also to the paper by Ornitz (p. 112).

dreaming advanced our knowledge of dreaming as a psychological experience?

Many investigators—in fact, most contemporary sleep and dream researchers—have proceeded as if the riddles of dreaming could be resolved by an ever-intensifying concentration on the physiology of REM sleep. Thus over the past decade we have seen a successive shift in emphasis from peripheral physiology to neurophysiology to neurochemistry. The unspoken assumption seems to be that once the physiological beachheads could be made completely secure penetration to the hinterlands of consciousness would constitute no great problem.

There are, however, dissenters from the physiological position. A minority, though a vocal one, speaks as if the physiological studies of dreaming were mainly exercises in futility. Hall [3], for example, feels we are in danger of physiologizing the dream out of existence and states that ". . . the night dream has been lost sight of in laboratories filled with expensive and complicated equipment . . . ."

Malcolm [7], the philosopher, also expresses dissenting views—he considers the electrophysiological studies of dreaming as largely irrelevant to the study of the dream as a psychological experience and advocates "holding firmly to waking testimony as the sole criterion of dreaming."

At this point, the veteran sleep researcher—someone who has lost a good deal of his own sleep while observing that of others—may be moved to ask: Surely, we have advanced a little in the past 15, or in the past 1500, years with respect to what we reliably know about the dream as a psychological experience! The position of the present writer is that we have indeed achieved some gains, and that these gains were made possible by a methodological innovation. Thus the viewpoint adopted here differs from both the previously described positions—the one emphasizing physiological data in the study of dreaming, the other stressing the verbal reports of subjects. We maintain that the combined use of physiological measures and verbal report—as in the REM studies of dreaming—represents a new strategy in the study of private events. Basically it is a strategy which has given us renewed credence in what subjects say about their dreams and has thus enhanced the status of dreams as phenomena suitable for scientific study.

We also maintain that this new strategy, the combined use of verbal report and physiological measures, is a method which need not be confined to dreaming but could, especially with the addition of information feedback procedures, be profitably extended to the study of certain types of waking mental activity as well. As an example of this extension of the basic method, I will discuss some recent work on the operant control of the EEG alpha rhythm. These studies employ electronic information feedback techniques which tell a subject at once whether he is showing alpha or non-alpha. Such an approach may be useful in exploring the particular state of consciousness associated with alpha and may be applicable in the case of other EEG rhythms as well.

Apart from its theoretical interest, feedback-acquired control of certain internal physiological events may also have some practical applications, in the sense that information feedback procedures may be useful in teaching control over certain physiological responses not normally under voluntary control, e.g., certain autonomic responses. Such training may prove useful in psychosomatic disorders.

BASIC LOGIC OF THE NEW APPROACH

Before pursuing the matter of practical applications, however, let us consider the basic logic of a new approach to the study of private events as exemplified in the REM-EEG studies of dreaming.

What essentially is the fundamental logic embodied in this new approach to the study of private events, in which combined physiological measures and verbal report are employed? In my estimation, it is the logic of converging operations, the essence of which is the selection or elimination of alternative hypotheses which might explain a given result.

As an example: Suppose we awaken subjects from REM sleep a great many times and we obtain dream recall 80 to 85 percent of the time. Can we be confident that REM sleep indicates the occurrence of dreaming? Not necessarily. The skeptic would point out that at least three different hypotheses capable of accounting for such a result could be proposed:

1. Verbal reports of dreaming from REM sleep reflect a reasonably accurate recall of a genuine dream experience.
2. Verbal reports of dreaming from REM sleep reflect an inaccurate recall of a genuine dream experience.
3. Verbal reports of dreaming from REM sleep represent fabrications concocted subsequent to awakening.

How do we determine which of these three hypotheses is correct? Simply repeating the original experiment will not allow us to reach a decision—although it would say something about the repeatability of the observation. What does permit a choice among the three hypotheses is the series of experiments performed early in the REM sleep era. In these experiments, positive correlations were noted between the density of REMs and the amount of physical activity in the dream report; between REM duration and the subjects' estimated length of the dream; between direction of REMs and direction of visual scanning movements recounted in the subsequent verbal report. These observations of agreement between the REM indicator and the subsequent verbal report of dreaming permit the elimination of hypotheses 2 and 3, leaving hypothesis 1 as the most likely interpretation. In other words, the verbal report of dreaming and the REM indicator support one another. Therefore REM reports of dreaming may be taken as reasonably accurate recall of actual dream experiences.

At first glance such supporting evidence, and the line of reasoning it makes possible, may not seem so important; but against the historical backdrop of the many objections raised against introspective evidence—and which have shaken our faith in such evidence—the high measure of agreement between a report of a consciousness process and a concurrent physiological measure assumes considerable significance. Looking specifically at the area of dreaming, what appears to have happened is that (given the validity of REMs as an indicator of dreaming and of localizing the dream process in time) it has proved possible for researchers to bring to light a whole body of new findings about dreaming, including the existence of qualitative differences in the type of mental activity recalled at various phases of the sleep cycle, effects of presleep stimulation on dream experience, and so forth.

With reference to the basic logic of this new approach in the study of private events, it is intriguing to note that similar proposals have arisen in other disciplines. Platt [10], for example, in examining the spectacular advancements in molecular biology and in high-energy physics, argues that the main impetus behind these advances has been the use of "strong inference." Basically this method involves (1) the explicit formulation of alternative hypotheses and ways of disproving them, and (2) "recycling the procedure, making sub-hypotheses or sequential hypotheses to refine the possibilities that remain . . . ."

Since they are amply described in other parts of this issue, the sleep-dream findings of recent years will not be dealt with in the present contribution. Instead in the remaining pages of this paper we will first briefly examine how the technique of combined physiological measures and the verbal report of some internal event need in no way be confined to the REM-dream area but could be more broadly applied in psychophysiological research. Secondly, we will examine how the basic research approach outlined in this paper, the combined use of verbal report and physiological measures, could —with the addition of information feedback procedures designed to teach individuals greater voluntary control over certain physiological events—prove of great practical significance for both psychology and psychiatry.

First, the question of extending the basic method. In addition to the dream area, another example of where a combination of verbal report and physiological measures could be profitably employed is in studying other states of psychophysiological interest, e.g., emotions such as anxiety and anger, the states of relaxation or sleep.

Also important to bear in mind are the remarkable instrumentation advances of the last few decades, which have dramatically expanded the range and sensitivity of measurements that can be made on the intact human subject. These advances seem likely to continue, thereby opening new possibilities for exploring relationships between verbal report and physiological measures. In particular one instrumentation—and conceptual advance—carries profound implications for the strategy for combined verbal report and physiological measures outlined in this paper. This is the principal of information feedback.

EXTENDING THE BASIC STRATEGY: MODIFICATION OF PHYSIOLOGICAL RESPONSES BY INFORMATION FEEDBACK

As Stoyva and Kamiya [13] pointed out, the combined use of verbal report and physiological measures need not be confined to the study of dreaming. Some recent work suggests that this general approach could, especially with the addition of information feedback procedures, be expanded in order to explore certain types of waking mental activity in addition to dreaming. This same work also suggests the possibility that man may learn to exercise greater control over certain mental events, specifically those mental events which are associated with controllable physiological events. An example will serve to make clear our position; namely, Kamiya's experiments [5] on the learned control of the EEG alpha rhythm.

In the late 1950's Kamiya asked himself what at the time seemed a decidedly far-fetched question: Could subjects learn to control their own alpha rhythms? In grappling with this problem, Kamiya hit upon a novel approach, one with far-reaching implications. The gist of this approach was to use information feedback procedures in order to make an individual aware of bodily events of which he is ordinarily not aware. In essence what Kamiya did was this: He attached electrodes to the occipital area of the brain, picked up the alpha waves, processed the signal through some electronic devices—amplifiers and filters—and devised circuits which would trigger a soft tone whenever the subject was showing the EEG alpha rhythm. The subject's task in this experiment was to produce more alpha. In other words, whenever the subject was showing alpha, he would hear a tone; as soon as he was *not* showing alpha, there would be *no* tone (the tone followed the alpha waves almost immediately, the time lag being in the order of 0.2 seconds).

Most subjects learned how to increase alpha above their base-line levels over the course of 4 to 10 separate training sessions. Thus, by means of information feedback procedures, these subjects acquired some ability to control their alpha brain wave rhythms.

In addition to changes in the amount of alpha, there was also evidence of changes in the subjects' state of consciousness. Typically, subjects reported that the mental state associated with alpha was characterized by an absence of visual imagery, was very tranquil and lacking in strong emotion, and could be described as a state of "blank mind." Many subjects described the experiment as an exercise in concentration and as a task which demanded quite a subtle and sustained response. (In my own alpha training experiences, I have noticed that any twinge of emotion, especially where there is a discernible visceral component, causes alpha to go away. The mental state associated with alpha, for about 50 percent of subjects, is that of a "content-free consciousness." For me, the "inner visual field" during alpha was like a flowing gray-black film with a luminous quality.)

In another experiment, Kamiya recruited subjects with considerable experience in meditation exercises—not too difficult to locate in San Francisco! These volunteers not only learned the alpha task very readily but reported that the alpha state was very similar to certain mystical states. The latter observation is of special interest because in both Zen and Yoga one of the major aims of the concentration exercises is to attain a "blank mind," an emptying of consciousness. This state is said to be quite difficult to achieve and may take years of training to acquire. Perhaps with information feedback techniques such abilities may be taught in a matter of months or even weeks.

Admittedly there are some controversies surrounding the alpha-control experiments (see Mulholland and Evans [9]). Nonetheless the alpha studies are useful in that they serve as a prototype for the use of information feedback procedures to modify and control certain internal events. The basic strategy, as Stoyva and Kamiya [13] have discussed, is that when the information feedback techniques have resulted in greater control over certain physiological events, there will presumably also be an increased degree of control over the mental events associated with the physiological events. Perhaps a new approach to the mind-body problem!

With the use of information feedback techniques, it is possible to proceed in either of two directions. One course of action is to use these techniques, such as the alpha training, in exploring a variety of conscious states. Kamiya [5], for example, wishes to condition a number of waves, e.g., alpha, beta, theta, alert rhythms, drowsy rhythms. Then he plans to examine the conscious state associated with each brain wave rhythm or with combinations of these brain wave rhythms. In this way he hopes to teach people to achieve a higher degree of discrimination and control over certain mental events. Eventually Kamiya would like to construct something akin to a "map of consciousness."

However, there is no reason why the feedback technique need be restricted to EEG rhythms. For example, both Yoga and Zen emphasize the importance of respiration, its frequency and depth, in the cultivation of certain mental states. Similarly, the European autogenic training emphasizes profound muscle relaxation. Why not train subjects with the feedback technique both in deep muscle relaxation *and* in controlling various aspects of respiration? Are there mental states reliably associated with each of these various parameters? What of a combination of these parameters, e.g., where an individual simultaneously shows an alpha EEG, slow and shallow respiration, and deep muscle relaxation? Is there a characteristic associated mental state? Perhaps such training on a combination of parameters could eventually help us to plot the physiological coordinates of a variety of mental states.

APPLICATION OF FEEDBACK TECHNIQUE TO BEHAVIOR THERAPY AND CERTAIN PSYCHOSOMATIC DISORDERS

In addition to its potential for the exploration of consciousness, the information feedback technique has a number of practical applications. For example, the possibility of controlling physiological responses through information feedback could be very useful in behavior therapy. In our own laboratory, Budzynski and Stoyva are using immediate feedback of electromyogram (EMG) activity, first of all, as a means of helping subjects obtain profound levels of muscle relaxation. Secondly, continuous EMG monitoring is employed during the desensitization phase of behavior therapy. As soon as a patient begins to tense up—indicated by rising EMG activity—he is told to stop visualizing that particular scene. No further visualization of the anxiety scene is attempted until the patient has regained a deep level of muscle relaxation.

In addition to behavior therapy, many psychosomatic disorders—where there seems to be a modifiable physiological component—seem promising candidates for a feedback approach. Pertinent in this respect is Jacobson's progressive relaxation technique and the German autogenic training. Both these therapies have one striking feature in common. At the core of each approach is a strong emphasis on deep muscle relaxation, which is said to be useful in diminishing anxiety, in producing drowsy, sleeplike states, and in treating a variety of stress-related psychosomatic disorders. It appears that muscle relaxation training has widespread effects on the organism; after such training, the pattern of high-arousal sympathetic discharge is replaced by a low-arousal parasympathetic pattern.

Complementary to the approach of Jacobson and the autogenic researchers, where the emphasis is on the whole organism, is the recent work of Miller [8] dealing with the instrumental conditioning of specific autonomic responses. In these experiments the animals were first curarized in order to rule out the possibility that the autonomic responses were simply mediated by skeletal muscle responses. The animals were then artificially respirated and reinforcement was accomplished through electrical stimulation of the Olds-Milner pleasure centers. Using such a preparation, Miller and his associates have been able to demonstrate operant conditioning of heart rate, stomach contraction, rate of urine secretion, blood pressure, blood flow to the ears, and intestinal contractions. Contrary to expectations, conditioning of autonomic responses proved more effective in the curarized animals than in animals with the skeletal musculature intact.

The practical implications of Miller's findings need not be labored. The crucial problem for the immediate future is how to apply such conditioning techniques to human subjects—intact and noncurarized. One line of attack is suggested by information feedback procedures. Engel and Hansen [1], for example, reported success with some subjects in using immediate information feedback of heart rate levels as a means of teaching human subjects to slow or accelerate their own heart rate. Similarly, Shapiro et al. [12] recently reported some success with information feedback procedures as a means of teaching subjects to lower their systolic blood pressure.

In our Colorado laboratory we are applying feedback procedures in the treatment of tension headache. Since the immediate cause of tension headache is an excessive and sustained contraction of the head and neck musculature [14], we surmised that training in systematic relaxation of the head musculature might be useful in alleviating this disorder. A single patient has so far received this training—immediate feedback of forehead EMG activity plus a "shaping" procedure. The patient, who has EMG electrodes placed on her forehead, hears a low-pitched tone whenever the frontalis is relatively relaxed, a high-pitched tone when the frontalis is not relaxed. As the patient progresses by deeply relaxing the frontalis the gain of the feedback loop is gradually increased, making the task more difficult since the patient must progressively decrease her level of EMG activity in order to keep the feedback tone at low frequencies. The patient's response is thus being "shaped" in the sense that the gain is carefully adjusted so as to maintain performance at the low-tone level approximately 85 percent of the time.

The results to date are most encouraging; with this patient, headaches have diminished both in frequency and intensity.

Another application, more in keeping with the focus in the present issue, is the possibility of applying feedback methods to the treatment of sleep-onset insomnia. In this context it is significant to note that although sleep research has been a remarkably fertile field of inquiry during the past decade, the practical yield has so far been disappointingly small. The situation is particularly glaring in the case of insomnia, probably the commonest of all sleep disorders. On this topic recent research has little to say.

There exists, however, a considerable body of evidence, chiefly in the older literature, that deep muscle relaxation can be very useful in dealing with sleep onset insomnia. Jacobson [4], for example, reported that insomnia was a disorder with which his progressive relaxation technique was particularly useful.

Less well known in this country is the German autogenic training, a muscle relaxation procedure which has been employed for a wide variety of stress-related disorders. In a considerable body of literature, most of it untranslated, there are numerous reports describing the use of autogenic training in cases of insomnia (see, for example, Schultz [11]). Levels of success reportedly range from 80 to 85 percent, although a serious shortcoming both in Jacobson's work and in that of the autogenic training school is the paucity of controlled outcome studies.

What could be accomplished with an information feedback approach? Actually there are a variety of maneuvers which might be attempted. One approach, following the lead of Jacobson and the autogenic training researchers, would be to train insomniacs in deep muscle relaxation by means of the feedback of EMG activity. When deep muscle relaxation has been achieved, reports of drowsiness are quite frequent. In our own work with feedback-induced relaxation, we have observed that deep relaxation of the head muscles is especially likely to produce strong feelings of drowsiness.

A parallel approach, which could readily be employed in conjunction with the EMG feedback technique, would be to train subjects in the operant control of the EEG alpha rhythm. The alpha state is a relaxed condition and is generally incompatible with vivid visual imagery—subjects frequently characterize the alpha condition as a state of "blank mind." Perhaps a combination of EMG training and operant control of alpha may develop as the most useful technique in dealing with insomnia. Support for this possibility is suggested by the fact that the two commonest complaints in insomnia are (1) an inability to relax the musculature—the patient is very tense, and (2) an inability to "switch off" one's thoughts, e.g., "when I try to go to sleep, my mind begins to race with thoughts" (cf. Geer and Katkin [2]). The techniques now at our disposal enable us to focus on both of these complaints, using either the EMG training or the alpha training, or some combination of these two methods.

An additional approach would be to attempt direct conditioning of EEG sleep rhythms such as was reported by Miller [8]. His curarized rats, reinforced by electrical stimulation in the pleasure centers when they showed the desired EEG pattern, learned to produce both drowsy and alert EEG patterns. Similar methods could be explored with humans, utilizing information feedback techniques.

Admittedly the foregoing suggestions do not constitute a solution to sleep-onset insomnia, a common affliction in our civilization, but at least they outline a mode of attack. Probably no single approach will prove universally effective in the treatment of this disorder; rather some combination of approaches may prove more generally useful.

SUMMARY

Finally, to summarize the arguments advanced in this paper: (1) We think that the combined use of physiological measures and verbal report, as in the REM studies of dreaming, represents a new strategy in the study of private events. Basically what is involved is the logic of converging operations: certain hypotheses about the dream experience can be *ruled out* on the basis of the physiological evidence. (2) The combined use of verbal report and physiological measures need not be confined to dreaming, but could—especially with the addition of information feedback procedures—be usefully extended to the study of certain types of waking mental activity as well. Such an extension is suggested by the recent experiments on the learned control of the EEG alpha rhythm. (3) The use of information feedback procedures has great practical potential and may prove extremely useful as a means of teaching people greater voluntary control over a number of physiological responses. The threefold approach outlined in this paper—precise measurement and amplification, information feedback, and shaping—seem potentially applicable to a wide variety of physiological events.

REFERENCES

1. Engel, B. T., and Hansen, S. P. Operant conditioning of heart rate slowing. *Psychophysiology* 3:176, 1966.
2. Geer, J. S., and Katkin, E. S. Treatment of insomnia using a variant of systematic desensitization. *J. Abnorm. Psychol.* 71: 161, 1966.
3. Hall, C. S. Process of fantasy. *Science* 153:626, 1966.
4. Jacobson, E. *Progressive Relaxation* (2d ed.). Chicago: University of Chicago Press, 1938. P. 419.
5. Kamiya, J. Conscious control of brain waves. *Psychology Today* 1:57, 1968.
6. Kammerer, T., Ritter, M., Botz, R. and Fétique, J. Utilisation du training autogène en groupe et en milieu psychiatrique. In W. Luthe (Ed.), *Autogenic Training: Correlationes Psychosomaticae.* New York: Grune & Stratton, 1965. Pp. 113–119.
7. Malcolm, N. *Dreaming.* New York: Humanities Press, 1959. P. 81.
8. Miller, N. E. Learning of visceral and glandular responses. *Science* 163:434.
9. Mulholland, T., and Evans, C. R. An unexpected artifact in the human electroencephalogram concerning the alpha rhythm and the orientation of the eyes. *Nature* 207:36, 1965.
10. Platt, J. R. Strong inference. *Science* 146:347, 1964.
11. Schultz, J. H. *Das Autogene Training: Konzentrative Selbstentspannung* (10 Auflage). Stuttgart: Thieme, 1960. P. 171.
12. Shapiro, D., Tursky, B., Gershon, E., and Stern, M. Effects of

feedback and reinforcement on the control of human systolic blood pressure. *Science* 163:588, 1969.

13. Stoyva, J., and Kamiya, J. Electrophysiological studies of dreaming as the prototype of a new strategy in the study of consciousness. *Psychol. Rev.* 75:192, 1968.
14. Wolff, H. G. *Headache and Other Head Pain*. New York: Oxford University Press, 1963.

Directions for Future Research

---

*What is the future of sleep-dream research? What studies are most needed in this field? What methods or tools are likely to be most useful?**

Methods for Research on Sleep Deprivation and Sleep Function

ROBERT T. WILKINSON

It was perhaps the early identification of REM sleep with dreaming which biased researchers toward clinical observation and projective tests in their attempts to discover the behavioral sequelae of losing REM sleep. Empirical studies now suggest that this emphasis was unfortunate. In the first place we know that dreaming or mental activity can be recalled from awakenings out of all stages of sleep, the difference between REM and NREM activity being more one of quality of recall than quantity.

It thus seems highly unlikely that REM deprivation can prevent dreaming as we are aware of it, or even reduce it to any considerable

* The reader interested in this question may wish to refer to papers by Hobson (p. 1), Kahn (p. 25), Karacan and Williams (p. 93), Skinner (p. 213), Ephron and Carrington (p. 269 and p. 344), Dewan (p. 295), and Hartmann (p. 308).

extent. This destroys the freudian-based rationale for expecting REM deprivation to result in increased psychopathology. In line with this is the empirical finding that in fact researchers have been singularly unsuccessful in demonstrating any such symptoms in subjects whose experimental REM deprivation has been well controlled. This lack of positive results has been clearly revealed in a review by Vogel [9].

It may be too early to reject completely the idea that the loss of REM sleep will disrupt personality, but there certainly seems to be a case for widening the net of behavioral tests in our search for the biological significance of the REM state. An obvious extension is the use of performance tasks. It is true that there have already been some studies of this [4, 7, 10] and the results, like those of the clinical assessments, have been negative. Thus, to use a well-known gambit, we have no evidence that REM deprivation has any effect upon performance; but it is quite possible that the reason for this is that no really searching performance procedures have been mounted.

The average term of REM deprivation, about 5 nights, causes a loss of about 8 hours of REM sleep. Only 30 hours of total sleep deprivation are required to produce an equivalent loss of whole sleep. Now it was not until 1958, 62 years after the first experiment on performance under sleep deprivation, that a significant effect of only 30 hours loss of sleep was demonstrated [11] and confirmed in similar tests [6, 15]. These and subsequent studies, which have been reviewed by Wilkinson [12], serve to outline the features which make a task vulnerable to total sleep deprivation. It should be (1) of long duration, (2) repetitive in nature, and (3) relatively low in interest and incentive. The performance tests used so far to investigate the effects of REM deprivation have failed to meet all these criteria, and particularly the first.

The reason for this is presumably that REM deprivation was expected to have an effect quite different in kind from that of total sleep deprivation, and therefore good tests of the latter would be inappropriate. This a priori rejection of the null hypothesis (that the two kinds of sleep are equivalent) is perhaps unwise, especially in light of a recent experiment by Donnell et al. [3] in which preliminary findings indicate that recovery sleep with REM excluded and recovery sleep with stage 4 excluded are equally effective in restoring performance following 2 nights of total sleep deprivation.

I shall start therefore with the thesis that, to begin with at least, the best criteria for the choice of performance tests for REM deprivation are those found most effective for tests of total sleep deprivation. I shall describe an experiment in which those criteria indicated were applied with greater rigor than before to achieve what has defeated sleep researchers hitherto [5, 8, 10], namely an effect on performance of reducing sleep (rather than witholding it completely) for 1 or 2 nights. The results of this experiment have already been reported in part [13, 14]. The point of this exposition is to emphasize the detail of the performance procedures involved.

The two tests involved were Vigilance and Adding, each of which continued without a break for 1 hour at a time. They are described in detail in the Appendix. The Vigilance test required subjects to monitor ½-second tones coming one every 2 seconds over a background of 85 decibels of white noise. Occasionally (40 times in 1 hour) one of the tones was shorter than usual (⅜ second) and had to be reported by pressing a key. Percent–Detections and Percent–False Reports were scored. The Adding simply presented the subject with books of sums to be added. Total Sums Done Per Hour and Percent Errors were scored.

At least as important as the tests themselves is the schedule in which they are administered. Enlisted men were available in groups of 6 for 6 weeks at a time. On the Wednesday and Thursday of each week they worked a full day of tests from 7:45 A.M. to 10:35 P.M. following the schedule shown in Table 1. The bulk of the work consisted of alternating 1-hour Vigilance and Adding tests, with the usual breaks between tests for meals and snacks. On each of the previous nights the subjects' sleep was "rationed," each man having one of six amounts: 7½ hours (control), 5, 3, 2, 1, and 0 hours. Thus on the first day of tests (Wednesday) 1 night had been passed on the particular sleep ration, and on the second day, Thursday, 2 nights. Each week the subjects rotated sleep rations so that by 6

TABLE 1. *Daytime program of work*[a] *following nights of reduced sleep*

Time	Activity	Time	Activity
A.M.		1:55– 2:55	Adding
6:30	Rise, have breakfast	3:00– 4:00	Coding[b] followed by tea
7:30	Leave unit of accommodation; walk to lab	4:05– 5:05	Vigilance
		5:10– 6:10	Evening meal at lab
7:40	Arrive lab	6:15– 7:15	Adding
7:45– 8:45	Vigilance	7:20– 8:20	Vigilance
8:55– 9:55	Adding	8:20– 8:30	Break for coffee
10:00–11:00	Coding[b] followed by coffee break	8:30– 9:30	Adding
		9:35–10:35	Vigilance
11:05–12:05	Vigilance	10:40	Walk to unit of accommodation
P.M.		11:00	7½-hours man to bed
12:05– 1:50	Leave lab; walk to unit of accommodation; lunch; walk to lab	A.M.	
		1:30	5-hours man to bed
		3:30	3-hours man to bed (and so on)

[a] Subjects worked in groups of 6, each subject being isolated in his own cubicle while working on the tasks. Vigilance and Adding tests were given alternately, and occasions on which the day's work began with vigilance or calculation were balanced over the whole 6 weeks.

[b] An unconnected test not reported on in this paper.

weeks each had experienced each ration. Summing over all subjects (24 minus 5 dropouts = 19) gives rise to Table 2, reflecting scores in each test after 1 or 2 nights on the particular sleep ration. Percent–Errors in Adding are not shown, as with reduced sleep this score showed only moderate changes in the direction of lower accuracy.

When one considers that previous studies have failed to demonstrate any significant effect on performance of 6 hours a night instead of 8 for one month [5], 3 hours a night for 8 days [10], or 2½ hours for 3 days [7], it is significant that the present routines have been able to discriminate a reduction of sleep to 2 hours on a single night and to 5 hours on 2 nights. This sensitivity is almost certainly due as much to the prolonged schedule of experimental sleep deprivation and testing as to the nature of the tests themselves. Good

TABLE 2. *Performance after 1 or 2 nights on each sleep ration*

Activity	Number of Nights	Sleep Ration (hours)					
		0	1	2	3	5	7½
ADDING							
Sums Done per Hour	1	175[a]	185[a]	199[a]	222[b]	228[b]	233[b]
	2	169[a]	152[a]	174[a]	201[ab]	219[ab]	229[b]
VIGILANCE							
Percent–Signals Detected	1	53.5[a]	58.5[a]	57.0[ab]	60.0[b]	62.0[b]	64.5[b]
	2	45.0[a]	50.5[ab]	53.0[ab]	57.0[ab]	62.5[ab]	67.0[b]
VIGILANCE							
Percent–False Reports	1	0.77	0.72	0.65	0.51[b]	0.67	0.73
	2	0.56	0.65	0.61	0.47[ac]	0.59	0.74

[a]Significantly different ($p < .05$ using the Wilcoxon Nonparametric Test) from 7½ hours.
[b]Significantly different ($p < .05$ using the Wilcoxon Nonparametric Test) from 0 hours.
[c]In Percent–False Reports only, significantly different from 1 hour ($p < .01$).

experimental control requires that nothing shall vary but the parameter under study. If a drug is being given, a placebo is used to ensure that any changes observed are due to the drug and not to the fact of being given a drug. This is commonplace in pharmacology; why should it be less valid in other areas? Yet few people consider what is the appropriate placebo for sleep deprivation. How do we ensure that the subject is responding to the sleep deprivation per se and not also to the fact of being experimentally sleep deprived? All we can do is to get him so used to the experience that he ceases to react to it as something special. In the case of sleep deprivation he ceases to regard it, perhaps, as a challenge to his powers of endurance and accepts it as normally as if it were due to a late night at the office or a party. This, to judge from comments from the subjects, is what the prolonged 6-week schedule achieves. Attitudes toward the test itself change similarly when a 1-hour test is only one of nine to be done during the day instead of the only one required. Finally there is less variability due to improvement with practice.

For all these reasons it is thought unlikely that similar effects of partial sleep deprivation would show in the same tests if they were presented only once or twice, even with some previous practice.

Nevertheless the 6-week schedule described above is a long and potentially costly one. It may well be asked, "Does it have to be *that* long?" To help answer this, an attempt has been made to show how the effects of the various sleep rations develop over successive tests and weeks of testing. As subjects changed rations every week, individual differences can obscure the trends. However, if the scores in each test across the whole 6 weeks are ranked within each subject, these ranks can then be used to compare the influence of the different sleep levels on performance at different stages of the experimental schedule. This is shown in Figure 1. In Vigilance and for 1 night on the sleep ration, the levels of sleep have not really separated until the third or fourth week of the procedure. With Adding, on the other hand, the separation is quite clear, even after only 1 night's sleep ration, by the end of the first 2 weeks. We may look within

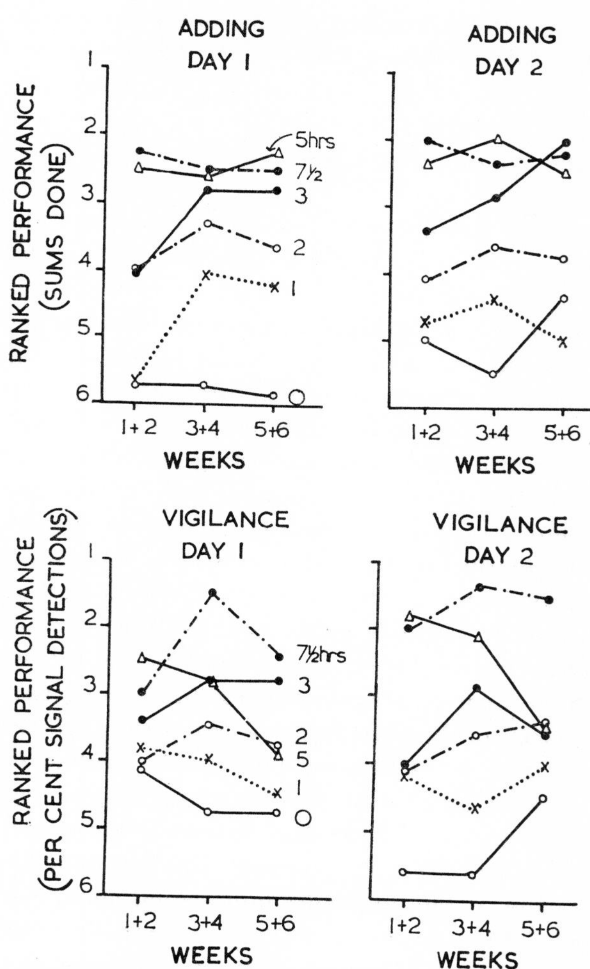

FIGURE 1. *The effect of sleep ration on Vigilance and Adding showing how this develops with successive 2-week periods on the performance schedule*

these 2 weeks again to see how far one has to go with the individual test sessions before performance separates according to the level of sleep. This is shown in Table 3, which gives for each test session of

TABLE 3. *Kendall's tau correlations between ranked performance in Adding (Sums Done) and sleep ration for individual 1-hour sessions during the first 2 weeks of testing*

	Day 1				Day 2			
Week	Test 1	Test 2	Test 3	Test 4	Test 1	Test 2	Test 3	Test 4
1	+0.40	+0.20	+0.73	+0.46	+0.60	+0.53	+1.00	+0.60
2	+0.06	+0.26	+0.73	−0.20	+0.73	+0.73	+0.86	+0.86

the first 2 weeks the correlation (Kendall's tau) between performance (Sums Done) and sleep ration. Notice that the effects of the partial loss of sleep are certainly not apparent after only two 1-hour sessions on Day 1 of Week 1, but have appeared by the second day of testing and sleep loss. It is particularly interesting that after a break in the procedure of 4 days, the initial tests of Week 2 (on Day 1) again have lost much of their ability to discriminate the sleep levels, but this has returned by the third 1-hour session of Day 1, Week 2, and is present in all the sessions of Day 2. The disparate point of Session 4, Day 1, Week 2 is unfortunate and hard to explain.

At a conservative estimate, then, it appears that the first 2 weeks of the 6-week program are sufficient for the Adding test to distinguish the effects of these six levels of partial sleep loss, not just for 2 successive nights but also for 1 only. The Adding test is thus superior in sensitivity to the Vigilance, as well as being easier to administer. Vigilance would probably not make the same discrimination until 3 or 4 weeks of the program had been completed. But, on the other hand, it can give more information about performance. In particular, Vigilance is a test in which trends in reporting both correct signal detections and false reports may be used to provide important information as to the *way* in which performance has been impaired. Normally, techniques of Theory of Signal Detection are used for this [1]. For the present it will suffice to say that when the pattern is one of declining detections accompanied by a reduction in false reports, this suggests a fall in the subject's willingness to report signals whether real or imaginary. On the other hand a decline in detections accompanied by no change or even an increase in false reports suggests that, in spite of being willing or keen to report signals (hence the many false reports), he cannot discriminate the signals well enough to maintain his score of detections. This implies a fall in his intrinsic ability to discriminate sensory events, something quite different from a reduced willingness to report signals either real or illusory.

Let me illustrate the possible application of this to the problems of REM deprivation. In the study of partial sleep deprivation which I have described, and from all that is known of all-night sleep profiles, the 3-hour ration of sleep must have excluded most of REM and much of stage 2, leaving stage 4 and most of stage 3 intact. As we have seen, there were significant effects of this upon performance in both Adding and Vigilance. But in Vigilance we can analyze the situation further with reference to the scores in Table 2 following 2 nights of rationed sleep. At the 3-hour point, when most of REM had been lost, Percent–Detections and Percent–False Reports had both fallen. This is the pattern of reduced willingness to respond, hardly similar to the hyperactivity reported for REM-deprived states in animals! Reducing sleep further to 0 hours removed stages 3 and 4. Referring again to Table 2, Percent–Detections fell still further, but Percent–False Reports rose from the low point of 3 hours sleep. This is the pattern of lowered ability to make sensory discriminations. It is the opposite of what has been claimed for both the cat [2] and man [4] when deprived of REM sleep alone. Thus the results of these studies of performance in depth following reduced sleep hardly bear out the conclusions of animal studies of the effects of REM deprivation on behavior; indeed, to some extent they suggest the opposite.

The weakness, of course, is that no direct EEG records were possible during the reduced sleep of the present experiment to confirm our estimates of how the balance of the sleep content was changed. It would be interesting to repeat the experiment with such records taken, or better still with REM and NREM deprivation substituted for the parametrically reduced sleep levels.

APPENDIX

Adding Test

The basic materials comprised the following: (1) A 30-page book, each page having 125 sums arranged in 5 rows of 25. Each sum consisted of five two-digit numbers to be added, the answer to be written at the foot of the sum in the usual way. (2) A book of answers for marking purposes.

Four separate 1-hour practice sessions were given before commencing the main series of experimental tests, each of which also comprised 1 hour of continuous adding. Subjects started one session from the point in the book at which they ended the last. A pen of a different color was used for each session so that the transition points could be distinguished.

When or if a subject had worked through a complete book, a second book was assembled using the same pages but in a different order.

The test was scored for the number of sums attempted in each session and the percentage of these incorrectly added.

The instructions were simply that the subject should add each column of two-digit numbers and write the answer in the space underneath. He should not omit any of the sums and should work as quickly as possible while doing his best not to get any of the answers wrong.

Vigilance Test

The Vigilance test was more complex than the Adding test, both administratively and in terms of equipment required. The basic test lasted 1 hour, during which the subjects listened to tones, ½-second in duration, coming at intervals of 2 seconds throughout the period. These tones were superimposed upon a background of white noise. There were a total of 1800 such tones during the 1-hour test. Forty of them, irregularly spaced in time, were slightly shorter than the others. The subject's task was to spot these and report them by pressing a button as soon as possible. Having done this, he had, at a little more leisure, to press one of three other buttons to indicate how confident he was that in fact it was a signal that he had heard.

The test materials were all recorded on standard ¼-inch magnetic tape and comprised the following: (1) A preliminary instruction tape, lasting about 20 minutes, which explained the nature of the test to the subjects, showed them the signal, and gave them some initial practice in learning to spot it. After that it explained the procedure for indicating their level of confidence, and finally it gave them a further short practice in responding in this way. (2) Two 1-hour practice tapes, the first of which was preceded by a short 3-minute familiarization run in which signals were presented at a comparatively high rate. The purpose of the latter was to revive the subject's memory of what the signals sounded like. (3) Ten 1-hour main test tapes which were identical to the two 1-hour practice ones except, of course, that different programs of signals were used in each.

Each subject was given the instruction tape and then the two practice tapes, followed by as many of the 1-hour main test tapes as the experimental design required, repeating them as necessary.

The Vigilance tapes were presented on a standard double channel (stereo) tape recorder operating at a speed of 3¾ inch per second and having independent gain controls for each channel on playback. The test material as described above was recorded on one channel of each tape and played through loudspeakers to the group of subjects, each in his separate cubicle. These subjects were thus isolated from each other visually and auditorily so that they were unable to tell from the responses of others when the signals had occurred. The gain of the tape recorder was adjusted so that the level of the white noise (minus tone) was about 85 decibels above threshold. This helped also to mask any auditory communication between the subjects.

The second channel of the tape recorder contained information for the experimenter. A voice proclaimed the start of the test and, coincident with the *end* of each shorter tone (the signal) on the subject's channel, a tone occurred on the experimenter's channel, so that he could record the subjects responses to the signal.

In General

An attempt was made to maintain a moderate level of incentive throughout the test procedures. The subjects' pay was not linked to their performance, but they were given feedback of knowledge of results on alternate 1-hour tests. This served to maintain a competitive spirit among the group.

Should the reader require further details of the Adding and Vigilance tests (e.g., apparatus, sample test materials) the author can supply them on written request.

REFERENCES

1. Broadbent, D. E., and Gregory, M. Vigilance considered as a statistical decision. *Brit. J. Psychol.* 54:309, 1963.
2. Dewson, J. H., Dement, W. C., Wagner, T. E., and Nobel, K. Rapid eye movement sleep deprivation: A central-neural change during wakefulness. *Science* 156:403, 1967.
3. Donnell, J., Lubin, A., Naitoh, P., and Johnson, L. Relative Recuperative Value of Sleep Stages After Total Sleep Deprivation: A Progress Report. Paper read at Association for the Psychophysiological Study of Sleep (APSS), Boston, 1969.
4. Greenberg, R., Pearlman, C., Fingar, R., Kantowitz, J., and Kawliche, S. The Effects of Dream Deprivation. Paper read at APSS, Denver, 1968.
5. Husband, R. W. The comparative value of continuous versus interrupted sleep. *J. Exp. Psychol.* 18:792, 1935.
6. Pepler, R. D. Warmth and lack of sleep: Accuracy or activity reduced. *J. Comp. Physiol. Psychol.* 52:446, 1959.
7. Sampson, H. Psychological effects of deprivation of dreaming sleep. *J. Nerv. Ment. Dis.* 143:305, 1966.
8. Smith, M. A contribution to the study of fatigue. *Brit. J. Psychol.* 8:327, 1916.
9. Vogel, G. REM deprivation. III. Dreaming and psychosis. *Arch. Gen. Psychiat.* (Chicago) 18:312, 1968.

10. Webb, W. B., and Agnew, H. W., Jr. Sleep: Effects of a restricted regime. *Science* 150:1745, 1965.
11. Wilkinson, R. T. The effects of sleep loss on performance. *Med. Res. Coun. Spec. Rep.* (London), Appl. Psychol. Res. Unit Report No. 323, 1958.
12. Wilkinson, R. T. Sleep Deprivation. In O. G. Edholm and A. L. Bacharach (Eds.), *The Physiology of Human Survival.* New York: Academic, 1965. Pp. 399–430.
13. Wilkinson, R. T. Sleep Deprivation and Behavior. In B. F. Riess and L. A. Abt (Eds.), *Progress in Clinical Psychology,* Vol. 8. 1968.
14. Wilkinson, R. T., Edwards, R. S., and Haines, E. Performance following a night of reduced sleep. *Psychonomic Sci.* 5:471, 1966.
15. Williams, H. L., Lubin, A., and Goodnow, J. J. Impaired performance with acute sleep loss. *Psychol. Monogr.* No. 14 (Whole No. 484), 73, 1959.

Study Wakefulness. Study the Rest-Activity Cycle. Don't Just Study Sleep!

NATHANIEL KLEITMAN

In the many published studies of sleep, the wakefulness phase, with which it alternates, is somehow taken for granted. Where wakefulness is treated, it is only to point out its qualitative and quantitative differences from sleep. The explanation is obvious: We are familiar with the events transpiring during our waking state—as against the oblivion of sleep—and familiarity breeds contempt. Thus one hears of the mystery of sleep, but not of the infinitely more complex nature of the analytical and integrative performance of the nervous system during wakefulness. As Oscar Wilde's Lord Henry put it to Dorian Gray, "The true mystery of the world is the visible, not the invisible."

The question of whether sleep is a cessation of wakefulness, or the other way around, like the question of the chicken and the egg, is bound up with the demonstration of the existence of sleep center(s), wakefulness center(s), or both [1]. It may be considered as established that both mechanisms operate in the sleep–wakefulness alternation, but the sleep centers are subsidiary to the wakefulness ones. Similarly, one can localize centers for vasoconstriction reflexes and vasodilatation reflexes in the medulla, but cutting the spinal cord just below the medulla leads to a profound drop in blood pressure, indicating the dominance of the vasoconstrictor mechanism.

There are many reports on the changes in incidence and duration of sleep periods in the human infant, but only one study by Parmelee [3], on one infant, furnished data on the progressive increase in wakefulness. For this infant, the daily *average* longest wakeful period increased from 2.0 to 2.5 hours in the first five weeks of life, to 4.0 to 4.1 hours in the thirty-third to thirty-fifth weeks; and the *absolute* longest wakeful period, during the same time stretch, about doubled from 3.0 to 6.5 hours. The *total* sleep per 24 hours for this infant decreased from 17.8 hours in the first week to 14.3 hours in the thirty-fifth, but the average and absolute longest periods of sleep were 4.4 hours and 5.5 hours in the first week and rose to 11.7 hours and 13.0 hours, respectively, in the twenty-ninth week. Thus there was a consolidation of both sleep and wakefulness, but the increase in wakefulness capability was relatively small. In the course of acculturation to the 24-hour rhythm of existence, it often takes an infant only 5 to 7 weeks to sleep through the night, but as much as 5 to 7 years for the child to attain an unbroken period of wakefulness by giving up the afternoon nap.

Is a high wakefulness capability—expressed as the ability to "get along" on 4 or 5 hours of sleep per night—evidence of mental superiority? Many persons boast of how little they sleep, but one seldom hears of the opposite. Does the afternoon nap habit denote a return to childhood conditions? Or would everyone enjoy a postprandial relaxation, if he or she could afford it? Answers to these questions will come from studies of wakefulness as well as of sleep.

Wakefulness capability may be related to a number of physiological and psychological variables that go to make up one's "personality." In an analysis of sleep pattern differences between good and poor sleepers, Monroe [2] found that poor sleepers not only slept less than good ones, but also awakened more often and moved more. Most striking was a statistically significant difference in the body temperature curves of the two groups of sleepers, poor sleepers showing a higher temperature curve during sleep and also in the presleep half hour. This suggests a lesser ability to relax one's musculature on the part of the poor sleepers, and personality inventory scales revealed greater psychosomatic and emotional disturbances in that group.

Another carry-over from sleep to wakefulness is the variation in the frequency of the alpha EEG pattern under different conditions. There is a 24-hour curve of alpha frequencies, with the lowest values prevailing at 4 to 6 A.M. when the body temperature is at its lowest and when it is hardest to keep awake. Slower alpha patterns are also associated with low-level conscious states, such as hypothyroidism, alcoholic intoxication, and senility [1]. Longitudinal studies of alpha frequencies—perhaps as components of periodic health examinations—may lead to the development of an objective method of determining a physiological, as different from a chronological, retirement age, reached when, along with a decrease in performance on a variety of physiological and psychological tests, there is a critical decrement in one's relaxed wakefulness alpha pattern frequency.

The operation of the basic rest-activity cycle—first discovered as a cyclic variation in the sleep pattern—during the waking hours also merits, and is getting, further attention from investigators.

Although there are many facets of the sleep state that have not been completely elucidated, the taken-for-granted state of wakefulness is the real mystery to be unravelled—both from the theoretical viewpoint, as a contribution to knowledge, and from practical needs of adjusting our mode of living to the physiological capabilities of the organism.

REFERENCES

1. Kleitman, N. *Sleep and Wakefulness* (rev. ed.). Chicago & London: University of Chicago Press, 1963.
2. Monroe, L. J. Psychological and physiological differences between good and poor sleepers. *J. Abnorm. Psychol.* 72:255, 1967.
3. Parmelee, A. H., Jr. Sleep patterns in infancy: A study of one infant from birth to eight months of age. *Acta Paediat. Belg.* 50:160, 1961.

Suggestions for Urgently Needed Research

ARTHUR SHAPIRO*

Two kinds of studies are urgently needed in the immediate future, and they are closely related to each other. The first of these is the systematic review of empirical data already available for the purpose of developing a theoretical framework and testable hypotheses concerning the nature and function of sleep and dreaming. In particular, such theories and hypotheses should seek to account for the average phenomena such as 90-minute cycles; stage 1 REM sleep in humans associated with irregular breathing, faster heart rate, and penis erection in men; tendency to make up for lost REM time on recovery nights after REM sleep deprivation and for stages 3 and 4 time after stages 3 and 4 sleep deprivation; tendency to report dreams after awakening from REM sleep.

But a useful theory should also account for the deviant phenomena such as individual sleep cycles lasting 20 to 120 minutes; REM sleep without irregular breathing, penis erections, or faster heart rate, and NREM sleep with these accompaniments; little or no REM sleep recovery in the early part of the recovery nights after REM sleep deprivation, even on the second and third recovery nights, and even when a marked increase in REM time is present

* Deceased.

in the later part of the same nights; reports of dreaming after some awakenings from NREM sleep and failure to report dreams, especially by some subjects, after some awakenings from REM sleep.

Such a theory should also deal with phylogenetic aspects of sleep with emphasis not only on what seems to be present across different species, but even more significantly on the specific differences noted between different species and how they correlate with behavioral and neuroanatomical differences.

Along with the theoretical analysis there is also a need for detailed empirical studies concerning the nature and functions of different kinds of sleep and of dreaming. In particular, techniques must be developed for studying changes in the observed behavior and reported experiences of subjects or patients who have been exposed to various kinds of spontaneous or induced, specific or total, sleep deprivation. Studies on various aspects of clinical insomnia may well provide the "missing link" for the solution of this problem.

Since humans as well as animals are very resistant to any attempts at prolonged prevention of natural sleep, it is nearly impossible, reliably, to separate the effects of prolonged sleep-preventing procedures from the effects of the sleep loss itself. To get around this difficulty, a number of experimental techniques are possible. In the first place, evaluation procedures must be developed to show the consequences of relatively short periods of total or specific (i.e., REM, stage 3 and 4) sleep deprivation. If these studies can be conducted in an environment in which the subject pursues his normal life activities, but with some abnormally long work periods maintained by adequate motivation, it may well be possible to detect the consequences of a few hours of total sleep deprivation or even less than an hour of REM sleep deprivation.

A possible setting for such a study might perhaps be a civilian or military airport radar installation where an on-the-job study is conducted of physiological patterns monitored by radiotelemetry during work periods, rest periods, and sleep. Actual control panels can be monitored so as to measure response behavior, and function tests can be given during off-duty rest periods. Natural sleep can be monitored at home by radiotelemetry and data-phone, and awakenings scheduled within the framework of normal life situations. The electronic techniques for such a study have already been developed in our laboratory, but the functional tests needed for it are proving to be more difficult to develop.

Nevertheless, staying up late is a normal experience and most human beings can detect the consequences of their having had too little sleep the night before. In such conditions, it should be possible to distinguish between the consequences of "staying up all night" to finish an interesting novel, to study for an examination, to finish an important job, to worry, or in response to an awakening stimulus given automatically within a few minutes of falling asleep. Suitable tests of behavior and attitude should be able to define the differences between the sleep-depriving effects of these different experiences or to establish that the differences are irrelevant.

There are also numerous anecdotal reports of the "healing power" of sleep. We need more experimental studies to investigate the effects of different kinds of sleep, of presleep procedures, and of life situations on such phenomena.

The neuroanatomical and neurophysiological studies on animal sleep which have been so actively and fruitfully pursued in the past must be continued for their own sake. But the kind of understanding which will make it possible to use our knowledge of sleep and dreaming for predicting future behavior and attitudes, as well as for the treatment of physical and mental illness, can come only from an active experimental attack on the problems of the nature and functions of sleep and dreaming.

The Scientific Study of Sleep and Dreams

CAROLYN J. HURSCH

Fortunately for the future of sleep research, it is one of the few fields of scientific investigation where the accumulation of data has preceded the expounding of theory. Doubtless this is at least partly due to the fact that sleep research represents a new field of inquiry. Its birth in the twentieth century makes it immediate heir to the technological luxury of the times. The present-day scientist, no matter what professional field issued his credentials, is much more likely to think in terms of hard data and machinery than was his counterpart in previous centuries.

Therefore sleep research emerges as a burgeoning field of inquiry, cutting across many disciplines, characterized now by a vast outpouring of fact—generated by little or no theory. True, authors of new publications in the field generally use some portion of their factual reporting space to put forth favorite ideas and guesses about some aspect of sleep. But as Webb [10] has commented about his own theoretical remarks, "These thoughts are launched with the fuel of only hints from current data mixed with a considerable portion of imagination."

This state of affairs is, in many respects, a happy one. The history of science is already overloaded with accounts of infamous theories which guided believers into long, blind alleys—alleys which could have been avoided by some responsible data collecting. Some such excursions may have been due to the lack of appropriate technology. Yet one can hardly assume that the absolute zenith of technology has been reached in the present era. Doubtless by the standards of the twenty-first century, our equipment will look feeble.

The important tool which differentiates the armchair philosopher of yesterday from the laboratory scientist of today is scientific method—an instrument which cuts as incisively in one century as in the next.

And scientific method is the tool of the twentieth century. To some extent this may be because it turns out better hardware. And to some extent it may be due to the invasion of once erudite disciplines by the common man, whose heritage lies in the production of concrete objects rather than in the production of the ethereal concepts toyed with by eighteenth- and nineteenth-century philosophers. One can hardly imagine Kant's labored doctrine of a priori knowledge being produced today, nor is it likely that it would command much attention now. It seems reasonable that Fleming's contribution does.

Yet what is the role of theory? Does it have any place in today's mad rush of data collecting? Was it a useless pastime engaged in by the articulate but lethargic philosophers of past eras? Do our data tell all, or could we use a modern-day Kant, a Leibnitz or two, and a couple of Schopenhauers?

The thesis of this chapter is that at the very least, sleep research has an immediate opening for a vigorous Linnaeus. After that, a Mendeleyev would bring some welcome organization to the field, and a David Hume would contribute law and order. It would then be ready for a Von Neumann.

In the meantime, it might be well to look more closely at the common man flailing around with his scientific method. While sleep research is largely devoid of formal theory, it is doubtful that any data are ever collected without the impetus of hunches, guesses, and pet notions about the variables being investigated. The researcher is often reluctant to put forth his hunch in the form of a theory, but such hunches do direct the research, do determine what variables are examined, and do shape the ultimate direction of the field.

Therefore an area growing as fast as is the current field of sleep research could profit from having its directions shaped by meaningful theoretical guidelines rather than by the confusion of eclecticism. Such guidelines, of course, impose no obligation on the research directions of any investigator. They would, however, give greater meaning to work already done and would serve to integrate programs of research that now appear unrelated. Without a logical network of theory, an important study can get overlooked or forgotten before its place in the scheme of things is realized. In fact, without the guidance of theory, there is no "scheme of things"; there are only isolated collections of facts.

At the same time, theory must arise through the application of the same principles of scientific method that generate the data. Theories postulate networks of relationships between collections of data. Good theories do so in such a way that each of the relationships in the network has been derived empirically, or can be so derived.

Current sleep research is largely concerned with description on several different levels. What is lacking is the logic necessary to tie these levels of description together and give them cohesion and meaning. This logic would constitute the theory.

We may view the research process as the construction of building blocks which are then assembled into a scientific edifice. Each level of description provides another dimension in this construction. First-order descriptions break down the phenomenon being investigated into a static set of variables which define it. For example, sleep is now defined by certain types of brain waves on an electroencephalograph. The phenomenon is sleep, and the different types of brain waves are the variables. Second-order descriptions state the ranges of variation of these variables, i.e., the normal amounts of each type of brain wave to be found in different species, in the same species at different ages, in different segments of the sleep period, and so on. Third-order descriptions state the relationships between changes in brain waves and changes in other variables, for example, the relationship between EEG changes and changes in blood pressure, biochemistry, disease state, or experimental conditions. Fourth-order descriptions are statements of the general principles governing the relationships between sleep variables and other sets of variables. For example, if specific items in an organism's biochemistry change reliably in response to a change in one or more of the sleep variables, then a general principle might be that one of the functions of sleep is to control these biochemical processes. Whether or not the principle were correct under all conditions and across all species would be a matter for further research to confirm or deny. The collection of such fourth-order descriptions, and all that they imply, would constitute the theory.

Each level of description is dependent on all the levels below it for its accuracy. In other words, if the sleep variables are not operationally defined (first order of description) to begin with, then it would be impossible to make any meaningful statements about relationships between sleep variables and variables from other systems. Likewise, if the principles (fourth-order descriptions) are not logically stated, with the conclusions following from the premises, then it would be impossible to verify their truth or falsity.

A scientific inquiry can start with theory but, in order to generate science, it must at some time proceed down through the levels of description and establish the validity of its principles. Conversely, a science may start out with operational definitions of variables, establish parameters for these variables under different conditions, and determine their relationship to other variables. But as the volume of these data increases, there will be no logical reason to examine more relationships or more variables, unless some general laws either arise directly from the data or are postulated by a theory.

With these considerations in mind, let us evaluate where we are now in sleep research.

We know from data emerging during the past two decades that sleep is not a simple blocking out or holding state of the organism. Instead it is a complex pattern of changing neurological and biological states. Or is it?

Our EEG machine tells us that the brain engages in several different types of electrical activity during sleep, the usual number agreed upon being five: stage 1 with rapid eye movement and stages 1 through 4 without REM. One can imagine that the researcher of the twenty-first century will have a machine which will detect a dozen different types, or perhaps a hundred. For the moment, we are busy enough with these five—measuring their length, their periodicity, their percentages of total sleep, their suppression during, preceding, or following unusual conditions, their constancy, their variation across age groups, their occurrence in other species, and their responses to various chemical, biological, and psychological agents.

But what do we really have? A highly sensitive amplifier and recorder at one end. At the other, a sleeping subject with electrodes secured to the skin of his scalp and to his eye muscles, or an animal with electrodes permanently implanted in his brain. The EEG records show only the amplitude and frequency of electrical activity. This is first-order data about sleep. It describes the sleeping states in EEG language. Everything emanating from this is a product of the ingenuity of the sleep researcher. This product may be a deduction, an induction, a correlation, an inference, a coincidence, or pure fiction, depending upon how it was derived.

The five stages are the result of current agreement based on convenience, although some researchers find it more convenient to combine stages 3 and 4, while others are further subdividing stage 1-REM according to its density. The decision to use five stages is an arbitrary one. An EEG record, run at a speed of 15 mm. per second, for an 8-hour night of sleep is nearly 1500 feet long. One cannot classify every rise and fall of the pen. Therefore certain amplitudes and frequencies have been singled out according to how accurately they can be distinguished from other amplitudes and frequencies. All these miles of EEG recordings, then, have been reduced to five sleep stages and one waking stage.

We have merely dissected the EEG record and given different names to the parts that look different. Whether or not this is a useful classification system will depend on whether or not these names are (1) mutually exclusive and (2) exhaustive. If they are mutually exclusive, then there will be no chance of finding the same segment of EEG tracings recorded under two different stages (given, of course, an expert EEG scorer). If they are exhaustive, then everything on the EEG record can be classified as one of the five sleep stages or the waking stage.

The current practice of combining stages 3 and 4 indicates that these two stages are probably not mutually exclusive. Too often it is difficult for the scorer to determine whether a certain segment of the record belongs in stage 3 or stage 4. At the extremes, these stages are different, yet there is a gray area of uncertainty where it is impossible to differentiate them. The only solutions possible, then, are (1) to combine 3 and 4 into one stage, or (2) to separate out the gray area and call it another stage.

Also, the original stage 1 was not exhaustive. This became apparent when the observation was made that sometimes REM occurs during this stage and sometimes it does not. Therefore this was separated into two categories, stage 1 and stage 1 with REM.

Density measurements which are now being closely viewed by many researchers [3] will gradually separate the general phenomenon of REM sleep into some number of different types of REM sleep.

Hartmann [7] has proposed that since the REM period is "not merely a different stage or depth of sleep, but a qualitatively different kind of sleep . . . different from ordinary sleep and from waking" that it be separated out and defined as "the D-state: a biological state concomitant with dreaming." He also offers a complete description of this state based on research to date.

This process of reclassification is the result of closer observation and finer measurements. Habit, practice, and one's investment in things as they are have impeded such necessary changes in science as well as many other areas of human effort, ranging from the work of Galileo to that of Rickover. In sleep research the investment in the classification of alpha, beta, gamma, and delta waves has more or less given way to the present numerical listings of stages. This listing should also give way, expand, or contract, as increasingly fine and abundant measurements are made which indicate a logical necessity for doing so.

Still in the realm of first-order description are the arbitrary groupings and summaries of the basic data, but these groupings and summaries will be affected by the rigor of our basic classification system. For example, consider the temporal sequences of the arbitrarily designated sleep stages: If there are discernible changes in defined amplitudes and frequencies of the EEG tracings, then we may state that stage 1 was followed by stage 2, and so on, and obtain frequency counts of the number of times that this happened. These changes are currently given the name *stage shifts* and require nothing but objective criteria defining each of the stages. Obviously the accuracy of the measurement of stage shifts depends on the mutually exclusive and exhaustive properties of the definitions of the stages. If these criteria have not been met, then error will be built into any measure of stage shifts.

These first-order descriptions give answers only to the question, "What is sleep?" Answers will continue to come in for a long time because of technological improvements in measuring instruments. Methodological improvement in the definition of the variables, the reliability of the measurements, and the standardization of research procedures will also contribute answers, with or without advanced technology.

Improved methodology is also mandatory for accurate second-, third-, and fourth-order descriptions, i.e., the descriptions which answer the questions: What are the ranges of the sleep variables? To what other variables are they related? What are the role and purpose of the sleep system? It is probably safe to state that everyone in the field of sleep research has these questions, in some form, at the root of his efforts. Measuring the length of REM periods and comparing them with changes in blood pressure probably has some intrinsic interest of its own; but more likely the researcher is probing at the question of whether REM periods cause blood pressure changes, or blood pressure changes cause REM periods. This bears on other questions, such as: Is sleep a cause or an effect? Or is it sometimes one and sometimes the other, or perhaps just part of a continuing sequence of events? Does it play different roles under different conditions, or are some of its roles constant over all conditions? Is its loss to be lamented, as Macbeth lamented the sleep deprivation threat, or is its approach to be feared, as Hamlet feared his REM periods? These are higher-ordered questions, all of which depend on the answers to the lower-ordered ones. But where is the theory necessary to postulate answers to these questions which will take into account the many bits and pieces of descriptive data already available?

The sleep researcher, busy with his voluminous data, finds it more feasible to continue to examine sleep under different conditions and to keep his theoretical tendencies in check, than to close down his laboratory for a couple of years while he considers the logical implications of the data on hand. He knows, too, that every other sleep researcher is also producing data by the mile. Construction of the theoretical framework on which to hang all these data is largely left to chance.

What then does the randomly forming structure of the body of sleep research look like? What directions is it taking?

A listing of the abstracts of papers presented to the annual meeting of the Association for the Psychophysiological Study of Sleep should provide answers. This listing is shown for the years 1967 and 1968 in Table 1.

In 1967 the Association grouped the 94 papers presented at its annual meeting under no less than 11 topics, which includes 7 papers in a category called "Varied Topics" and 25 papers relegated to "Miscellaneous." In 1968 the number of topics jumped to 15 for 129 papers presented, of which only 10 were relegated to the miscellaneous pile. Closer examination of the lists of topics for the two years also reveals that only 4 of the topics used in 1967 were used again in 1968, and this includes "Miscellaneous." Therefore, if we exclude "Varied Topics," we find that in the course of two successive annual meetings of the APSS, papers were presented under a total of 22 different topics. Quite a range of activity when one realizes that this constitutes only 223 different papers!

The above by no means indicates a criticism of the Association or its program chairmen. In fact, a perusal of the abstracts themselves indicates that without some organizational effort, these 22 subgroups could quite reasonably have been split into double that number.

The topics covered range all the way from Ontogeny of Penile Erections During Sleep in Infants [9] to Sleep and Dreaming in the Elephant [8]. The research was conducted on both humans and animals; investigators looked at sleep in connection with such variables as age, schizophrenia, response to drugs, aggressive behavior,

TABLE 1[a]. *Abstracts of papers presented to the 1967 and 1968 annual meetings of the Association for the Psychophysiological Study of Sleep*

1967		1968	
Topic	Number of Abstracts	Topic	Number of Abstracts
1. Environmental effects	9	1. Environmental effects	12
2. Dream content	13	2. Dream content	21
3. Neurophysiology	4	3. Neurophysiology	5
4. Autonomic functions	4	4. Phylogeny	5
5. Varied topics	7	5. Theory	6
6. Developmental, circadian	2	6. Drug effects	12
7. Symposium, EEG scoring	1	7. Neurochemistry	8
8. Biochemistry	7	8. Mental retardation	5
9. REM deprivation	13	9. Computer analysis	3
10. Sleep pathology	9	10. Biological rhythms	6
11. Miscellaneous	25	11. Physiology	6
		12. Ontogeny and pregnancy	11
		13. Psychopathology	7
		14. Deprivation	12
		15. Miscellaneous	10
Total	94	Total	129

[a]See references [1] and [2].

pregnancy, biological rhythms, selective deprivation, neuro-humoral mechanisms, smoking, dream recall, placebo effects, wakefulness, asthmatic attacks, bruxism, hypothalamic lesions, mental retardation, noise, temperature, and oxygen availability, to list just a few of the topics within topics. Animals studied include the crocodile, cat, field frog, tree frog, monkey (*Macaca nemistrina*), monkey (*Macaca mulatta*), hedgehog, elephant, rat, mouse, and the spiny anteater.

The above, of course, is not all of the sleep research being conducted, since only some unknown portion less than 100 percent of ongoing sleep research is reported at such meetings. The 1969 meeting of the APSS brought forth additional topics, subtopics, and species. Clearly the above serves to illustrate the fact that sleep research is being attacked from all directions at once.

In the midst of this welter of topics, one finds a slim total of 6 papers under the heading of Theory. It seems that despite the diversity, or perhaps because of it, it is much easier to find out what sleep researchers are doing than it is to find out why they are doing it. Therefore the first task is obvious: a taxonomy of sleep data into meaningful categories, subdivisions, and types in order to classify data already collected. Variables being investigated in all species could be defined, and the changes in these variables under different conditions could be listed.

Once this classification is accomplished, it would become obvious that some areas have been neglected, some overstudied. Such classification would indicate possible relationships between categories of information already on hand. Bodies of related data would begin to emerge. For example, normative values for sleep parameters appear in many unrelated pieces of sleep research, but where is there a standard list of normative values for the amounts, percents, lengths, and periodicity of each of the five sleep stages in human beings, let alone the spiny anteater? True, there are articles in print setting forth norms for certain age groups of human subjects [5], but the groupings are broad, they are not usually separated by sex, the results are based on small numbers of subjects, and some age groups are missing. The missing groups and the sex differences may be filled in by reference to other pieces of research—research done at another time, in another place, using slightly different measures and terminology, and for another purpose.

In short, in this electronic age, the accuracy with which a capsule is sent out into space and returned to earth is considerably greater than the accuracy with which the required sleep parameters of its occupants can be stated. This is true largely because no one has set out to record, standardize, and list the necessary measurements for all relevant groupings of subjects.

Next, it is obvious from the topics listed by the APSS that current research in sleep is first-, second-, and third-order research, with perhaps the largest effort in second-order research, and the next largest in third-order research. This means that before there is a clear definition of the important variables of sleep under different conditions, investigators are attempting to relate the sleep system to other systems. There is no necessary stipulation that all research should be completed on one level before the next level is attempted. It is quite possible to clock the speed of two different automobiles at the same time, even though one knows nothing about the mechanical attributes of either automobile. But this assumes that someone *does* know the mechanical attributes in detail, and that comparing these two cars is a reasonable thing to do. If not, then the comparison could be pointless—as for instance, if one has a motor designed to pull heavy loads, and the other is built solely for speed. Trial and error comparisons will, of course, produce data: we can test for speed, then ease of handling, then endurance, power, load capacity, and so forth. But this is not an economical way to do research. A more detailed knowledge of the component parts of each of the automobiles would make it possible to find many of the answers by simple computations rather than costly test runs.

To some extent, the same is true of sleep research. In some cases it is inefficient to compare the sleep system with another set of variables when the sleep variables involved are still ill-defined and their range and variation under different conditions are unknown. For example, it would be pointless to conduct an investigation of the use of sleep-inducing drugs during the course of some pathological condition if the sleep patterns under that same condition without the drug were unknown.

Therefore a compendium of the entire range of measurements on the standardized set of sleep variables under all relevant conditions would be useful to any investigator attempting to correlate the sleep system with some other system. Obviously such correlations should not have to wait until this compendium is complete, but if the established data were systematized, then there would be empty cells waiting for all new data uncovered. The periodic table of elements did not halt research in chemistry; it did organize information already available and indicate where the gaps were. Such organization is obviously needed in sleep research at this point.

A similar development on the relationships of sleep with other body processes would likewise serve to inventory what has already been done, what still awaits investigation, and what studies should be repeated for verification of results. Correlations are performed in the absence of reasons to assume cause and effect relationships. But when strong correlations are found, it is then reasonable to test for whether or not one of the variables is actually dependent upon the other, or if a third variable is influencing both. There are enough data emanating from research on the concomitant variation of different systems during sleep for some theoretical postulations to emerge regarding such relationships. This would direct the choice of dependent variables and result in more efficient studies. Sleep research is too expensive for trial and error experiments.

In contrast to the rest of the field of sleep research, the whole matter of dreams is heavily burdened with theory, most of which could be more accurately described as folklore. Hartmann's recent work [7] does bring together in one well-organized volume what is currently known about the biological concomitants of stage 1-REM. But his discussion, "The Functions of the D-State," makes it clear that current "theories" about the phenomenon of dreaming itself, apart from the biological changes of stage 1-REM, are for the most part untested, or untestable, as they now stand.

Unlike the sleep stages, which can be recorded directly from subject to EEG paper, untouched by time lag or human interpretation, dreams can be obtained only in retrospect and in response to the experimenter's question. Enough has been written at this point about the effect of the experimenter on the subject's responses to make it clear that with properly directed questioning, one can govern the amount and content of dream reporting, whether or not one intends to. In addition there are great individual differences in recall and in ability to verbalize thoughts and feelings. There are also differences in motivation, depending upon the rapport between subject and experimenter. Literally, the experimenter is at the mercy of the subject in this situation.

Therefore adherence to rigorously standardized procedures and measurements is mandatory in order to avoid the introduction of extraneous variables—such as the subject's motivations or the experimenter's.

The amount of dream research presently being conducted and the general regression toward simplicity has a tendency to transform suggestion into fact as follows: Aserinsky and Kleitman's discovery [4] of the correlation between REM periods and dreaming, and the corroboration of this finding by many investigators since then, has gradually led to an equating of REM with dreams. The result is that the two terms are becoming synonymous, and the REM period is often referred to as the dream period. But the findings by Aserinsky and Kleitman, and everyone since then, actually were that a correlation existed, not that REM caused dreams or dreams caused REM, or that all dreams occurred during REM, or that all REM periods contained dreams. In fact the Dement and Kleitman [5] findings stated that 80 percent of REM awakenings and 7 percent of NREM awakenings resulted in dream reports. Since dreams themselves cannot be monitored, all we really know is that there is more dream reporting during REM than during NREM. This still leaves open the possibility that the increased autonomic activity of the REM period stamps more into memory than does the relative quiescence of the NREM periods. For all we know, dreams may occur uniformly throughout the night, with REM dreams being more readily recalled than NREM dreams; or perhaps the subject is more verbal immediately after REM than after the deeper stages of NREM. But the practice of awakening the subject for dream recall only during or after an REM period is becoming built into the technology of sleep research. This can result in what may be a well-constructed fallacy, i.e., that REM equals dreaming. Even if this equation turns out to be true, the fact is being neglected that sometimes NREM equals dreaming. A theory of dreaming based entirely on REM periods will still have this fact to explain.

Lack of precise methodology in dream research is also allowing other fallacies to slip through unnoticed, such as the implication that longer dream reports indicate longer dreams, when it could easily be illustrated that one could contemplate in a second what would take several hundred words to describe; that more detailed dream reports indicate more detailed dreams, when no check of the difference in subjects' verbal ability has been made; that a night of little dreaming is followed by a night of increased dreaming, thus "proving" a need for dreaming. (This is only true if REM equals dreams, which has not yet been proved. All we know is that REM deprivation is followed by increased REM. Since the subject can and does dream during NREM, the "need" could just as well be attributed to some other REM-linked activity.)

In short, dream research has two urgent needs at the present time: (1) rigorous elimination or control of all extraneous variables which could in any way bias the subject's reporting of dreams, followed by careful manipulation of independent variables, one at a time, in order to determine their effects on dream reports, and (2) consistent theory which bears directly on rigorously collected data.

As in all aspects of sleep research, or any scientific endeavor, theories about dreams must be testable. An untestable theory contributes little more than a convenient repository for unexplained events. It also contributes the feeling that the matter has been "explained," and it thereby impedes the research for a true explanation.

Consider, for example, a theory which states that dreams wipe out useless thoughts of the day. To begin with, it would be impossible to define a "useless thought" since no one can judge, especially for someone else, what random thoughts of the day just might come in handy the next day. Even if such thoughts could be defined, how can it be determined that they have been "wiped out"? If dreams really wiped out a "useless thought," then the subject could never report the useless thought that was wiped out. If we were to ask the subject to list for us all useless thoughts before going to bed, this procedure in itself would probably determine that he would recall most of them the next day.

But armed with this "theory," we can safely say that any trivia that is not remembered the next day was wiped out the night before by dreams, because it will be impossible for anyone to either confirm or deny such a statement. Therefore, the "theory" stands—not because it has any validity, but because it is untestable. But of what use is it? Can we safely pour "useless thoughts" into a subject, fully confident that he will have been relieved of them by the following day? How does the somnolent subject manage to make this fine discrimination between useful and useless thoughts when he is apparently incapable of doing so while he is awake? And how does the thought get "wiped out"? We do not even know yet how memories get stamped in, much less how they are removed.

The theory does not submit to any test because the variables with which it deals are undefined and undefinable. Since it cannot be proved wrong any more than it can be proved right, it remains as a hunch to be tossed in as a solution to the mystery of why people dream. But the mystery remains unsolved.

A completely new approach to the problems of dream research is needed: one which strips away the weight of baroque theories which are patently untestable, one which operationally defines the variables it seeks to measure, and one which eliminates the contamination of other variables. It is too late in the history of science for such a well-engineered discipline as sleep research to have one of its most interesting appurtenances—the dream—supported by archaic methodology.

In general then the field of sleep research needs what any new field of science needs as the data begin to pour in—organization. This organization will bring into focus the conflicting reports of different investigators and will force standardization and operational definition of the variables. This will have a sharpening influence on research. Relationships now being sought will have a higher probability of being found—if they are there. It is difficult to state exactly when theory should enter a field of inquiry and exert its structuring influence. But the avalanche of data now pouring out of sleep laboratories leaves little doubt that for this field, formal theory is already overdue; and for dream research, conjecture has posed as theory for too long. If dreams are to emerge from the provinces of the mystic, and take their place on the EEG machine along with stages 1 through 4, then the methodology and the theory applied to them must also emerge.

In short, in only two decades, sleep research with all of its concomitants has come of age. It is time for the puberty rites of re-evaluation. The next two decades should see it attain full stature as a science.

REFERENCES

1. *Abstracts of Papers Presented to the Sixth Annual Meeting of the Association for the Psychophysiological Study of Sleep.* The Society for Psychophysiological Research, Los Angeles, 1967.
2. *Abstracts of Papers Presented to the Seventh Annual Meeting of the Association for the Psychophysiological Study of Sleep.* The Society for Psychophysiological Research, Denver, 1968.
3. Aserinsky, E. Physiological Activity Associated with Segments of the Rapid Eye Movement Period. In S. Kety, E. Evarts, and H. L. Williams (Eds.), *Sleep and Altered States of Consciousness. Res. Publ. Ass. Res. Nerv. Ment. Dis.* 45:338, 1967.
4. Aserinsky, E., and Kleitman, N. Two types of ocular motility occurring in sleep. *J. Appl. Physiol.* 8:11, 1955.
5. Dement, W. C., and Kleitman, N. The relation of eye movements during sleep to dream activity: An objective method for the study of dreaming. *J. Exp. Psychol.* 53:339, 1957.
6. Feinberg, I., and Carlson, V. R. Sleep variables as a function of age in man. *Arch. Gen. Psychiat.* (Chicago) 18:239, 1968.
7. Hartmann, E. *The Biology of Dreaming.* Springfield, Ill.: Thomas, 1967.
8. Hartmann, E., Bernstein, J., and Wilson, C. Sleep and Dreaming in the Elephant. *Abstracts of Papers Presented to the Seventh Annual Meeting of the Association for the Psychophysiological Study of Sleep* 4:3:389, 1968.
9. Karacan, I., Marans, A., Barnett, A., and Lodge, A. Ontogeny of Penile Erection During Sleep in Infants. *Abstracts of Papers Presented to the Seventh Annual Meeting of the Association for the Psychophysiological Study of Sleep* 4:3:363, 1968.
10. Webb, W. B. *Sleep: An Experimental Approach.* New York: Macmillan, 1968.

Knowledge is Power

Knowledge is power. All power corrupts. Are there signs of corruption in this field of knowledge? Can knowledge from sleep-dream research be misused?

No answers received. Silence.

*Appendix A**

THE D-STATE†*: A Review and Discussion of Studies on the Physiologic State Concomitant with Dreaming*

ERNEST HARTMANN

Throughout recorded history man has been fascinated by his dreams, whether he considered them the voyages of his soul, the conveyors of messages from the gods, the perverse products of a poorly oxygenated brain, the psychoses of the sane man or the *via regia* to the unconscious. Even after Freud's[1] great work on dreams, and after it had been accepted that dreams had a meaning in terms of the unconscious wishes of the dreamer, dreaming was considered a fleeting, probably instantaneous phenomenon superimposed on the solid physiologic state of sleep; likewise, the various properties of dreaming, in almost all psychologic and psychoanalytic formulations, were based on the properties of the state of sleep.

Recent work, to be reviewed in this article, casts doubt on this formulation. It had been known for some time that there were several different electroencephalographic configurations, all associated with behavioral sleep, and these had been numbered from one to four, the numbers supposedly representing sleep depth, since stage 1, a low-voltage, fast cortical pattern, was seen at the onset of sleep and resembled the electroencephalogram of the waking state, whereas stage 4, consisting of large slow waves, usually developed only after a few minutes of sleep, and looked the least like an encephalogram with the subject awake. However, it was not until 1953 that Aserinsky and Kleitman[2] discovered, in a series of original studies, that four or five periods during an average night's sleep were characterized by rapid conjugate eye movements, as

* Reprinted with permission from the *New England Journal of Medicine* 273:30–35, 87–92 (July 1 & 8), 1965.

† From the Department of Psychiatry, Tufts University School of Medicine, and the Boston State Hospital.

well as by a stage-1 electroencephalogram, and that subjects awakened during these periods almost always reported that they had been dreaming. Thus, sleep was found to be cyclical (Fig. 1), with regular periodic "emergence" to stage 1 with eye movements, occurring predictably four or five times a night, and with fairly regular intervals between these periods.[3-5] The first such period never occurs under ordinary conditions until fifty to ninety minutes after the onset of sleep. The association of these periods with dream reports is impressive but, of course, not perfect (Table 1).

Accordingly, it seems likely that people dream not for brief moments while awakening, nor all the time, but at specified periods during the night totaling about ninety minutes in an average night's sleep. Recent studies, which will be reviewed in greater detail later, demonstrate that these periods, associated with dreaming in human beings, probably occur in all mammalian species, and have a distinct physiology—including not only eye movements and low-voltage fast electroencephalograms but also characteristic changes in pulse, blood pressure, respirations and muscle potential—and have a distinct neurophysiology, including the activity of a specific pontine center.[16-19]

This state accompanying dreaming has been called light sleep, since the electroencephalographic pattern looks like that of light sleep, but it has also been referred to as deep sleep, since in most species it is hardest to wake the animal from this state, and since the resting muscle potential, which is lowered during "slow-wave" sleep, drops out entirely during this "dreaming sleep." Present evidence makes it more reasonable to call this state not light or deep sleep, but a qualitatively different kind of sleep, as suggested by Oswald et al.[20] and Jouvet,[17] or (since it basically resembles ordinary sleep as little as it resembles waking) a third organismic state, as suggested by Snyder.[19] Accordingly,

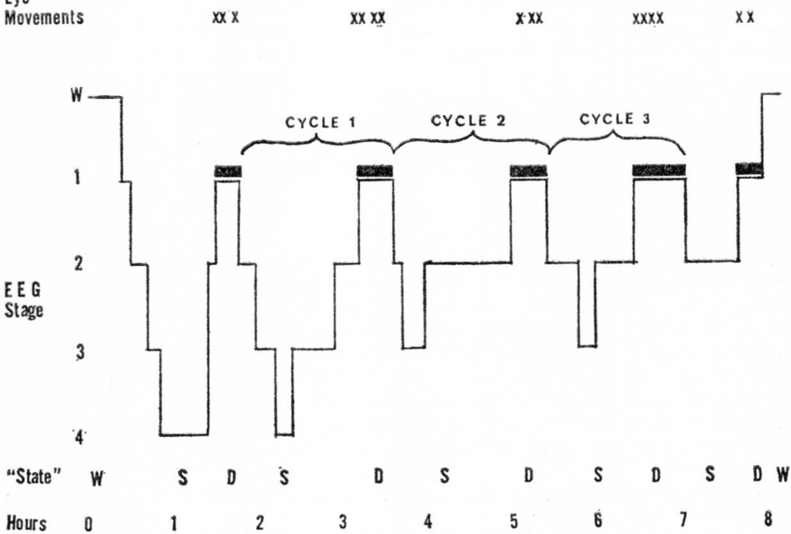

FIGURE 1. *Typical night's sleep in a young adult*

TABLE 1. *Periods of "emergence" (D-state) in relation to dream reports.**

Source of Data	No. of Subjects	Total No. of Awakenings	Criteria of Dream Recall	Percentage of Dream Recall: D-state Awakenings	Percentage of Dream Recall: S-state Awakenings
Aserinsky & Kleitman[3]	10	50	Definite recall of dream content	74	7
Dement[6]	10	70	Vivid recall of content	88	0
Dement & Kleitman[5]	9	351	Coherent, fairly detailed description	79	7
Wolpert & Trosman[7]	10	91	Detailed recall of complete drama	85	0
Goodenough et al.[8]	16	190	A dream recalled in some detail	69	34
Jouvet et al.[9]	4	50	Not specified	60	3
Snyder[10]	16	237	Content recalled in some detail	62	13
Wolpert[11]	8	88	Not specified	85	24
Kremen[12] (Series II)	9	57	Subject's impression of dreaming, regardless of content	75	12
Rechtschaffen et al.[13]	17	282	Some specific content	86	23
Foulkes[14]	8	244	Specific content	82	54
Orlinsky[15]	25	908	Any specific content	86	42

* Adapted from Snyder.[10]

the term "D-state" will be used here to designate this physiologic state, which has been variously referred to in the literature as "Rapid Eye Movement Sleep," "Emergent stage 1," "Stage 1-REM," "Activated sleep," "Rapid sleep," "Light sleep," "Deep sleep," "Rhombencephalic sleep" and "Paradoxical phase."

The remainder of this review will attempt to summarize and organize the large number of recent studies investigating the properties of the D-state.

PHYLOGENY OF THE D-STATE

This third state, unrecognized until ten years ago, has now been described in the opossum,[21] the mouse,[22] the rat,[22,23] the rabbit,[22,24] the cat,[9,16] the dog,[25] the sheep,[26] the goat,[27] the monkey,[28] the chimpanzee[29] and, of course, man. It does not require any great speculative leap, therefore, to postulate that the D-state is found in all mammalian species, especially since there are no reports of failure to find it when the proper techniques have been used. It must be admitted that the aquatic mammals, whales and dolphins, have not yet been studied in this light. According to one report by Jouvet[30] on chickens, it is possible that birds have very brief periods resembling the D-state in mammals, but this has not been adequately confirmed. Despite several attempts, no one has as yet found any evidence of this state in reptiles or "lower" forms.[30,31]

There are differences between the various mammalian species in such properties of the D-state as the amount of hippocampal theta rhythm, the increase or decrease in mean pulse rates and others, but at present it appears that the similarities greatly outweigh the differences and that the D-states in different species are truly homologous.

The amount of time spent in the D-state varies considerably, from about 2 per cent of total time asleep in the adult sheep[26] to 20 to 60 per cent of time asleep in the adult cat[9] (Table 2). The significance of these differences is not known. The cycle length, or the average length of time from the beginning of one D-period to the beginning of the next, varies from three or four minutes

TABLE 2. *D-state in various mammalian species (young adult animals)**

Species	Average Length of D-Period *min.*	Average Cycle Length *min.*	D-Time as Percentage of Total Sleep
Man	14	80–90	20–24
Monkey	4–10	40–60	11–20
Cat	10	20–40	20–60
Sheep	—	—	2–3
Rabbit	—	24	1–3
Rat	4–7	7–13	15–20
Mouse	—	3–4	—
Opossum	5	17	22–40

* Based on data taken from work of many authors.

in the mouse[22] to about ninety minutes in adult man. There does seem to be a rough relation of cycle length with other characteristics of the species—apparently, the larger animals with a longer life-span and a lower metabolic rate tend to have longer cycles.

ONTOGENY OF THE D-STATE

One of the most fascinating aspects of these studies is the finding that, at least in the species investigated from this point of view (man, cat and sheep), the very young always seem to spend more time in the D-state than the adult of the species.[26,32,33] A compilation of the studies of a number of laboratories (Table 3) shows that a young human adult spends 20 to 25 per cent of his total

TABLE 3. *Ontogeny of the D-state*

Subject	Time Spent in D-State as Percentage of Total Time Asleep
Premature infant	50–80
Neonate (1–15 days)	45–65
Infant <2 yr. old	25–40
Child 2–5 yr. old	20–30
Child 5–13 yr. old	15–20
Adolescent 13–18 yr. old	15–20
Young adult 18–30 yr. old	20–25
Adult 30–50 yr. old	18–25
Older adult 50–70 yr. old	13–18

sleep time in the D-state; this amount decreases to about 15 per cent in older subjects, but the most remarkable finding is that the figure is as high as 30 to 40 per cent in young children, about 50 per cent in neonates[33] and apparently even higher in premature infants.[34] (It should be mentioned that the electroencephalogram is not a very reliable index in neonates or premature infants, so that in these cases the presence of the D-state is judged mainly by eye movements, muscle potential and pulse and respiratory changes.) Taken in conjunction with the fact that neonates spend about 75 per cent of their total day asleep, and premature infants even more, it is obvious that a tremendous amount of time is spent in the D-state at this age, probably more than is spent in either the waking (W) state or the nondreaming sleep (S) state. One might speculate that the fetus *in utero* spends most or all of its time in the D-state, or at least in a state that later develops into "dreaming sleep." Jouvet[32] has lent some support to this possibility by his finding of up to 100 per cent D-time in the newborn kitten.

It is hard to believe that the newborn child or kitten has well-formed dreams as adult human beings know them (although some interesting speculations about the dream content could no doubt be made), and yet it appears that the D-state, which later in life is associated with dreaming, is ontogenetically an earlier, more primitive state than the states that later mature into "waking" or "nondreaming sleep."

PERIPHERAL PHYSIOLOGY OF THE D-STATE

Vegetative Function

A wide variety of functions have been studied in human beings, and a few of these also in cats and other species. The respiratory rate is one of the best studied: most workers have found a higher mean respiratory rate in the D-state than in the rest of sleep (S-state), but the respiratory irregularity, the change in rate from one minute to the next, is more characteristic of the D-state than the change in mean respiratory rate.[2,9,35,36] The pulse rate behaves in a similar fashion: in man at least the mean pulse rate is increased during the D-state, but the irregularity is far more striking than the increase in mean rate.[19] Blood pressure has not been studied as thoroughly because of the technical difficulties of all-night recording, but again the principal finding appears to be greatly increased irregularity and variability from one minute to the next.[37] One might suppose that such shifts in blood pressure might be quite dangerous to a patient with cardiac disease, and in this connection it is interesting that as early as 1921, before any of this work was known, MacWilliam,[38] pondering the sudden deaths during sleep of patients with heart disease, speculated that it was probably caused by blood-pressure changes associated with dreaming; he took some random single recordings on some of his patients and on a few occasions did find high levels, quite outside the range usually associated with sleep.

The galvanic skin response, one of the psychophysiologists' favorite measures, has, of course, been studied during sleep, but there are difficult technical problems in long-term recordings, and up to now the results have not been clear. Several studies show no consistent pattern of changes of galvanic skin response during the D-periods.

An interesting recent finding is that in human males, full or partial penile erections almost always accompany D-periods.[39] These have been found to occur in all subjects studied, in over 90 per cent of the D-periods and apparently regardless of the manifest content of the dream.

In summary, one might say that almost all measures of autonomic activity are different, and are in a sense activated, during D-periods—as opposed to nondreaming sleep, during which the respiratory rate, pulse and blood pressure all remain at a steady low level and there are probably no penile erections. The differences are sufficiently marked so that it is almost as easy to pick out D-periods from an all-night record of pulse and respirations as from the more commonly employed records of electroencephalogram and eye movements. In these respects the D-state is much more active even than quiet waking (lying in bed) and bears more resemblance to an active waking state.

Muscular System

The rapid eye movements have already been mentioned. These are very characteristic conjugate movements of the eyes, the actual movement usually taking one-tenth to two-tenths seconds. These are almost never found in nondreaming sleep, but they are very similar and perhaps identical in normal adults to conjugate movements of the eyes when following an object during the waking state. Although these eye movements are very useful in differentiating D-periods from nondreaming sleep they do not occur constantly during D-periods, but rather sporadically and in bursts. This is probably related to dream content and will be further discussed below.

Gross movements of the body are quite common during human sleep; these are generally found toward the beginning or the end of D-periods, but they sometimes occur at other times and are not pathognomonic of the D-state. Various minor sporadic movements of the facial muscles and of the paws in cats and dogs have been noted; these generally seem to be associated with D-periods, but this has not been studied in great detail. Human infants have especially prominent movements that include smiling, stretching, grimacing and sucking during D-periods[33]; the amount of movement decreases gradually with age.

However, the major change in the muscular system during the D-state is a distinct decrease or even a complete cessation of tonic muscle potential. This was first noted in the dorsal neck muscles of the cat[40] and is so clear cut in these muscles that in some laboratories the dropout of muscle potential is used instead of the electroencephalogram as an indicator of D-periods. This finding appears most prominently in the antigravity muscles, but is found to some extent in most striated muscles. The dropout of muscle potential has been noted in man, but appears somewhat less clear cut, and the results depend greatly on what muscles are studied.[41] It has been found that certain reflexes are greatly diminished during during the D-state,[42] and this may be due to a diminished sensitivity of the motor neurons.

NEUROPHYSIOLOGY OF THE D-STATE

A series of imaginative and careful studies, chiefly in the laboratory of Michel Jouvet, has greatly increased our knowledge of what is going on in the brain during the D-state, as opposed to S-state sleep, and of what regions are involved in initiating and maintaining the D-state.[17,18,43] His group first observed that not only the cortex but also many other parts of the brain show an "activation" during the D-state. The diencephalon and mesencephalon tend to show a low-voltage, fast activity; the pons shows occasional spindle-like activity of 6 to 8 per second, and the hippocampus is characterized by a striking activity of 5 to 6 per second similar to that found in an active waking state. This work was done in the cat, but similar results have been reported by others in the rat[22] and the opossum.[21]

Jouvet's group then did a series of brain transection studies in the cat, aimed at localizing an area responsible for the D-state. They found that a decorticate animal, or an animal with a complete transection through the anterior border of the mesencephalon, still showed recurrent D-periods, identified by rapid eye movements and dropout of muscle potential, both of which are controlled from below the level of the lesion. Cortical activation, of course, no longer occurred during D-periods in these animals. They next studied a series of animals with complete transections through the middle of the mesencephalon ("cerveau isolé" preparations) or through the anterior border of the pons; in these animals recurrent D-periods were still noted, although now identified only by muscle-potential dropout (and respiratory changes), since the nuclei of the third, fourth and sixth cranial nerves were above the level of the lesion. Then, they studied a group of animals with transections at the lower border of the pons, and in these animals no evidence of D-periods was seen. Thus, it appeared that a pontine structure was responsible, and for this reason some workers usually refer to what is here called the D-state as pontine or rhombencephalic sleep. Jouvet's group confirmed this localization by a series of coagulation studies. They found that by entirely destroying a nucleus in the central pons (nucleus reticularis pontis caudalis), they obtained an animal with no evidence of the D-state, although it continued to show periods of waking and of slow-wave sleep (S-state).[18] Thus, it appears that the D-state is controlled, or at least initiated, by a center in the pons, one of the most primitive parts of the brain. A number of laboratories have been investigating the pathways whereby this center transmits its impulses upward to achieve activation of the cortex and downward to achieve inhibition of muscle potential and decreased sensitivity of the motor neurons; these pathways, however, have not yet been established.

There have been some important neurophysiologic experiments using microelectrodes to study single units (neurons) in various parts of the brain. For instance, Huttenlocher[44] has reported that many units in the mesencephalon of the cat show a very high spontaneous activity during the D-state, much higher than in S-state sleep, but that evoked potentials in the same neurons are lower during D. Likewise, Evarts[45] has observed high spontaneous activity in single units in the visual pathways and the visual cortex during the D-state, much higher than in S-sleep and about similar to spontaneous activity in an active waking state. Incidentally, this provides the best evidence available at present that cats probably experience visual dreams.

One group of researchers has found that cortical blood flow is about 30 to 50 per cent higher during D than during S[46]; the significance of this is not yet clear, but it certainly adds to the impression that almost anything one can measure is different during the D-state and that the D-state represents a distinctly different neurophysiologic organization from that found in ordinary sleep. The studies reviewed above, which establish the existence of a pontine center specifically responsible for the initiation of D-periods, supply the best support for this thesis.

NECESSITY FOR THE D-STATE

In 1886 W. Robert[47] wrote that dreams are a safety valve of the mind, allowing the tensions accumulated during the day to be discharged. He further stated, ". . . a human being deprived of the possibility of dreaming would have to become mentally disturbed after some time. . . ." Interestingly enough, a number of recent experiments have lent strong support to this formulation; however, it must be remembered that the modern studies refer to the effects of deprivation of the entire D-state, not only deprivation of the psychic experience of dreaming. Dement[48] described a classic experiment on "dream deprivation" in 1960. Using 5 normal human subjects, he first deprived them of "dreaming" for five nights in a row, by the simple device of awakening them whenever their electroencephalographic and eye-movement records indicated that they were entering the D-state. Such a procedure could not be expected to deprive them completely of D-periods, but it did succeed in reducing their D-time per night by 80 to 90 per cent. He then allowed the subjects to sleep in the laboratory for five "recovery" nights, without awakenings. He noted three very significant findings. In the first place, it required more and more awakenings to keep the subjects from having D-periods. During the first night of deprivation four or five awakenings were sufficient, one at the start of the usual four or five nightly D-periods; however, by the fifth night of deprivation the subjects made increasingly frequent attempts to have D-periods, so that twenty to thirty awakenings were required. Secondly, during the "recovery nights" the D-time was markedly increased, often taking up 30 to 40 per cent of total sleep time; it appeared that the subjects were trying to "make up for" lost D-time. Finally, in the daytime, during the deprivation period, the subjects were noted to be unusually tense and irritable, acting as though they had been deprived of a great deal of sleep, although actually they had slept six to seven hours a night. In a control study done later on the same 5 subjects, in which they were subjected to the same number of awakenings, but during S-state sleep, none of these three results occurred: clearly the effects were not due merely to the stress of being awakened frequently at night. These findings certainly suggest a "need for dreaming" or at least a need for the D-state. The recovery-after-deprivation effect has also been found by Jouvet[17,18] in cats—even those in which the entire brain above the pons has been removed and the experience of "dreaming" is highly unlikely. In these experiments, of course, only the first and second of Dement's effects were looked for and found—the increase in awakenings necessary and the increased D-time during recovery periods; there was no attempt to judge increased irritability in the cat.

Very recently Dement[49] has done further studies on 3 human subjects, involving up to fifteen nights of dream deprivation. He found all the effects previously mentioned, but to an increased extent: it became so hard to awaken subjects toward the end of the fifteen-day period that premedication with dextroamphetamine sulfate (Dexedrine) was necessary to allow the experiment to continue. The recovery periods showed a few nights of extremely high D-values—up to 60 per cent of total sleep. And perhaps most interesting, not only did the subjects become irritable during the daytime, but 2 of them showed distinct personality changes, one in a paranoid direction, and the other in the direction of levity and giggling quite unusual for the subject, thus fulfilling Robert's original prediction.

In any event a very definite need for the D-state has been established, and it may be that the D-state is the really necessary portion of sleep, since the psychologic effects of "dream deprivation" so closely resemble those found in other reports of total sleep deprivation.[50-52] However, it seems most likely that there is a need for the S-state as well as for the D-state, since subjects deprived of sleep often catch up on stage 4 (deep S-sleep) even before they catch up on lost D-time,[50] and in addition a preliminary study on "Stage 4 sleep deprivation"[53] showed some tendency for recovery of "lost" stage 4 sleep, although the effect was much less striking than that found in "dream deprivation."

PHARMACOLOGY AND THE D-STATE

A great many data, mostly from small informal studies, are available concerning the effect of drugs on the D-state, but as yet no definite pattern has emerged. A number of substances decrease the amount of time spent in the D-state. This is true in man for phenobarbital and several other barbiturates studied so far.[20] Phenothiazines likewise tend to decrease D-time; trifluoperazine

(Stelazine) has some confusing early effects[54] but probably actually decreases D-time like the others.[55] Alcohol has been shown to cause a decrease in D-time,[56] and in fact it has been suggested that delirium tremens may represent a state of acute "rebound" from dream deprivation—that is, the patient has had his D-time suppressed over a prolonged period while drinking, and the vivid hallucinatory state when he finally stops drinking represents an effort to "catch up" on D-time.[57,58] The authors present evidence for increased D-time after withdrawal from alcohol, but this is, of course, during sleep: the delirium-tremens condition is certainly not a typical D-period but might be seen as the condition of a "waking dreamer" in whom somehow both the mechanisms underlying the D-state and those underlying waking are operating at once.

Since hypnogenic and tranquilizing drugs have been shown to decrease D-time, it was thought that stimulants such as caffeine or the amphetamines might have the opposite effect. However, this does not turn out to be the case: caffeine apparently has little effect[56]; dextroamphetamine sulfate definitely reduces D-time, when it allows the subject to sleep at all.[59]

These studies have been done on man, but it appears that in general these groups of drugs have the same effect on cats; in addition it has been shown that large doses of atropine effectively suppress D-periods in cats[18] and rats.[60]

Thus, a variety of drugs appear to be able to depress D-time; it would certainly be useful to have a drug that would increase D-time or at least provide sound sleep with a normal amount of D-time, in view of the dangers of dream deprivation, but no such drug has yet been found. However, large doses of eserine, an acetylcholinesterase inhibitor, have a tendency to increase the length of D-periods in cats although total D-time is not definitely increased.[18] Lysergic acid diethylamide (LSD) has been found to have little effect, or if anything to decrease D-time in cats,[61] but a recent study shows that within a very narrow dosage range, it may lengthen at least one D-period during the night in man, without increasing total D-time for the night.[62]

Although there are no drugs that definitely increase D-time, one may with reasonable ease achieve a night of increased D-time pharmacologically by administering for a time, and then withdrawing, either phenothiazines, alcohol or dextroamphetamine sulfate.

Altogether, the pharmacologic findings do not point to any clear-cut conclusions as yet, except perhaps the conclusion that the D-state is quite fragile in the sense that it can be suppressed fairly easily either by drugs that increase sleep (S-sleep) or by those that increase wakefulness. In addition, the findings on atropine and the acetylcholinesterase inhibitors suggest that a cholinergic mechanism may be involved. This is supported, though only indirectly, by a number of reports on the effect of DFP (a potent cholinesterase inhibitor) in man[63]; one of the most common effects noted is "excessive dreaming" although, of course, this refers only to dream reports, since no electroencephalographic studies were done.

NEUROCHEMISTRY OF THE D-STATE

This is a field of inquiry that does not yet exist, but in my opinion it must make its appearance soon, since a recurrent, regular, basic biologic state such as the one under discussion, characterized by a well-defined neurophysiologic picture, almost certainly must have central chemical changes underlying it. And there are certain tentative indications of what neurochemical substances or mechanisms may be implicated.

Jouvet[18] has reported, though this has not been confirmed by other investigators, that it is possible to set off a D-period of fifteen to twenty minutes in cats by a very brief electric stimulation of the central pons during S-sleep and that after such a D-period there is a refractory period lasting for ten to fifteen minutes during which one cannot set off another D-period. Of course, this must be interpreted cautiously: it may mean only that one can set off a D-period by stimulation at just about the time another period would have appeared spontaneously. However, if one accepts these findings, the length of time involved suggests a neurohumoral mechanism; taking into account the previously mentioned findings on atropine, eserine and di-isopropyl fluorophosphate (DFP), one might conclude that acetylcholine is probably involved, at least in the discharge of the D-periods. This is hardly a very novel suggestion, however, since acetylcholine discharge is involved in many, or most, multineuron events in the nervous system.

Several kinds of evidence suggest that, in addition to this mechanism, there may be some substance that gradually accumulates during waking and nondreaming sleep and is then discharged or metabolized during D-periods; acetylcholine itself does not behave in this way, but another substance might build up and at a certain level act to stimulate certain areas and release acetylcholine. Evidence for this possibility comes first of all from the dream-deprivation studies mentioned previously[48]; it certainly appears in these studies that a "need to dream" builds up during the deprivation period. This is also supported by the informal finding in many laboratories that a patient who gets to bed much later than usual, or has slept poorly the night before, tends to have his first D-period much sooner after falling asleep than usual, as though he had built up a "need to dream." A study of the relation between the length of a non-dreaming sleep (S) period and the length of the subsequent D-period also bears this out: the finding is a positive correlation between the length of the S-period and of the following D-period, with the subject, time of night and other conditions held constant, but there is no correlation between a D-period and the following S-period.[64] This again implies that a "need to dream," actually a need for D, builds up during S, so that, other things being equal, a longer S period is followed by a longer D-period. Jouvet's cats with a complete destruction of the pontine nucleus (RPC nucleus) are also relevant here: these animals, as mentioned, continued to have ordinary-looking waking states and S-states but no longer had D-periods. They lived only a few months, during which they manifested a condition characterized by increasing tachycardia, agitation and episodes during which the cats looked about curiously, wiped nonexistent objects with their paws and appeared to the observers to be probably hallucinating.[18,30] The cats finally died in an apparently toxic condition after a period of coma. Again, this suggests the possibility that something that eventually became toxic to the animal was gradually accumulating during the prolonged time without D-periods.

All these studies, of course, only indicate the existence of an accumulable "tendency to have D-periods"; there is no present evidence that this "tendency" is actually represented by a chemical substance although this is perhaps the simplest explanation. Certainly, a combination of substances, the lack of a substance or altered sensitivities of certain cell groups might explain the facts as well. But to speculate further and assume that the accumulation of one or more substances is involved, are there any hints of what substance it might be? Two possibilities come to mind, both of them substances that are found in the central nervous system, that might build up in the way hypothesized and could act as neuromodulators—a term used by Freedman[65] to describe a substance that is not directly released at nerve endings, as true neurotransmitters are, but whose level in the nerve cell somehow influences events at the nerve endings and synapses. One is GABA, gamma-aminobutyric acid, and its claim to consideration comes from the tentative finding that gamma-butyrolactone, a closely allied substance, causes sound sleep with normal D-periods[30] and a recent report that the administration of sodium butyrate, very close to GABA in structure, may induce D-periods in cats.[66]

The other possibility is serotonin. The effects of LSD previously referred to, some very recent work on the effects of tryptophane[64,67] and reserpine[64] on the sleep-dream cycle and a great deal of indirect evidence[64] lend support to the possibility that serotonin is involved. Several of the so-called "paradoxical effects" of serotonin (for instance the fact that substances that increase brain serotonin levels seem to produce first a period of slow-wave electroencephalographic patterns, followed after a few minutes by low-voltage, fast activity) can perhaps be explained on the basis that increased brain or brainstem serotonin levels produce a "tendency to have D-periods" rather than either general "excitation" or "depression." But this is a very complex question that cannot be discussed in detail here and will, it is hoped, soon be elucidated by work in progress. This section has been intended only to indicate one field of inquiry that will probably become important in the near future, and some speculation has necessarily been involved.

D-STATE AND MENTAL ILLNESS

Hughlings Jackson wrote: "Find out about dreams and you will find out about insanity."[68] Jung[69] said, "Let the dreamer walk about and act like one awakened, and we have the clinical picture of dementia praecox." Freud,[1] of course, carried the same idea farther in his conception of primary process thinking. Therefore, when it was first discovered that one could determine objectively, by the electroencephalogram and eye movements, when a person was dreaming, it was believed that this would provide a key to the study of schizophrenia, or at least an excellent diagnostic test. It was clear that the amount of "dream time" should be very different in schizophrenia, though a good a priori argument could be made for changes in either direction. It was predicted that schizophrenic patients might not have dream periods at all during sleep since they "did their dreaming" while awake; on the other hand it was predicted that they obviously had a tremendous "need for dreaming" and thus should show far more D-time than other people. The facts, unfortunately, do not support either speculation, at least in the extreme forms cited above. Studies by Dement,[6] Feinberg et al.[70] and others on large mixed groups of schizophrenic patients have shown a mean D-time of about 20 to 25 per cent—the same as that in normal subjects. A further disappointment was that even hallucinating schizophrenic patients had normal D-times, as did those with very acute schizophrenia, at least in the series reported by Koresko, Snyder and Feinberg[71] and Feinberg and his associates.[70] A group of 6 middle-aged depressed patients likewise showed normal D-time.[20]

However, these negative results may not represent the entire picture: Rechtschaffen and Verdone[72] have reported a slight but significant correlation between anxiety, measured by the Taylor Manifest Anxiety Scale, and D-time in a population of college students. Fisher and Dement[73] mention a group of borderline patients whom they studied who consistently show a D-time of about 29 per cent, well above normal levels. They also report a case of a paranoid patient who normally had fairly high levels, around 30 per cent, whose D-time rose to over 50 per cent one night as he was becoming psychotic. Unfortunately, the patient had received trifluoperazine that day, which produces a confusing electroencephalographic picture when first administered, and therefore the actual D-time for that night was probably much lower than reported. However, these studies do give some reason to suspect that a high D-time may be associated with stress or certain forms of stress. A study of identical twins, discordant for schizophrenia, showed a much higher D-time, about 30 per cent, in the schizophrenic twin, although twins were expected to show quite similar records.[55] One long-term study of individual psychotic patients under standardized conditions, attempting to relate several measures of D-time with various ratings and measures of psychologic state, has also been conducted.[74] One manic-depressive patient in this study showed definitely high D-time when he was very depressed, with a gradual fall to normal as he improved; he did not have any manic periods during the twelve months of the study. Results on 2 other patients, 1 of whom was definitely schizophrenic and 1 borderline, did not show such a straightforward correlation.

Thus, the relation between mental illness or stress and amount of D-time is far from clear although there are a few positive hints that D-time may be related to stress or depression. Of course, it cannot be certain that one is really dealing with something significant when merely D-time is studied—perhaps some persons can somehow achieve twice as much "dreaming" or "discharge" in a given time as others; however, the work on D-deprivation and on length of D- and S-periods suggests that time spent in D is an important variable. There have been studies of other characteristics of the sleep-dream records of psychotic patients, such as the actual number of eye movements within D-periods, but these have not been very productive. One finding that has struck me as well as others is that the D-periods are not as clearly demarcated in schizophrenic patients as in normal persons. It is hard to decide from the record just where a D-period starts or ends since there are transitional periods sometimes marked both by signs of D, such as rapid eye movements, and signs of S-sleep, such as spindles. However, this is probably not specific to schizophrenia since it appears to some extent in the records of anxious subjects and those sleeping in the laboratory for the first time.

It was also thought that if indeed schizophrenia resembles dreaming, perhaps some of the electroencephalographic and physiologic criteria of the D-state could be found in schizophrenic patients while they were awake. The results so far have been entirely negative,[75] but this may be because only very crude and peripheral measures that can be applied to human subjects are available.

One other possible relation to mental illness concerns the onset of psychotic episodes. In these situations a patient is anxious and disturbed for a variety of reasons: he is unable to sleep or sleeps poorly and thus probably deprives himself of D-time to some extent; this makes him feel worse—more anxious; and a vicious circle may be set up. Furthermore, a patient in a prepsychotic state often has frightening dreams that quickly awaken him, thus farther depriving him of D-time even if superficially he appears to be getting enough sleep. The possibility should be considered that some of the symptoms associated with acute psychosis, such as excessive fantasies and visual hallucinations, are actually a result of superimposed D-deprivation, rather than part of the underlying psychiatric problem. Here, a drug is badly needed that will tranquilize and allow sleep, but without depriving the patient of further dreaming.

D-STATE AND DREAM CONTENT

Now that much of the work on the D-state, the physiologic organismic state concomitant with dreaming, has been reviewed and commented on, the discussion may return to the starting point, the dream itself, and consider what light these studies have shed on the experience of dreaming.

There have been a large number of such studies on dream content, stimulated by the ability to tell objectively when a subject is dreaming, and they cannot all be reviewed here. What this review will do is consider some of the most frequent and most interesting questions about dreaming and indicate what answers have been found or are being sought by work in progress.

One abvious question is whether the characteristics of the D-state, such as the eye movements, pulse, blood pressure and respiratory changes, have anything to do with the dream content. Do the dreamer's eyes move back and forth constantly if he is dreaming of watching a tennis match, for example, and does he stop breathing for a few seconds when he sees something startling or frightening in his dream? The answer at present is a tentative "yes." As far as the eye movements are concerned, there are various informal reports of dreams that involved a great deal of motion and were also found to include many eye movements on the record. One study has been done, involving only a few subjects, however, in which highly verbal, intelligent subjects were awakened from a D-period and asked to describe carefully just what they were looking at for the minute before awakening. From this report, judges who had not seen the records tried to predict how the subjects' eyes should have moved if they had indeed watched the scenes described for one minute. There was a very good corrspondence between the predicted eye movements and the subjects' actual recorded eye movements.[76] Incidentally, this study also strongly supports the present point of view that dreaming takes time—about as much time as watching the same events in waking life, in fact—and that one does not have a long dream in an instant.

The evidence for the other physiologic changes is not so good as that for the eye movements. Again, there is anecdotal evidence about very exciting dreams associated with large changes in pulse or respiratory rate; the only systematic study so far found a significant but not a very strong general relation between respiratory variability and the vividness or emotionality of the dream.[77]

However, it must be remembered that eye movements and changes in pulse and respirations also occur in decorticate cats and human beings,[18,78] in whom there is almost certainly no subjective experience of dreaming. Thus, perhaps the best formulation at present would be to say that a primitive state, the D-state, necessary to all mammals, involves eye movements and a general autonomic outflow, whether or not accompanied by the subjective experience of dreaming, but when this experience is present, it is somehow synchronized with the physiologic changes. The various possible patterns of feedback between activity in the visual cortex, which is presumably concomitant with the visual dream experience, and the physiologic changes and eye movements, cannot be discussed here.

Another interesting question is whether there are systematic differences between dreams at different times of night. It appears at present, from studies by Rechtschaffen et al.,[13] that there are such differences—specifically that dreams occurring later in the night, or nearer morning, tend to be more vivid, more emotional, more bizarre or, in other words, more "dreamlike." Further work is in progress to determine whether such vivid dreams are primarily associated with time of day, with amount of previous time in bed or with low body temperature.

A further question in this area would be whether the content of the four or five dreams on the same night is related in some way. Again, there are many anecdotal reports of content relation and some more formal studies[79,80] indicating that often the same content reoccurs or, more frequently, that the same problem is dealt with in successive dreams. At times the expression of the problem becomes more and more direct in successive dreams on the same night.

Another question of interest is whether external events can influence dreams or initiate dreams. It appears that an external stimulus, such as a sound, a light or a jet of water on the skin, can indeed be incorporated into the dream content, in about 20 to 60 per cent of the cases, if introduced during a D-period.[81] This has been confirmed informally in a number of laboratories, and it is possible that the percentage of incorporations would be higher if symbolic or greatly distorted incorporations were considered as well as the direct incorporations usually sought. Thus, a stimulus presented during a D-period can definitely be incorporated into the dream content; however, it has never been possible to initiate a D-period by introducing any kind of external stimulus during nondreaming sleep.

One final question, since all human beings under normal conditions spend approximately the same amount of time dreaming (about ninety minutes a night in young adults), is what is responsible for the tremendous differences in how much dreaming people claim to experience—a range all the way from "I've never had a dream in my life" to "I dream every night, sometimes several times a night."

The difference apparently does not lie in the amount of subjective experience accompanying the D-periods as they occur, since even someone who claims never to dream finds, to his surprise, that upon being put to sleep in the laboratory and awakened during a D-period, he does generally remember a dream that seems very like the dreams of others who normally recall their dreams.

Evidently, the differences must lie in the ability to remember one's dreams under ordinary conditions. There have been several studies comparing groups of "recallers"—subjects who frequently recall their dreams—and "nonrecallers."[8,82] It appears that "recallers" may have a little more D-time, on the average, but these differences are very slight. More important, there are general differences in personality between the two groups: chiefly it seems that the "recallers" are more introspective, more interestd in the workings of their minds and more tolerant of ambiguity than the "nonrecallers." In addition, more superficial, often conscious factors also obviously play a part in the recall of dreams. For instance, it is well known that a patient in psychoanalysis, whose analyst asks him about his dreams, will usually begin to recall more dreams; likewise, a conscious interest in dreams, in someone doing research on sleep and dreams, for example, is usually associated with increased dream recall. Also, frequent awakenings during the night are associated with greater recall, since a dream will generally be remembered if an awakening of at least a few minutes in length occurs during or soon after a D-period. Some persons claim that they dream only when they are ill or upset; this phenomenon is almost certainly the result of increased dream recall due to frequent awakenings during the night.

CONCLUSIONS

The D-state has been examined from a number of points of view, and conclusions have generally been drawn as the discussion progressed. It is clear that dreaming is associated with a basic biologic state, here called the D-state. Knowledge in this field is rudimentary, but it is growing rapidly and in many directions at once, like a young octopus. This discussion has attempted to indicate some of the directions of growth and what the tentacles seem to be grasping.

A few words should perhaps be said about the function of the D-state since the question of function always arises sooner or later. The answer is simple: the function of the D-state is not known, but in the context of present knowledge, the question does not seem a very useful one. It is much like asking the function of sleep or of waking, states that are much better known and whose function can still be argued endlessly. Certainly, it appears that the D-state is necessary for life, as are presumably the states of waking and sleeping, and in this sense its function is to keep the organism living; this is not a very specific or useful answer, however. One will probably achieve more by not asking for one basic function but by examining the various functions or roles of this state in the integrated functioning of the organism's chemistry, physiology and psychology. Even if it should be definitely proved, as seems possible, that there is a chemical substance that is somehow used up or destroyed during D and is toxic if not destroyed, one should not be satisfied with the formulation that *the* function of the D-state and of dreaming is to destroy a toxin.

One more comment on function is suggested: all the studies mentioned so far provide no grounds for accepting or rejecting Freud's basic thoughts on the dream itself—the formulation of the meaning of the dream as the fulfillment of an unconscious wish and the language of the dream as primary process. However, Freud's theory that the function of the dream is the preservation of sleep is open to question, since in fact stimuli threatening to disturb sleep and wake the sleeper never appear to initiate a dream. In this sense the dream or the D-state functions only to preserve itself. Also, the psychoanalytic formulations implying that certain aspects of the dream are due to the prevailing state of sleep should perhaps be re-examined in view of the present concept that the dream does not really occur in the state of sleep, but in a state of its own, the D-state.

It has been said that the study of dreams is a fool's errand, but it appears possible that this fool's errand will eventually lead the patient fool through the tortuous pathways of insanity, along the royal road to the unconscious and even across the shaky bridge between mind and body.

REFERENCES

1. Freud, S. Interpretation of dreams. In *Standard Edition of the Complete Psychological Works of Sigmund Freud.* 24 vol. Vol. 4. Edited by J. Strachey. London: Hogarth, 1953.
2. Aserinsky, E., and Kleitman, N. Regularly occurring periods of eye motility and concomitant phenomena during sleep. *Science* 118:273, 1953.
3. *Idem.* Two types of ocular motility occurring in sleep. *J. Appl. Physiol.* 8:1–10, 1955.
4. Dement, W., and Kleitman, N. Cyclic variations in EEG during sleep and their relation to eye movements, body motility, and dreaming. *Electroencephalog. & Clin. Neurophysiol.* 9:673–690, 1957.
5. *Idem.* Relation of eye movements during sleep to dream activity: objective method for study of dreaming. *J. Exper. Psychol.* 53:339–346, 1957.
6. Dement, W. Dream recall and eye movements during sleep in schizophrenics and normals. *J. Nerv. & Ment. Dis.* 122:263–269, 1955.
7. Wolpert, E., and Trosman, H. Studies in psychophysiology of dreams. *Arch. Neurol. & Psychiat.* 79:603–606, 1958.
8. Goodenough, D. R., Shapiro, A., Holden, M., and Steinschriber, L. Comparison of

"dreamers" and "nondreamers": eye movements, electroencephalograms, and recall of dreams. *J. Abnorm. & Social Psychol.* 59:295–302, 1959.

9. Jouvet, M., Michel, F., and Mounier, D. Analyse électroencephalographique comparée du sommeil physiologique chez le chat et chez l'homme. *Rev. neurol.* 103:189–205, 1960.
10. Snyder, F. Organismic state associated with dreaming. Presented at Conference on Psychoanalysis and Current Biological Thought, University of Wisconsin, Madison, June 13–15, 1963.
11. Wolpert, E. Studies in psychophysiology of dreams. II. Electromyographic study of dreaming. *Arch. Gen. Psychiat.* 2:231–241, 1960.
12. Kremen, I. Dream reports and rapid eye movements. Unpublished doctoral dissertation, Harvard University, Cambridge, Massachusetts, 1961.
13. Rechtschaffen, A., Verdone, P., and Wheaton, J. Reports of mental activity during sleep. *Canad. Psychiat. A. J.* 8:409–416, 1963.
14. Foulkes, W. Dream reports from different states of sleep. *J. Abnorm. & Social Psychol.* 65:14–25, 1962.
15. Orlinsky, D. Psychodynamic and cognitive correlates of dream recall. Unpublished doctoral dissertation, University of Chicago, Chicago, Illinois, 1962.
16. *Idem.* Occurrence of low voltage, fast electroencephalogram patterns during behavioral sleep in cat. *Electroencephalog. & Clin. Neurophysiol.* 10:291–296, 1958.
17. Jouvet, M. Telencephalic and rhombencephalic sleep in cat. In *Ciba Foundation Symposium on the Nature of Sleep.* Edited by G. E. W. Wolstenholme and M. O'Connor. 422 pp. Boston: Little, Brown, 1961.
18. Jouvet, M. Recherches sur les structures nerveuses et les mécanismes responsables des différentes phases du sommeil physiologique. *Arch. ital. biol.* 100:125–206, 1962.
19. Snyder, F. New biology of dreaming. *Arch. Gen. Psychiat.* 8:381–391, 1963.
20. Oswald, I., et al. Melancholia and barbiturates: controlled EEG, body and eye movement study of sleep. *Brit. J. Psychiat.* 109:66–78, 1963.
21. Snyder, F. Unpublished data.
22. Weiss, T. Sleep cycles in rodents. Report to Association for Psychophysiological Study of Sleep, Palo Alto, California, March 27–29, 1964.
23. Michel, F., Klein, M., Jouvet, D., and Valatx, J. Étude polygraphique du sommeil chez le rat. *Compt. rend. Soc. de biol.* 155:2289–2290, 1961.
24. Khazan, N., and Sawyer, C. Rebound recovery from deprivation of paradoxical sleep in rabbit. *Proc. Soc. Exper. Biol. & Med.* 114:536–539, 1963.
25. Shimazono, Y., et al. Correlation of rhythmic waves of hippocampus with behavior of dogs. *Neurol. medico. chir.* 2:82–88, 1960.
26. Jouvet, D., and Valatx, J. L. Étude polygraphique du sommeil chez l'agneau. *Compt. rend. Soc. de biol.* 156:1411–1414, 1962.
27. Ruckebusch, Y., and Bost, J. Activité corticale au cours de la somnolence et de la rumination chez la chèvre. *J. de physiol.* 54:409–410, 1962.
28. Weitzmann, E. Note on EEG and eye movements during behavioral sleep in monkeys. *Electroencephalog. & Clin. Neurophysiol.* 13:790–794, 1961.
29. Adey, W. R., Kado, R. T., and Rhodes, J. M. Sleep: cortical and subcortical recordings in chimpanzee. *Science* 141:932, 1963.
30. Jouvet, M. Studies on rhombencephalic sleep. Report to Association for Psychophysiological Study of Sleep, Palo Alto, California, March 27–29, 1964.
31. Snyder, F. Observations concerning REM-state in "living fossil." Report to Association for Psychophysiological Study of Sleep, Palo Alto, California, March 27–29, 1964.
32. Jouvet, D., Valatx, J., and Jouvet, M. Étude polygraphique du sommeil du chaton. *Compt. rend. Soc. de biol.* 155:1660–1664, 1961.
33. Roffwarg, H., Dement, W., and Fisher, C. Preliminary observations of sleep dream patterns in neonates, infants, children, and adults. In *Problems of Sleep and Dream in Children.* Edited by E. Harms. 147 pp. New York: Pergamon, 1964. (No. 2, *Monographs on Child Psychiatry.*) Pp. 60–72.
34. Parmelee, A., Akiyama, Y., Wenner, W., and Flescher, J. Activated sleep in premature infants. Report to Association for Psychophysiological Study of Sleep, Palo Alto, California, March 27–29, 1964.
35. Kamiya, J. Behavioral, subjective and physiological aspects of sleep and drowsiness. In *Functions of Varied Experience.* Edited by D. W. Fiske and S. R. Maddi. 501 pp. Homewood, Illinois: Dorsey Press, 1961. Pp. 145–174.
36. Snyder, F., Hobson, J., Morrison, D., and Goldfrank, F. Changes in respiration, heart rate and systolic blood pressure in relation to electroencephalographic patterns of human sleep. *J. Appl. Physiol.* 19:417–422, 1964.
37. Snyder, F., Hobson, J., and Goldfrank, F. Blood pressure changes during human sleep. *Science* 142:1313, 1964.
38. MacWilliam, J. A. Some applications of physiology to medicine. III. Blood pressure

and heart action in sleep and dreams: their relation to hemorrhages, angina, and sudden death. *Brit. M. J.* 2:1196–1200, 1923.
39. Fisher, C., Gross, J., and Zuch, J. Cycle of penile erection synchronous with dreaming (REM) sleep. *Arch. Gen. Psychiat.* 12:29–45, 1965.
40. Jouvet, M. Sur l'existence d'un système hypnotique ponto-limbique: ses rapports avec l'activité onirique. In *Physiologie de l'hippocampe (Colloques Intern. du C.N.R.S. No. 107)*. Edited by P. Passouant. 512 pp. Paris: Editions C.N.R.S., 1962. Pp. 297–330.
41. Jacobson, A, Kales, A., Lehman, D., and Hoedemacher, F. Muscle tonus in human subjects during sleep and dreaming. *Exper. Neurol.* 10:418–424, 1964.
42. Hodes, R., and Dement, W. Abolition of electrically induced reflexes (EIRs or "H-reflexes") during rapid eye movement periods of sleep in normal subjects. Report to Association for Psychophysiological Study of Sleep, Brooklyn, New York, March 30–31, 1963.
43. Jouvet, M., and Michel, F. Recherches sur l'activité électrique cérébrale au cours du sommeil. *Compt. rend. Soc. de biol.* 152:1167–1170, 1958.
44. Huttenlocher, P. R. Evoked and spontaneous activity in single units of medial brainstem during natural sleep and waking. *J. Neurophysiol.* 24:451–468, 1961.
45. Evarts, E. Activity of neurons in visual cortex of cat during sleep with low voltage past EEG activity. *J. Neurophysiol.* 25:812–816, 1962.
46. Kansow, E., Krause, D., and Kühnel, H. Die Vasomotorik der Hirnrinde in den Phasen desynchronisierter EEG-Aktivität im natürlichen Schlaf der Katze. *Arch. f. d. ges. Physiol.* 274:593–607, 1962.
47. Robert, W. *Der Traum als naturnotwendigkeit Erklart.* 53 pp. Hamburg: H. Seippel, 1886.
48. Dement, W. Effect of dream deprivation. *Science* 131:1705–1707, 1960.
49. *Idem.* Paper presented at meeting of American Academy for Psychoanalysis, New York, December 7–9, 1963.
50. Berger, R., and Oswald, I. Effects of sleep deprivation on behavior, subsequent sleep, and dreaming. *J. Ment. Sc.* 108:457–465, 1962.
51. Tyler, D. Psychological changes during experimental sleep deprivation. *Dis. Nerv. System* 16:293–299, 1955.
52. West, L., Janszen, H., Lester, B., and Cornelisoon, F. Psychosis of sleep deprivation. *Ann. New York Acad. Sc.* 96:66–70, 1962.
53. Agnew, H., Webb, W., and Williams, R. Effects of stage four sleep deprivation. Report to Association for Psychophysiological Study of Sleep, Palo Alto, California, March 27–29, 1964.
54. Fisher, C. Personal communication.
55. Hartmann, E., and Verdone, P. Sleep and dream patterns of pair of identical twins discordant for schizophrenia. Report to the Association for the Psychophysiological Study of Sleep, Washington, D. C., March 26–28, 1965.
56. Gresham, S., Webb, W., and Williams, R. Alcohol and caffeine: effect on inferred visual dreaming. *Science* 140:1226, 1963.
57. Greenberg, R., and Pearlman, C. Delerium tremens and dream deprivation. Report to Association for Psychophysiological Study of Sleep, March 27–29, Palo Alto, California, 1964.
58. Gross, M., et al. Observations of sleep in acute alcoholic psychoses. EEG and behavioral aspects. Report to Association for Psychophysiological Study of Sleep, March 27–29, Palo Alto, California, 1964.
59. Rechtschaffen, A., and Maron, L. Effect of amphetamine on sleep cycle. *Electroencephalog. & Clin. Neurophysiol.* 16:438–445, 1964.
60. Weiss, T. Bohdanecky, Z., Fifkova, E., and Roldan, E. Influence of atropine on sleep cycle in rat. *Psychopharmacologia* 5:126–135, 1964.
61. Hobson, J. Effect of LSD on sleep cycle in cat. *Electroencephalog. & Clin. Neurophysiol.* 17:52–56, 1964.
62. Muzio, J., Roffwarg, H., and Kaufman, E. Alterations in young adult human sleep EEG configuration resulting from d-LSD-25. Report to Association for Psychophysiological Study of Sleep, March 27–29, Palo Alto, California, 1964.
63. Grob, D., Lilienthal, J., Harvey, A., and Jones, B. Administration of DFP to man. *Bull. Johns Hopkins Hosp.* 81:217–244, 1947.
64. Hartmann, E. Unpublished data.
65. Freedman, D., and Giarman, N. Brain amines, electrical activity, and behavior. In *EEG and Behavior*. Edited by G. Glaser. 406 pp. New York: Basic Bks., 1963.
66. Matsuzaki, M., Takagi, H., and Tokizane, T. Paradoxical phase of sleep: its artificial induction in cat by sodium butyrate. *Science* 146:1328, 1964.
67. Oswald, I. Personal communication.

68. Jackson, J. *Selected Writings of Hughlings Jackson*. Edited by J. Taylor, G. Holmes and F. Walshe. Vol. 2. 1010 pp. New York: Basic Bks., 1958. P. 25.
69. Jung, C. *The Psychology of Dementia Praecox*. 150 pp. New York: Journal of Nervous and Mental Disease Publishing Company, 1944.
70. Feinberg, I., Koresko, R., Gottlieb, F., and Wender, P. Sleep electroencephalographic and eye-movement patterns in schizophrenic patients. *Compr. Psychiat.* 5:44–53, 1964.
71. Koresko, R., Snyder, F., and Feinberg, I. 'Dream time' in hallucinating and non-hallucinating schizophrenic patients. *Nature* (London) 199:1118, 1963.
72. Rechtschaffen, A., and Verdone, P. Amount of dreaming: effect of incentive, adaptation to laboratory, and individual differences. *Perceptual & Motor Skills* 19:947–958, 1964.
73. Fisher, C., and Dement, W. Studies on psychopathology of sleep and dreams. *Am. J. Psychiat.* 119:1160–1168, 1963.
74. Hartmann, E., Verdone, P., and Snyder, F. Sleep and dream patterns in psychiatric patients: longitudinal clinical study. Report to Association for Psychophysiological Study of Sleep, March 27–29, Palo Alto, California, 1964.
75. Rechtschaffen, A., Schulsinger, F., and Mednick, S. Schizophrenia and physiological indices of dreaming. *Arch. Gen. Psychiat.* 10:89–93, 1964.
76. Roffwarg, H., Dement, W., Muzio, J., and Fisher, C. Dream imagery: relationship to rapid eye movements of sleep. *Arch. Gen. Psychiat.* 7:235, 1962.
77. Hobson, J., Goldfrank, F., and Snyder, F. Respiration and mental activity in sleep. Report to Association for Psychophysiological Study of Sleep, March 27–29, Palo Alto, California, 1964.
78. Jouvet, M., Pellin, B., and Mounier, D. Étude polygraphique des différentes phases du sommeil au cours des troubles de conscience chronique (comas prolongés). *Rev. neurol.* 105:181, 1961.
79. Offenkrantz, K., and Rechtschaffen, A. Clinical studies of sequential dreams. *Arch. Gen. Psychiat.* 8:497–508, 1963.
80. Trosman, H., Rechtschaffen, A., Offenkrantz, W., and Wolpert, E. Studies in psychophysiology of dreams: relations among dreams in sequence. *Arch. Gen. Psychiat.* 3:602–607, 1960.
81. Dement, W., and Wolpert, E. Relation of eye movements, body motility, and external stimuli to dream content. *J. Exper Psychol.* 55:543–553, 1958.
82. Antrobus, J., Dement, W., and Fisher, C. Patterns of dreaming and dream recall: EEG study. *J. Abnorm. Soc. Psychol.* (in press).

Appendix B

Glossary

ALPHA ACTIVITY See ALPHA WAVES.

ALPHA-DELTA SLEEP Stage 4 sleep including obvious visual signs of alpha waves; rare in normal subjects, it is reported to occur in some pathological conditions.

ALPHA WAVES (ALPHA RHYTHM, ALPHA ACTIVITY) EEG activity with a frequency of 8 to 13 cycles per second. Found in most subjects during relaxed waking.

BASIC REST-ACTIVITY CYCLE (BRAC) A basic rhythmicity occurring in many bodily systems in mammals, noted most easily as the "sleep-dream cycle" at night. It has a length of about 90 minutes in man.

BETA WAVES or BETA ACTIVITY EEG activity at a frequency of over 13 cycles per second.

BIPOLAR RECORDING Recording electropotential between 2 "active" electrodes—for instance, between two points on the human scalp.

BRAC See BASIC REST-ACTIVITY CYCLE.

CAT ON AN ISLAND See D-DEPRIVATION.

CIRCADIAN RHYTHM A rhythm whose cycle length is approximately 24 hours.

CONJUGATE EYE MOVEMENTS Synchronous movements of the two eyeballs as when following an object during waking life.

D-DEPRIVATION (DREAM DEPRIVATION or REM DEPRIVATION) The selective deprivation of the D-state of sleep or REM sleep. This is usually achieved in humans either mechanically by awakening the subject every time his EEG indicates he is entering a D-period or chemically by use of the appropriate pharmacological agents. In animal studies a technique has been developed known as the "island technique," "rat on an island," "cat on an island," or other term, which involves the animal's standing on a small flower pot or block of wood surrounded by cold water. This allows him to obtain relatively normal waking periods and S-periods, but the onset of a D-period with its dropout of muscle potential causes the animal to fall into the water and waken. In fact the animals very quickly condition themselves to wake at the beginning of each D-period so that they seldom actually fall into the water.

DEEP SLEEP See LIGHT SLEEP.

DELTA SLEEP See SLOW WAVE SLEEP.

DELTA WAVES EEG activity with a frequency of less than 4 cycles per second. Characteristic of stages 3 and 4 sleep (sometimes called *delta sleep*) and of certain kinds of anesthesia and coma. In human sleep scoring, a minimum amplitude for scoring delta waves is usually established at 50, 75, or 100 µv. 75 µv (peak to peak) has been recommended as a standard.

DESCENDING STAGE 1 A low voltage, random, desynchronized EEG pattern found at sleep onset or during transition from waking to stage 2. See STAGES OF SLEEP.

DESYNCHRONIZED SLEEP D-state. A term used especially in animal studies where two kinds of sleep are distinguished: S or synchronized sleep, and D or desynchronized sleep.

D-PERIOD (or REM PERIOD) A single continuous or almost continuous stretch of time during which recordings indicate that the human or animal subject is in the D-state (REM state). A typical young human adult has 4 or 5 D-periods in the course of one night of sleep.

D-PRESSURE or REM PRESSURE Also sometimes referred to as D-tendency or *need for D*. This is a hypothetical construct which has been found useful in explaining many results in sleep research, although it will probably have to be discarded as more precise chemical and physiological mechanisms are uncovered. It is based on a hydraulic model which implies that a mammal has a certain requirement for D-time every day and that if this requirement is not fully met, the deficit accumulates, producing an increased "need" or "pressure" which then must be equalized or discharged. "D-pressure" has gained currency far more than, for instance, "sleep pressure," because there is a much more quantitative recovery of lost D-time than of lost sleep as a whole. It is probably the phasic events of the D-period which have this quasi-hydraulic property; thus it has been estimated that the cat somehow requires or manages to obtain a "quota" of 12,000 PGO spikes per 24 hours.

DREAM DEPRIVATION Generally refers to D-deprivation (REM-deprivation), although evidence that "dreams" can occur during sleep onset and sometimes during S-sleep make it unlikely that a subject deprived totally of D-time is also deprived totally of dreams.

DREAM WORK The psychic process involving condensation, displacement, and representability, which forms the dream (manifest dream) from the latent dream.

D-STATE (or REM STATE, REM SLEEP) One of two qualitatively different biological states comprising sleep. It is characterized by low voltage random EEG (stage 1), almost completely absent muscle potential, occasional rapid conjugate eye movements, and other phasic events; in man, awakenings from the D-state usually result in dream reports. Thus the D-state is the biological state (desynchronized sleep) concomitant with the psychological experience of dreaming. Also called REM sleep, emergent stage 1, desynchronized sleep, dreaming sleep, paradoxical sleep, rhombencephalic sleep.

D-TENDENCY See D-PRESSURE.

D-TIME The length of time spent in the D-state. Usually expressed in minutes per night. D-time percent refers to D-time as a percentage of the total night's sleep time; e.g., in a typical young adult, D-time is 100 minutes per night, D-time percent is 22 percent.

ECT Electroconvulsive therapy. The passage of enough electric current through the head to produce a convulsion. Used as treatment for certain severe depressions. Sometimes this term is used loosely to apply also to electroconvulsions produced for experimental purposes in animal studies.

EEG Electroencephalogram. A recording of electrical potentials from the scalp and the moment-to-moment change in these potentials.

EMERGENT STAGE 1 Low voltage, random, desynchronized EEG activity found without a previous awakening, i.e., after a period of stages 2, 3, and 4. Such periods of stage 1 activity are D-periods—i.e., associated with rapid eye muscle potential, eye movements, and so on; therefore one of the names given to D-periods has been emergent stage 1. See D-STATE.

EMG Electromyogram. A recording of electrical activity from the muscular system. Clinically this usually involves small needle electrodes placed directly in the muscles. In all-night human sleep studies this would be both painful and impractical, so the usual human EMG recording involves surface electrodes, similar to those used for scalp recordings, placed at two points over the submental musculature. These small muscles under the chin have been found empirically to produce the most reliable results in terms of a reduction of resting muscle potential between waking and S-state and a further dropout during D-state. In studies on cats and rats, EMG is usually recorded from electrodes permanently implanted in the dorsal neck muscles.

EOG Electro-oculogram. A recording of the electrical potential generated by movement of the eyeball, i.e., the fundocorneal dipole of the eye; usually measured by electrodes placed at the outer canthi of the eyes.

EST Electroshock therapy. See ECT.

FIRST-NIGHT EFFECT (or ADAPTATION EFFECT) Term used to describe the fact that on a subject's first (and sometimes second or third) night in the laboratory his recorded sleep is different from later nights. Specifically there is less D-time and often less total sleep and more awakenings.

HIPPOCAMPAL THETA Theta activity (4 to 8 cycles per second) seen very prominently in recordings from the hippocampus of some species, especially rodents, during D-periods, and therefore used to identify D-periods in these species. Though less prominent, this activity is also found at times during waking, especially during motor activity and perhaps learning.

HYPNAGOGIC IMAGERY Images occurring during sleep onset—chiefly in descending stage 1.

HYPNOPOMPIC IMAGERY Imagery during awakening from sleep.

ISLAND TECHNIQUE (OF DEPRIVATION) See D-DEPRIVATION.

K-COMPLEX A rapid, high amplitude, spikelike wave followed usually by a very brief period—about ½ second—of spindle activity. The exact significance of the K-complex is unknown; it frequently occurs spontaneously during stage 2 of human sleep and to some extent during stages 3 and 4; it can also often be elicited by an external stimulus, such as noise, not powerful enough to awaken the sleeper.

LATENT DREAM The meaning of the dream as arrived at by dream interpretation; the day-residues, thoughts, wishes forming the basic material which the dream work uses to construct the manifest dream.

LIGHT SLEEP (and DEEP SLEEP) Terms used frequently by laymen but rarely by sleep researchers because of their ambiguity. In terms of the appearance of the EEG, descending stage 1 → 2 → 3 → 4 represents increasing sleep depth and the D-state (Stage 1–REM) looks like "light sleep." However, in terms of muscle potential or body posture, it is not easy to differentiate descending 1, 2, 3, 4; but D-state is clearly "deeper" than all of these, i.e., there is *least* muscle potential. In terms of arousal threshold, 1 → 2 → 3 → 4 represents increasing depth; D-state is variable—usually, however, closer to stage 4 than to descending stage 1.

In animals it is difficult or impossible to distinguish four stages in S-sleep, but S and D are clearly differentiable. Again S looks deeper than D in terms of the surface EEG and most forebrain EEG patterns, but D is definitely deeper than S in terms of muscle potential and arousal threshold.

Thus at present the terms *deep* and *light* can be confusing and should be avoided unless the measure referred to is precisely specified.

MANIFEST DREAM The dream as experienced, as opposed to latent dream. See LATENT DREAM.

MONOPOLAR RECORDING Recording of the electrical potential between one active and one inactive electrode, for instance a parietal (active) electrode referred to a mastoid or ear lobe (presumably inactive) electrode.

NARCOLEPSY A condition characterized chiefly by sleepiness and a sudden inability to remain awake during the daytime; these are the simple sleep attacks of narcolepsy. In addition narcolepsy may be characterized by cataplexy, a sudden loss of muscular tone so that the patient collapses to the floor, sometimes however without actually losing consciousness; sleep paralysis, an inability to move or to use the muscular system while being subjectively awake and conscious—this occurs usually in the morning on awakening from sleep in certain narcoleptics; and nocturnal hallucinations, vivid dream-like hallucinatory images occurring usually during a drowsy state at night.

NEED FOR D See D-PRESSURE.

NREM SLEEP (NONRAPID EYE MOVEMENT SLEEP) See S-STATE.

ORTHODOX SLEEP S-state or NREM sleep.

PARADOXICAL SLEEP D-state or REM sleep.

PGO SPIKES Ponto-geniculo-occipital spikes. Sharp spikelike activity found especially in the cat—in the pons, lateral geniculate, and occipital area, i.e., the visual pathways—during D-periods. These are among the most prominent phasic events of the D-state. See PHASIC EVENTS.

PHASES OF SLEEP See STAGES OF SLEEP.

PHASIC EVENTS Neurophysiological or other events occurring sporadically during the course of a D-period. These include movements of the external ocular muscles and other small muscle groups, sporadic presynaptic inhibition of spinal motoneurons, and PGO spikes.

PRIMARY PROCESS A presumably primitive type of mental functioning characterized by condensation, displacement, and wishful thinking and by relatively massive, poorly controlled "energy" discharge.

RAT ON AN ISLAND See D-DEPRIVATION.

REBOUND or REBOUND INCREASE The increase in D-time found after a period of D-deprivation.

REM DENSITY Number of REMs (rapid eye movements) per unit of time during a REM period (D-period).

REM PROPENSITY See D-PRESSURE.

REM(s) Rapid eye movement(s).

REM SLEEP See D-STATE.

REM TENDENCY See D-PRESSURE.

REM TIME The amount of time spent in REM sleep (D-state), sometimes expressed as a percentage of total sleep.

SECONDARY PROCESS The presumably advanced type of mental functioning characterized by logical, realistic, controlled thinking and by relatively small, controlled shifts of "energy."

SEM(s) Slow eye movement(s). Usually refers to conjugate rolling movements of the eyes, frequently seen at sleep onset.

SLEEP-DREAM CYCLE The recurrence of S and D throughout a night of sleep or period of sleep. The length of one cycle, usually defined as the time from the end of one D-period to the end of the next, is 95 minutes in man, about 30 minutes in the cat, and 15 minutes in the rat. See also BASIC REST-ACTIVITY CYCLE.

SLEEP SPINDLES See SPINDLES.

SLOW WAVE SLEEP Sleep characterized by low frequency waves (1 to 4 per sec.), also called delta waves. In human sleep, slow wave sleep is equivalent to stage 3 plus stage 4 of sleep. In animal recordings, where the sleep stages are usually not distinguished, slow wave sleep is sometimes used synonomously with S-state (synchronized sleep, NREM sleep).

SOMNAMBULISM Sleep walking.

SPINDLES or SLEEP SPINDLES Electroencephalographic activity occurring at a frequency of 13 to 17 cycles per second and with great regularity, allowing for easy visual identification. Spindles are usually 1 to 2 seconds in length, and the activity sometimes waxes and wanes so as to give the entire complex a spindlelike appearance. Spindle activity is most clearly visible during stage 2 of human sleep but persists during stages 3 and 4 although obscured for visual scoring by the delta waves.

S-STATE (S-SLEEP, NREM SLEEP) One of two qualitatively different biological states comprising sleep. It is characterized in animals by relatively high voltage slow activity and a resting muscle potential lower than that of waking but higher than that of the D-state. In man, the total of descending stage 1, stage 2, stage 3, and stage 4 of sleep. Also called synchronized sleep, slow wave sleep, nonrapid eye movement sleep, orthodox sleep, telencephalic sleep.

STAGE 1, 2, 3, 4 See STAGES OF SLEEP.

STAGES OF SLEEP A convenient although probably arbitrary method of classifying patterns seen during sleep in the human EEG.

Stage 1 is dominated by low voltage, desynchronized, random-appearing EEG activity. This is seen at sleep onset (descending stage 1) and during D-periods (sometimes called emergent stage 1).

Stage 2 is characterized by a background similar to stage 1 but also including sleep spindles—activity of 13 to 17 cycles per second lasting 1 to 2 seconds—and K-complexes, and usually defined as including not over 20 percent delta waves (1 to 4 per sec.) activity.

Stage 3 is characterized by the presence of spindles and so on, similar to stage 2, except for the presence of more delta waves (1 to 4 per sec.); usually defined as a segment of record containing 20 to 50 percent delta waves.

Stage 4 is a segment of record consisting of more than 50 percent delta waves.

Stages of sleep has been meaningfully applied only to human records so far. Animal records are usually divided into W, S, and D (waking, synchronized sleep, and desynchronized sleep). In the editor's opinion, W, S, and D represent true qualitative differences, while stages 1 to 4 are somewhat arbitrary divisions within a continuum during S-sleep. Nonetheless some such divisions may be useful, since delta sleep —stages 3 and 4 but not stage 2—appears to have certain biological functions, such as recovery from physical fatigue.

SYNCHRONIZED SLEEP S-state; term used often in animal studies where two states of sleep are distinguished: S, or synchronized, and D, or desynchronized.

THETA WAVES EEG activity with a frequency of 4 to 8 cycles per second. Sometimes found at sleep onset in man. Very characteristic of D-state hippocampal activity in rodents.

TONIC EVENTS Those neurophysiological and peripheral physiological events which characterize an entire D-period, such as stage 1 EEG, dropout of resting muscle potential, and so on (as opposed to phasic events).

ULTRADIAN RHYTHM A rhythm with a frequency greater than one cycle per 24 hours—i.e., with more than one peak per 24 hours.

W, S, D Some evidence indicates that the S-state and D-state actually differ as much from each other as each does from waking (W). Thus, rather than consider that the organism exists in two major states, waking and sleeping, with the latter subdivided into S and D, the suggestion has been made that there are three qualitatively different organismic states: W, S, and D (or W, NREM sleep, and REM sleep).

Index